Encyclopaedia of Food and Nutrition

Encyclopaedia of

Food and Nutrition

SANDHYA TRIVEDI

ANMOL PUBLICATIONS PVT. LTD.

NEW DELHI - 110 002 (INDIA)

ANMOL PUBLICATIONS PVT. LTD.

H.O.: 4374/4B, Ansari Road, Darya Ganj,
New Delhi-110 002 (India)
Ph.: 23278000, 23261597

B.O.: No. 1015, Ist Main Road, BSK IIIrd Stage
IIIrd Phase, IIIrd Block
Bangalore - 560 085 (India)
Visit us at: www.anmolpublications.com

Encyclopaedia of Food and Nutrition

ISBN 978-81-261-3388-8

PRINTED IN INDIA

Printed at Mehra Offset Press, Delhi.

Preface

The Encyclopaedia of Food and Nutrition is the perfect guide for those studying, either at university level or anyone interested in food and nutrition.

This volume provides clear and lucid definitions of terms associated with all aspects of food nutrients and various aspects of food science such as diets, food values, different types of foods and various processing techniques. The aim of this Encyclopaedia is also to satisfy the immediate needs of the user. Concepts are presented in a clear and lucid manner. In terms of its broader objectives, the present book may be viewed as an outline or compendium of Food ideas correlated with a large collection of specialized items.

In preparation of this book, the author has freely consulted large number of books and journals so no authenticity is claimed. Author is especially thankful to Anmol Publications Pvt. Ltd., New Delhi for shaping this book in its final form. Suggestions for further improvement of this book are welcome.

Author

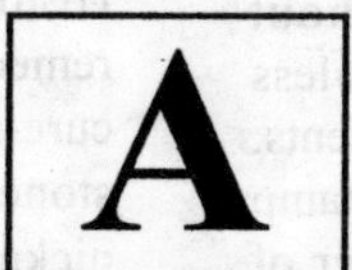

Ababai Ababai comes from the Caricacae family of fruits, which also contains the Mau Mau, and some forms of papaya. It is considered an exotic fruit in the United States. It is imported from Chile, as Chile is the only country in the world that exports this luscious fruit. Very few countries grow Ababai and then only for their local market. It is a protected fruit in Chile and was only recently available for export. Fresh off the tree, ababai has a thin skin and looks like a small papaya. It is never eaten fresh due to its high enzyme content. It is first cooked for several minutes and then jarred. Its pale yellow colour turns to a brilliant gold after processing. It is one of the few fruits that will not dissolve when cooked. It is superb for sauting with vegetables, broiling on fish, and grilling on the barbecue (shish kebob). The seeds look like small raisins. The male and female seeds of the fruit cannot be distinguished before planting, and there is also a hermaphrodite seed. Several seeds are planted with the prospect of growing one successful Ababai tree. Ababai trees grow for 7 1/2 to 8 years and only bear fruit for 5 years. The tree is then cut down, recycled, and must be replanted on virgin soil.

Abaisee A French term that describes puff pastry that has been rolled very thin or sponge cake that has been cut very thin for dessert preparation.

Abalone Abalone are shellfish of the univalve family, meaning they only have one shell, unlike bivalves such as clams that consist of two shells. This edible gastropod belongs to the same family as the sea slug and is related to the snail. Out of its shell, it resembles a large scallop. They are found in United States, Japan, Australia, Mexico, and Indo-Pacific Region. On the Pacific coast, they are found on rocky inter-tidal and sub-tidal areas from Baja California to Alaska, as each species prefers a particular habitat, which appears related to the local sea temperature.

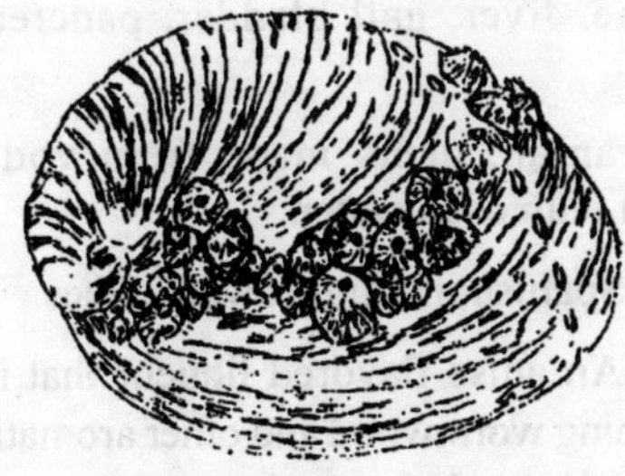

Fig. Abalone

They are also called ear shells, or sea ears (as their shape resembles the human ear). Also called Awabi in Japanese cuisine and Loco in South American cuisine. Since the abalone has been over-harvested, it is very expensive when available. History: Abalone has lived along the Pacific coast of North America for millions of years. Fossilized shells have been found in sediments that are approximately 100 million years old. In more recent times, abalone were important in the economy of all native American peoples who dwelled in California's coastal areas. Native Americans were using abalone for food, implements, and decoration long before the arrival of Europeans in North America

ABAWDs Able-Bodied Adults Without Dependents. This term is applied to jobless individuals aged 18 to 50 without dependents. ABAWDs are limited to 3 months of food stamp benefits in a 36-month period unless either of the following two exemptions apply. Individuals are exempt if he or she is: 1. employed or participating in an approved work or training program at least half time; or

2. participating in federal workforce programs for the required number of hours. States can apply for a waiver to this rule for areas that: 1. have an unemployment rate which exceeds 10 percent; or

2. do not have a sufficient number of jobs to provide employment for the individuals.

Abboccato Italian; medium sweet wines.

Abdomen Area between the chest and the hips that contains the stomach, small intestine, large intestine, liver, gall bladder, pancreas, and spleen.

Abdug Iranian; drink made from vodka and yoghurt with soda water.

Abocada Spanish; medium sweet wines.

Absinthe An anise-flavored liqueur that is made by steeping wormwood and other aromatic herbs (hyssop, lemon balm, and angelica) in alcohol. The drink is distinguished by its dazzling blue-green clarity due to its chlorophyll content. It was traditionally served with water and a cube of sugar; the sugar cube was placed on an "absinthe spoon" and the liquor was drizzled over the sugar into the glass of water. The sugar helped take the bitter edge from the absinthe, and when poured into the water the liquor turned milky white. Absinthe was believed to raise the drinker's consciousness, insights, and emotional experience to another level altogether. Unfortunately, it also caused terrible hallucinations, permanent neural damage, as seen in the dazed condition of dedicated drinkers, and even its own diseases, known as absinthism, recognized as early as the 1850s. History Dr. Pierre Ordinaire as an all-purpose remedy invented Absinthe in 1792. Used as a cure-all for epilepsy, gout, drunkenness, kidney stones, colic, headaches, and worms, it was nicknamed "La Fee Verte" meaning The Green Fairy. In 1797, the heirs of Dr. Ordinaire sold the recipe to Henri-Louis Pernod. Pernod opened the first absinthe distillery in Switzerland and then moved to a larger one in Pontarlier, France in 1805. After the Algerian War (1844-1847), the demand for absinthe rose dramatically. The soldiers had developed a taste for absinthe, as they were given rations of absinthe along with their drinking water as a bacterial deterrent, and began drinking it after the war. At the beginning of the 20th century, the drinking of absinthe was so popular that the cocktail hour in France was called "l'heure verte," meaning the "green hour." Absinthe was exported to New Orleans and reached the same popularity in the United States. It was a drink considered ladylike and women freely enjoyed it in the coffee houses, where it was commonly served. In New Orleans, as well as in the rest of the United States, it became banned in 1912. Absinthe is still available in other areas of the world where it is not illegal.

Absolute alcohol Pure ethyl alcohol.

Absorb 1. To take something in, as through the skin or the intestine.

2. To react with radiation and reduce it in intensity, as with a dose of radiation or transmitted light.

Acarbose The name of a group of complex carbohydrates (oligosaccharides) which inhibit the enzymes of starch and disaccharide digestion; used experimentally to reduce the digestion of starch, and so slow the rate of absorption of carbohydrates. It has been marketed for use in association with weight-reducing diet regimes as a 'starch blocker', but there is no evidence that it is of any use whatsoever in weight reduction.

Acaricides Pesticides used to kill mites and ticks (the biological family Acaridae) which cause animal diseases and the spoilage of flour and other foods in storage.

Accelase A mixture of enzymes which hydrolyse proteins, including an exopeptidase from the bacterium Streptococcus lactis, which is one of the starter organisms in dairy processing. The mixed enzymes are used to shorten the maturation time of cheeses and intensify the flavour of processed cheese.

Acceptable Daily Intake (ADI) The amount of a food additive that could be taken daily for an entire life-span without appreciable risk. Determined by measuring the highest dose of the substance that has no effect on experimental animals, then dividing by a safety factor of 100. Substances that are not given an ADI are regarded as having no adverse effect at any level of intake. See also no effect level.

Accoub Edible thistle (Goundelia tournefortii) growing in the Mediterranean region and Middle East. The cooked flower buds have a flavour resembling that of asparagus or globe artichoke; the shoots can be eaten in the same way as asparagus and the roots as salsify.

Accra Caribbean; heavy batter fritters with salt cod; also known as stamp-and-go, bacalaitos.

Accuncciata Corsican; goat, lamb, or mutton stew with potatoes.

Acesulfame K Acesulfame potassium, is a low calorie sweetener approved for use in the United States in 1988. It is an organic salt consisting of carbon, nitrogen, oxygen, hydrogen, sulphur and potassium atoms. It is 200 times sweeter than sucrose, has a synergistic sweetening effect with other sweeteners, has a stable shelf life and is heat stable. It is excreted through the human digestive system unchanged, and is therefore non caloric.

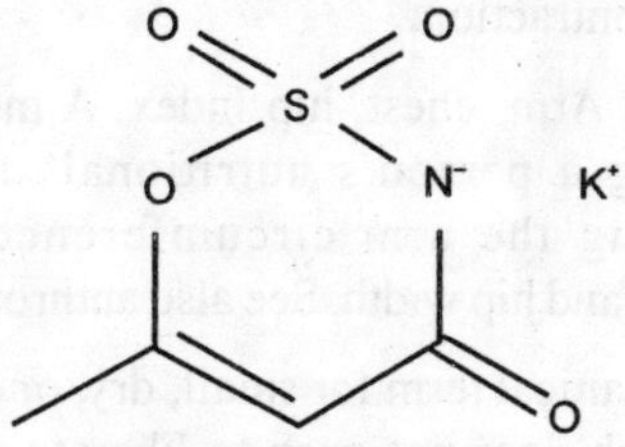

Fig. Acesulfame K

Acetic acid One of the simplest organic acids, also known systematically as ethanoic acid, chemically it is CH_3COOH. It is the acid of vinegar (which is a solution of acetic acid in water), and is formed, together with lactic acid, in the fermentation (pickling) of foods.

Aceto dolce Italian; pickles eaten as an appetizer.

acetoin A precursor of the compound diacetyl, which is one of the constituents of the flavour of butter. Chemically acetyl methyl carbinol.

Acetobacter A genus of bacteria which oxidize ethyl alcohol to acetic acid, used in the manufacture of vinegar. They also grow as a film on the surface of beer wort, pickle brine, and fruit juices, when they are commonly known as 'mother of vinegar'.

Acetomel A mixture of honey and vinegar that produces sweet-sour syrup. Traditionally used to preserve fruits.

Acetomenaphthone Synthetic compound with vitamin K activity; vitamin K3, also known as menaquinone-0.

Acetone One of the ketone bodies formed in the body in fasting. It is a metabolically useless side-product of fat metabolism, but detection of acetone in blood, urine, or breath may be clinically useful in cases of diabetes, as a means of detecting ketosis. Also used as a solvent, e.g. in varnishes and lacquer.

Acetylcholine The acetyl derivative of choline, produced at some nerve endings (cholinergic nerves) both in the brain, where it acts as a chemical transmitter, and at the junctions between nerves and muscles, where it stimulates muscle contraction.

ACH index Arm, chest, hip index. A method of assessing a person's nutritional status by measuring the arm circumference, chest diameter, and hip width. See also anthropometry.

Achene Botanical term for small, dry, one-seeded fruit which does not open to liberate the seed, e.g. a nut.

Achlorhydria Deficiency of hydrochloric acid in gastric digestive juice. See also anaemia; gastric acidity.

Achondroplasia An inherited problem with the growth of cartilage in the long bones and skull; characterized by short stature

Achromotricia Loss of the pigment of hair. One of the signs of pantothenic acid deficiency in animals, but there is no evidence that pantothenic acid affects loss of hair colour in human beings.

Acid Chemically, compounds that dissociate (ionize) in water to give rise to hydrogen ions (H+); they taste sour. Mineral acids such as hydrochloric, sulphuric, and nitric are more or less completely dissociated and so are strong acids. Organic acids are generally weak since they are not completely dissociated. See also alkali; amino acids; buffers; esters; fatty acids; pH; salt.

Acid drops Boiled sweets with sharp flavour from tartaric acid (originally acidulated drops); known as sourballs in USA.

Acid foods, basic foods These terms refer to the residue of the metabolism of foods. The mineral salts of sodium, potassium, magnesium, and calcium are base-forming, while phosphorus, sulphur, and chlorine are acid-forming. Which of these predominates in foods determines whether the residue is acidic or basic (alkaline); meat, cheese, eggs, and cereals leave an acidic residue, while milk, vegetables, and some fruits leave a basic residue. Fats and sugars have no mineral content and so leave a neutral residue. Although fruits have an acid taste due to organic acids and their salts, the acids are completely oxidized and the sodium and potassium salts form an alkaline residue.

Acid number, acid value (of a fat) A measure of its rancidity due to hydrolysis, releasing free fatty acids from the triacylglycerol of the fat; serves as an index of the efficiency of refining since the fatty acids are removed during refining and increase with deterioration during storage.

Acid, gastric The acid in the gastric secretion is hydrochloric acid; see also achlorhydria; gastric acidity.

Acidify To add acid (lemon juice or vinegar) to a culinary preparation to made a dish slightly acid, sour, or piquant.

Acidophilus milk Resembles yoghurt but is more astringent in taste and cultured only with Lactobacillus acidophilus; claimed to enhance the growth of beneficial bacteria in the intestine. acidophilus therapy A treatment for constipation based on the consumption of milk containing a high concentration of viable Lacrobacillus acidophilus, although the milk itself is unfermented. The effect is believed to be due to the implantation of the organisms in the intestine.

Acidosis An increase in the acidity of blood plasma to below the normal range of pH 7.3-7.45, resulting from a loss of the buffering capacity of the plasma, alteration in the excretion of carbon dioxide, excessive loss of base from the body or metabolic overproduction of acids.

Acids, fruit Organic acids such as citric, malic, tartaric, etc. which give the sharp or sour flavour to fruits; often added to processed foods for taste.

Acidulated water Water that has been made slightly acidic by the addition of an acid substance such as lemon juice or vinegar (about one teaspoon to half a litre of water). Peeled fruit and vegetables such as apples, pears, celeriac, globe artichokes and salsify are immersed in acidulated water to prevent them from discolouring. It can also be used for cooking. Cauliflower, for instance, will be snowy white if boiled in acidulated water.

Ackee The fruit of the Caribbean tree Blighia sapida. The fruit is toxic when unripe because it contains the toxin hypoglycin.

ACNE Inflammatory pustular skin eruption occurring around sebaceous glands, especially around the time of puberty. Not known to be caused or exacerbated by diet, although a low-fat diet is sometimes recommended. Severe persistent acne may be treated by topical application of retinoids (synthetic vitamin A derivatives).

Acorn Fruit of the oak tree (Quercus spp.), used both for animal feed and (especially in Spain) to make a flour for baking. Roasted acorns have been used as a coffee substitute (German: ersatz Kaffee).

Acrodynia A specific type of skin lesion (dermatitis) seen in animals which are deficient in vitamin B_6. There is no evidence for a similar dermatitis in deficient human beings.

Acrolein An aldehyde formed when glycerol is heated to a high temperature. It is responsible for the acrid odour and lachrymatory (tear-causing) vapour produced when fats are overheated.

Acronize Trade name for the antibiotic chlortetracycline; 'acronized' is used to describe products that have been treated with chlortetracycline, as, e.g. acronized ice.

Active oxygen method A method of measuring the stability of fats and oils to oxidative damage by bubbling air through the heated material and following the formation of peroxides. Also known as the Swift stability test.

Actomyosin The combination of the two main contractile proteins in muscle, actin and myosin.

Additive Any compound not commonly regarded or used as a food which is added to foods as an aid in manufacturing or processing, or to improve the keeping properties, flavour, colour, texture, appearance, or stability of the food, or as a convenience to the consumer. The term excludes vitamins, minerals, and other nutrients added to enrich or restore nutritional value. Herbs, spices, hops, salt, yeast, or protein hydrolysates, air and water are usually excluded from this definition. Additives may be extracted from natural sources, synthesized in the laboratory to be chemically the same as the natural materials (and hence known as nature-identical), or may be synthetic compounds that do not occur in nature.

In most countries only additives from a permitted list of compounds which have been extensively tested for safety may legally be added to foods. The additives used must be declared on food labels, using either their chemical names or their numbers in the EU list of permitted additives (E-numbers). Some additional compounds, numbered in the same sequence but without the preface E-, are permitted in the UK.

See also Acceptable Daily Intake and Appendix VIII.

Adenine A nucleotide, one of the purine bases of the nucleic acids (DNA and RNA). The compound formed between adenine and ribose is the nucleoside adenosine, and can form four phosphorylated derivatives important in metabolism: adenosine monophosphate (AMP, also known as adenylic acid); adenosine diphosphate (ADP); adenosine triphosphate (ATP) and cyclic adenosine monophosphate (cAMP). See also ATP; energy metabolism.

NH2 NH N N N

Fig. Adenine

Adipectomy Surgical removal of subcutaneous fat.

Adipose tissue Adipose tissue is an anatomical term for loose connective tissue composed of adipocytes. Its main role is to store energy in the form of fat, although it also cushions and insulates the body. Obesity in animals, including humans, is not dependent on the amount of body weight, but on the amount of body fat - specifically adipose tissue. In mammals, two types of adipose tissue exist: white adipose tissue (WAT) and brown adipose tissue (BAT). Adipose tissue also serves as an important endocrine organ[1] by producing recently-discovered hormones such as leptin, resistin and TNFα.

Adirondack bread American baked product made from ground maize, butter, wheat flour, eggs, and sugar.

Adlay The seeds of a wild grass (Job's tears, Coix lachryma-jobi) botanically related to maize, growing wild in parts of Africa and Asia and eaten especially in the south-east Pacific region.

Adoucir French; to reduce the bitterness of food by prolonged cooking, or to dilute a dish with milk, stock, or water to make it less salty.

Adrenal glands A pair of ductless glands located above the kidneys. Through hormonal secretions, the adrenal glands regulate many essential functions in the body, including biochemical balances that influence athletic training and general stress response.

Adrenaline A hormone secreted by the medulla of the adrenal gland, especially in times of stress or in response to fright or shock. Its main actions are to increase blood pressure and to mobilize tissue reserves of glucose (leading to an increase in the blood glucose concentration) and fat, in preparation for flight or fighting. Derived from the amino acids phenylalanine or tyrosine.

Adrenocorticotrophic hormone (ACTH) A hormone secreted by the anterior part of the pituitary gland which stimulates the adrenal gland to secrete corticosteroids.

Adulteration The addition of substances to foods etc. in order to increase the bulk and reduce the cost, with intent to defraud the purchaser. Common adulterants are starch in spices, water in milk and beer, etc. The British Food and Drugs Act (1860) was the first legislation to prevent such practices.

Adverse Reaction Monitoring System (ARMS) A system operated by FDA which monitors and investigates all complaints by individuals or their physicians that are believed to be related to a specific food, food and colour additives or vitamin and mineral supplements. The ARMS computerized database helps officials decide whether reported adverse reactions represent a real public health risk associated with food so that appropriate action can be taken.

Advocaat Dutch; liqueur made from brandy and eggs.

Aerate Aerate means the same as "sift." To pass dry ingredients through a fine-mesh sifter so large pieces can be removed. The process also incorporates air to make ingredients like flour, lighter.

Aerobic 1. Aerobic micro-organisms (aerobes) are those that require oxygen for growth; obligate aerobes cannot survive in the absence of oxygen. The opposite are anaerobic organisms, which do not require oxygen for growth; obligate anaerobes cannot survive in the presence of oxygen.

2. Aerobic exercise is physical activity which requires an increase in heart rate and respiration to meet the increased demand of muscle for oxygen, as contrasted with maximum exertion or sprinting, when muscle can metabolize anaerobically, producing lactic acid, which is metabolized later, creating a need for increased respiration after the exercise has ceased (so-called oxygen debt).

Aerobic exercise Aerobic exercise refers to the kind of fast-paced activity that makes you "huff and puff." It places demands on your cardiovascular apparatus and, over time, produces beneficial changes in your respiratory and circulatory systems.

Aerosol cream Cream sterilized and packaged in aerosol canisters with a propellant gas to expel it from the container, giving conveniently available whipped cream. Gelling agents and stabilizers may also be added.

Aesculln A glucoside of dihydroxycoumarin found in the leaves and bark of the horse chestnut tree (Aesculus hippocastanum) which has an effect on capillary fragility.

AFD Accelerated freeze drying, see freeze drying.

Afferent nerves Nerve fibers (usually sensory) that carry impulses from an organ or tissue toward the brain and spinal cord (central nervous system), or the information processing centres of the enteric nervous system, which is located within the walls of the digestive tract.

Afferent pathways Nerve structures through which impulses are conducted from a peripheral part (e.g., the gut or intestines) toward a nerve centre (e.g., the central nervous system).

Aflatoxins A group of mycotoxins formed by the mould Aspergillus flavus, which can grow on peanuts and cereal grains when they are stored under damp and warm conditions. Several different aflatoxins are known; in addition to being acutely toxic, many, especially aflatoxin B 1, are potent carcinogens. Fungal spoilage of foods with A. flavus is a common problem in many tropical areas, and aflatoxin is believed to be the cause of much primary liver cancer in parts of Africa. Aflatoxins can be secreted in milk, so there is strict control of the level of aflatoxins in cattle feed.

After taste Taste which returns to the mouth after ingestion of certain foods and beverages.

Agalactia Failure of the mother to secrete enough milk to feed a suckling infant.

Agar-agar Processed seaweed, grayish white in colour and comes in sticks, flakes, granules or powder. It is a vegetarian gelatin. After it is soaked in cold water, it becomes bouncy, resilient, and crisp. It is used mostly for cold oriental dishes that contain chicken, meat, and vegetables. In the old days, before the introduction of gelatin, agar-agar was also used as a thickening agent in making cold jellied dishes. Once soaked in boiling water, it melts into a gelatinous substance. The Chinese use this paste to make their famous delicacy called "bird's nest soup." Agar-agar is commonly referred to as Chinese gelatin.

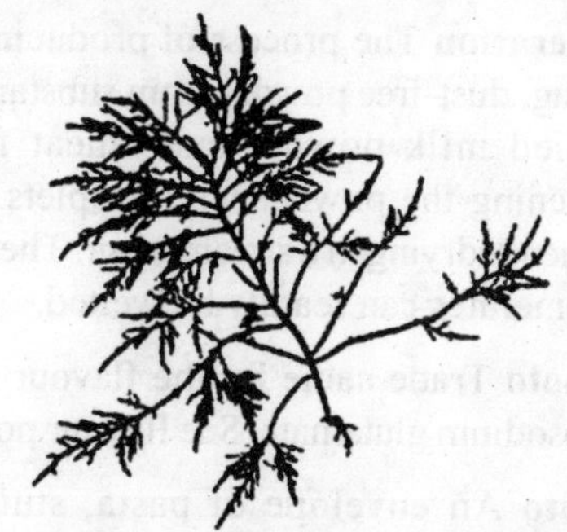

Fig. Agar-agar (A Vegetarians gelatin)

Ageing 1. As wines age, they develop bouquet and a smooth mellow flavour, associated with slow oxidation and the formation of esters, as well as losing the harsn yeasty flavour of young wine.

2. The ageing of meat by hanging in a cool place for several days results in softening of the muscle tissue, which stiffens after death (rigor mortis). This stiffening is due to anaerobic metabolism leading to the formation of lactic acid when the blood flow ceases.

3. Ageing of wheat flour for bread making is due to oxidation, either by storage for some weeks after milling or by chemical action. Freshly milled flour produces a weaker and less resilient dough, and hence a less 'bold' loaf, than flour which has been aged. Chemicals that are used to age flour include ammonium persulphate, ascorbic acid (vitamin C), chlorine, sulphur dioxide, potassium bromate, and cysteine. In addition, nitrogen peroxide or benzoyl peroxide may be used to bleach flour, and chlorine dioxide both bleaches and ages

flour. The use of these chemicals, and the amounts that may be used, is controlled by law in most countries.

Agene Nitrogen trichloride, used at one time as a bleaching and improving agent for wheat flour in bread making. It can react with the amino acid methionine in proteins to form the toxic compound methionine sulphoximine, and is no longer used.

Ageusia Loss or impairment of the sense of taste.

Agglomeration The process of producing a free-flowing, dust-free powder from substances such as dried milk powder and wheat flour, by moistening the powder with droplets of water and then redrying in a stream of air. The resulting agglomerates can readily be wetted.

Aginomoto Trade name for the flavour enhancer monosodium glutamate. See flavour potentiator.

Agnelloto An envelope of pasta, stuffed with minced meat, cheese, or vegetables, cut into a half-moon shape, and so differing from ravioli, which is cut into squares.

Agneshka churba Bulgarian; whole spring lamb stuffed with rice, offal, and raisins, then roasted. A traditional Easter dish.

Agrochemicals Term for artificially produced chemicals (such as feed additives, pharmaceuticals, fertilizers or pesticides) used in agriculture to improve crops or livestack production.

Ahi Ahi tuna is simply yellow fin tuna. It is a term used in Hawaii to describe this variety of tuna, which is distinguished from the other variety of tuna, known as blue fin.

Aigre-douce French; sweet and sour. See acitomel.

aigrette French; small, light, fried flaky pastry biscuit.

Aiguillette A thin strip or slice of cooked poultry, meat, or fish.

Aollade French; prepared with garlic.

AIN American Institute of Nutrition.

Aioli The French word for garlic is "ail." Aioli is garlic-flavored mayonnaise made from pounded cloves of garlic, egg yolks, oil, and seasoning. Just before it is served, lemon juice and a little cold water are added. It is served as a sauce for a variety of garnishes and main courses.

Air classification A way of separating the particles of powdered materials in a current of air, on the basis of their weight and size or density. Particularly applied to the fractionation of the endosperm of milled wheat flour; smaller particles are richer in protein. Various fractions range from 3% to 25% protein.

Aitchbone Cut of beef from the upper part of the leg. Sometimes incorrectly called the edgebone.

Ajada Spanish; sauce made from bread steeped in water and garlic.

Akkra Caribbean (originally West African); fritter made from black-eyed peas or soya beans. Also known as calas, samsa.

Akni Indian; bouillon, made from water and herbs, used for cooking rice and vegetables.

Akutok Inuit (Eskimo); strips of dried caribou meat; the outer part has a crust, but the inside is only partially dry.

Akutaq Also known as aqutuk, ackutuk, or Eskimo Ice Cream. Not the creamy ice cream as we know it, but a concoction made from reindeer fat or tallow, seal oil, freshly fallen snow or water, fresh berries, and sometimes ground fish. Air is whipped in by hand so that it slowly cools into foam. It is eaten as a desert, a meal, a snack, or a spread. Traditionally it was made for funerals, potlatches, celebrations of a boy's first hunt, and any other celebration where food is brought. Today it is usually made with Crisco shortening instead of tallow and with raisins and sugar sometimes added

Akutok Inuit (Eskimo); strips of dried caribou meat; the outer part has a crust, but the inside is only partially dry.

Al dente Firm to the bite, applied to pasta and cooked vegetables (Italian: 'to the tooth').

Alderman's walk The name given in London to the longest and finest cut from the haunch of venison or lamb.

Al dente The only way to serve pasta! This is an Italian phrase meaning 'to the tooth'. It's used to describe the texture of pasta (and risotto rice) as tender or soft on the outside but with some resistance when bitten into. If you normally serve your pasta soft, try it this way and taste the difference. Every shape and brand of pasta cooks differently; only the taste test, not packet instructions, will tell when it's cooked perfectly.

Alactasia Partial or complete deficiency of the enzyme lactase in the small intestine, resulting in an inability to digest the sugar lactose in milk, and hence intolerance of milk and milk products.

Alanine A non-essential amino acid, found in all proteins. β-Alanine is an isomer of alanine in which the amino group is attached to carbon3 of the molecule rather than carbon-2 as in alanine; it is important as part of pantothenic acid, carnosine, and anserine.

Albacore A long-finned species of tunny fish, Thynnus alalunga, usually canned as tuna fish.

Albacore A long-finned species of tunny fish, Thynnus alalunga, usually canned as tuna fish.

Albedo The white pith (mesocarp) of the inner peel of citrus fruits, accounting for some 20-60% of the whole fruit. It consists of sugars, cellulose, and pectins, and is used as a commercial source of pectin.

Albert French name for English hot horseradish sauce.

Albigeolse, A l' French; garnish for meat consisting of stuffed tomatoes and potato croquettes.

Albion French; 1. Fish soup made with lobster quenelles and truffles;

2. Chicken broth with truffles, asparagus, chicken liver quenelles, and cocks' combs.

Albumen The white part of an egg. It contains virtually no fat and is high in protein. Egg whites have many uses in cooking. Whisking egg whites traps air. When whisked egg whites are folded into other ingredients which are then baked, the air remains trapped inside making the likes of meringues, mousses or soufflus light and airy. A good tip egg whites will whisk to a greater volume at room temperature than if they're chilled. Egg whites are also used in making sorbets because the protein stabilises the mixture during freezing, minimising the chance of ice crystals forming. When they're heated, the proteins in egg whites combine and coagulate - essential when making cakes, pancakes and batter puddings.

Albumin index A measure of the quality or freshness of an egg — the height: width ratio of the albumin when the egg is broken onto a flat surface. As the egg deteriorates, so the albumin spreads further, i.e. the albumin index decreases.

Albumin water Beverage made from lightly whisked egg-white and cold water, seasoned with lemon juice and salt.

Albuminolds Fibrous proteins that have a structural or protective rather than enzymic role in the body. Also known as scleroproteins. The main proteins of the connective tissues of the body. There are three main types: 1. collagens in skin, tendons, and bones are resistant to enzymic digestion with trypsin and pepsin, and can be converted to soluble gelatine by boiling with water;

2. elastins in tendons and arteries, which are not converted to gelatine on boiling;

3. keratins, the proteins of hair, feathers, scales, horns, and hoofs, which are insoluble in dilute acid or alkali, and are resistant to all animal digestive enzymes.

Alcohol Colourless liquid, which forms part of drinks such as wine and whisky, and which is formed by the action of yeast on sugar solutionsalcohol abuse or alcohol addiction = condition where a patient is addicted to drinking alcohol and cannot stopalcohol poisoning = poisoning and disease caused by excessive drinking of alcoholpure alcohol or ethyl alcohol or ethanol = colourless liquid, which is the basis of drinking alcohols (whisky, gin, vodka, etc.) and which is also used in medicines and as a disinfectantdenatured alcohol = ethyl alcohol (such as methylated spirit, rubbing alcohol, surgical spirit) with an additive (usually methyl alcohol) to make it unpleasant to drinkmethyl alcohol = wood alcohol (poisonous alcohol used for heating)alcohol rub = rubbing a bedridden patient with alcohol to help protect against bedsores and as a tonic.

Alcohol dehydrogenase 1. Alcohol dehydrogenases are a group of dehydrogenase enzymes that occur in many organisms and facilitate the conversion between alcohols and aldehydes or ketones. In humans and many other animals, they serve to break down alcohols which could otherwise be toxic; in yeast and many bacteria they catalyze the opposite reaction as part of fermentation.

2. The enzyme, present in most tissues of the body, that catalyses the oxidation of alcohol to acetaldehyde. There are several genetically determined forms of the enzyme, whose pattern differs among individuals.

Alcohol units For convenience in calculating intakes of alcohol, a unit of alcohol is defined as 8 g (10 mL) of absolute alcohol; this is the amount in ½ pint (300 mL) beer, a single measure of spirit (25 mL) or a single glass of wine (100 mL). The Royai College of Physicians of England has set upper limits of prudent consumption of alcohol as 21 units (= 168 g alcohol) per week for men and 14 units (= 112 g alcohol) per week for women.

Alcohol, denatured Drinkable alcohol is subject to tax in most countries and for industrial use it is denatured to render it unfit for consumption, by the addition of 5% methyl alcohol (methanol, CH_3OH, also known as wood alcohol), which is poisonous. This is industrial rectified spirit. For domestic use a purple dye and pyridine (which has an unpleasant odour) are also added; this is methylated spirit.

Alcoholic beverages Drinks made by fermenting fruit juices, sugars, and fermentable carbohydrates with yeast to form alcohol. These include beer, cider, and perry, 4-6% alcohol by volume; wines, 9-13% alcohol; spirits (e.g. brandy, gin, rum, vodka, whisky) made by distilling fermented liquor, 38-45% alcohol; liqueurs made from distilled spirits, sweetened and flavoured, 20-40% alcohol; and fortified wines (aperitif wines, madeira, port, sherry) made by adding spirit to wine, 18-25% alcohol. See also alcohol; proof spirit.

Alcoholism Physiological addiction to alcohol, associated with persistent heavy consumption of alcoholic beverages. In addition to the addiction, there may be damage to the liver (cirrhosis), stomach (gastritis), and pancreas (pancreatitis), as well as behavioural changes and peripheral nerve damage.

Alcool blanc French; white spirit (silent spirit) or eau de vie. Distilled spirits from fermented fruit juice.

Alderman's walk The name given in London to the longest and finest cut from the haunch of venison or lamb.

Aldosterone A steroid hormone secreted by the adrenal cortex which controls the excretion of salts and water by the kidneys.

Aleatico A grape variety widely used for wine making, although not one of the classic varieties; makes fragrant sweet red wines.

Alecost An aromatic herbaceous plant, Tanacetum (Chrysanthemum) balsamita, related to tansy, used in salads and formerly used to flavour ale.

Aleurone layer The single layer of large cells under the bran coat and outside the endosperm of cereal grains. About 3% of the weight of the grain, and rich in protein, as well as containing about 20% of the vitamin B_1, 30% of the vitamin B_2 and 50% of the niacin of the grain. Botanically the aleurone layer is part of the endosperm, but in milling it remains attached to the inner layer of the bran.

Alewives River herrings, Pomolobus pseudoharengus, commonly used for canning after salting.

Alexander A cocktail; usually gin, crµme de cacao, and cream, although other spirits may be used.

Alfalfa Or lucerne, Medicago sativa, commonly grown for animal feed and silage; the seeds can be soaked in water to germinate and then eaten as sprouts.

Algae Simple (primitive) plants that do not show differentiation into roots, stems, and leaves. They are mostly aquatic — either seaweeds or pond and river-weeds. Some seaweeds, such as dulse and Irish moss, have long been eaten, and a number of unicellular algae, including Chlorella, Scenedesmus, and Spirulina spp. have been grown experimentally as novel sources of food (50-60% of the dry weight is protein).

Algerienne 1. Garnish for steak consisting of tomatoes and peppers simmered in oil.

2. Fried eggs served with a purιe of tomatoes, peppers, and aubergine.

3. Salad of courgettes, tomatoes, and cooked sweet potato.

4. Sautιed chicken and aubergine with sauce of tomatoes, garlic, and onions.

5. Cream soup made from sweet potatoes and filbert nuts.

Algin A compound which is extracted from algae and used in puddings, milk shakes and ice cream to make these foods creamier and thicker and to extend shelf life.

Alginates Salts of alginic acid found in many seaweeds as calcium salts or the free acid. Chemically, alginic acid is a non-starch polysaccharide Composed of mannuronic acid units.

Iron, magnesium, and ammonium salts of alginic acid form viscous solutions and hold large amounts of water. They are used as thickeners, stabilizers and gelling, binding, and emulsifying agents in food manufacture, especially in ice-cream and synthetic cream. Trade name Manucol.

Aligote A grape variety widely used for wine making, although not one of the classic varieties. Burgundy's second-ranking white grape; the wines need drinking within three years.

Alimentary canal The digestive tract, comprising (in man) the mouth, oesophagus, stomach, duodenum, and small and large intestines. See also gastro-intestinal tract.

Alitame A sweetener made from amino acids (L-aspartic acid, D-alanine, and a novel amide [a specific arrangement of chemical bonds between carbon, nitrogen and oxygen]). It offers a taste that is 2000 times sweeter than that of sucrose and can be used in a wide variety of products including beverages, tabletop sweeteners, frozen desserts and baked goods. Only the aspartic acid component of alitame is metabolized by the body. As a result, alitame contains 1.4 kcal/g. Since alitame is such an intense sweetener, however, it is used at very low levels and thus contributes negligible amounts of calories. It is highly stable, can withstand high temperatures in cooking and baking, and has the potential to be used in almost all foods and beverages in which sweeteners are presently used. FDA is currently considering a petition to approve its use in the United States food supply. Alitame has been approved for use in all food and beverage products in Australia, Mexico and New Zealand.

Alkali A compound that takes up hydrogen ions and so raises the pH of a solution; see also acid; buffers; salt.

Alkaloids Naturally occurring organic bases which have marked pharmacological actions in man and other animals. Many are found in plant foods, including potatoes and tomatoes (the Solanum alkaloids), or as the products of fungal action (e.g. ergot), although they also occur in animal foods (e.g. tetrodotoxin in puffer fish, tetramine in shellfish), and some are formed in the body (e.g. tryptamine, tyramine, phenylethylamine, and histamine are amines formed by the decarboxylation of amino acids). A number of alkaloids are used medically, e.g. morphine, colchicine, quinine, and atropine.

Alkannet A colouring obtained from the root of Anchusa (Alkanna) tinctoria which is insoluble in water but soluble in alcohol and oils. It is blue in alkali (or in the presence of lead), crimson with tin and violet with iron. Used for colouring fats, cheese, essences, and inferior port wine. Also known as orcanella.

Allantoin The oxidation product of uric acid which is the end-product of purine metabolism in most animals apart from man and apes, which excrete uric acid.

All-Bran Trade name for a breakfast cereal prepared from wheat bran, and hence a rich source of non-starch polysaccharide. A 60-g portion is a rich source of vitamins B_1, B_2, B_6, B_{12}, niacin, folate, iron, and copper; a source of protein; contains 1.5 g of fat of which 24% is saturated; provides 18 g of dietary fibre; supplies 160 kcal.

Allemande Classic French sauce, veloutı blended with egg yolks and cream. Also known as sauce blonde or parisienne. Named for its light colour, as opposed to sauce espagnole, which is dark.

Allergen An allergen is any substance (antigen), most often eaten or inhaled, that is recognized by the immune system and causes an allergic reaction.No comprehensive list of allergens is currently possible. Sensitivities vary from one person to another and it is possible to be allergic to an extraordinary range of substances. Dust, pollen and pet dander are all common allergens, but it is possible to be allergic to anything from chlorine to perfume. Food allergies are not as common as food sensitivity, but some foods such as peanuts (really a legume), nuts, seafood and shellfish are the cause of serious allergies in many people. A few people have even been recorded to be allergic to certain chemicals found in almost all water. Poison ivy (and other plants, like poison sumac or poison oak) is a plant that will cause an allergic reaction for anyone, given enough repeated contact — like any allergy, the human body must learn to fight the allergen, some bodies learn slower and will appear to be "immune" to poison ivy.

Allergy 1. A hypersensitivity of the body's immune system in response to exposure to specific substances (antigens), such as pollen, beestings, poison ivy, drugs, or foods. Anaphylactic shock is a severe form of allergy response which is a medical emergency. Symptoms of anaphylactic shock include dizziness, loss of consiousness, labored breathing, swelling of the tongue and breathing tubes, blueness of the skin, low blood pressure, and death.

2. An allergy can refer to several kinds of immune reactions including Type I hypersensitivity in which a person's body is hypersensitised and develops IgE type antibodies to typical proteins. When a person is hypersensitised, these substances are known as allergens. The word allergy derives from the Greek words allos meaning "other" and ergon meaning "work". Type I hypersensitivity is characterised by excessive activation of mast cells and basophils by immunoglobulin E resulting in a systemic inflammatory response that can result in symptoms as benign as a runny nose, to life-threatening anaphylactic shock and death.

Alliance French; sauce made from reduced (partially concentrated) white wine with tarragon vinegar and egg yolk.

Allicin A sulphur-containing compound partially responsible for the flavour of garlic.

Allinson bread A wholewheat bread named after Allinson, who advocated its consumption in England at the end of the nineteenth century, as did Graham in the USA (hence Graham bread). Now trade name for a wholemeal loaf.

Allodynia Pain due to stimuli that do not normally provoke pain.

Allostasis The ability of the organism to achieve stability through adaptation or change. This process, which is critical to our survival, involves the autonomic nervous system, the HPA axis, and the cardiovascular, metabolic, and immune systems which act to protect the body by responding to internal and external stimuli. Paradoxically, these same systems, when activated by stress, can protect and restore as well as damage the body.

Allotriophagy An unnatural desire for abnormal foods; also known as cissa, cittosis, and pica.

All-purpose flour All-purpose flour is made from a blend of high-gluten hard wheat and low-gluten soft wheat. It is a fine-textured flour milled from the inner part of the wheat kernel and contains neither the germ (the sprouting section) nor the bran (the outer husk). By law, in the United States, all flours not containing wheat germ must have niacin, riboflavin, and thiamin added. Most all-purpose flours are labeled "enriched," indicating that these nutrients have been added. All-purpose flour comes bleached and unbleached and they can be used interchangeably.

Allspice An aromatic spice that looks like a large, smooth peppercorn (about the size of a pea), allspice is the dried berry of the West Indian allspice tree. It's also called Jamaican pepper or pimento and is so called because its taste is said to resemble a combination of cinnamon, cloves, nutmeg and black pepper. Allspice can be bought whole or ground and is used in both sweet and savoury dishes including mulled drinks, Christmas pudding, pickles and marinades, and Jamaican jerk chicken.

Allumettes Potatoes cut into thin 'matchsticks' and fried, also known as straw potatoes. Also used sometimes for narrow fingers of pastry.

Ally methyl trisulfide, dithiolthiones A type of sulfide/thiol found in cruciferous vegetables which may provide the health benefits of lowering LDL cholesterol and of maintaining a healthy immune system.

Almond It is the kernel of the fruit of the almond tree that is native of the warmer parts of western Asia and North Africa. It belongs to the same group of plants as the rose, plum, cherry, and peach. The seed is rounded at one end and pointed at the other, and covered with a thin brown coat. The almond belongs to the same group of plants as the rose, plum, cherry, and peach. There are two types of almonds - sweet and bitter. Today, Americans give guests at weddings a bag of sugared almonds (representing children, happiness, romance, good health, and fortune). In Sweden, cinnamon-flavored rice pudding with an almond hidden inside is a Christmas custom (find it and good fortune is yours for a year).

Almond extract A solution of oil, bitter almonds, and alcohol (approximately 1%) that is used for a flavoring in baking.

Almond flour Almond flour or meal is the residue left after almond oil has been extracted from the kernels. It is entirely free from starch and is used in making bread and biscuits for diabetics.

Almond paste A mixture of sugar, almonds, and egg whites. Also called marzipan. It is widely used in dessert preparations. Almond paste and marzipan are both made from ground almonds. They differ mainly in their sugar content. Marzipan is made from almond paste and sugar and is used primarily in confections and decorations because it is more moldable and the almond flavor is less pronounced. Almond paste is used in pastries and other baked goods. They are not interchangeable in recipes.

Almorta Spanish; flour made from seeds of common vetch or tare, Vicia sativa.

Aloe Dried juice from the leaves of Aloe perryi, used in medicines. Contains a glycoside, aloe-emodin or rhabarberone, aloe oil, and aloin or barbaloin.

Alpha carotene A type of carotenoid found in carrots which provides the health benefit of neutralizing free radicals that may cause damage to cells.

Alpha lipoic acid An efficient antioxidant, Alpha-Lipoic Acid at high dose levels has been shown to increase glucose uptake, indicating potential utility in the management of blood glucose levels. In diabetics, proteins tend to bind with glucose, precipitating oxidative damage. Alpha-Lipoic Acid supplementation reduces glycation of proteins, thereby offering protection. Alpha-Lipoic Acid also protects against cholesterol oxidation and the consequent atherosclerosis in diabetics as well as in others at risk of cardiovascular diseases.

Alpha-Laval centrifuge A continuous bowl centrifuge for separating liquids of different densities and for clarifying. Widely used for cream separation.

Alpha-L-polylactate CytoSport's proprietary formula that provides a long-lasting source of carbohydrate energy and buffers lactic-acid production in the working muscles. The principal ingredient in Cytomax.

Alternative agriculture A range of technological and management option farms striving to reduce costs, protect health and environmental quality, and enhance beneficial biological interactions and natural processes. Alternative agriculture techniques cannot be uniformly applied across all commodities or all regions of the country. Such practices typically require more information, trained labor, time and management skills per unit of production than conventional farming.

Alum Alum is used as an ingredient in baking powder and is used to give crispness to pickles and maraschino cherries and to harden gelatin. Alum can be a dangerous substance when not used properly. Ingestion of 30 grams (1 ounce) has killed adults. Alum is legal to use in baking powders. In pickles and cherries, the amount left in the product amounts to less than 0.2 percent. According to USDA, if good quality ingredients are used in pickling and up-to-date methods are followed, alum is not needed for crisp pickles. If alum is used in pickling, it is used only in a soak solution. It should be washed off thoroughly before completing the recipe. Do not put alum in the final pickling liquid. Use only food-grade alum. (Douche alum is not food-grade.)

Aluminium The third most abundant element in the earth's crust (after oxygen and silicon) but with no known biological function. Present in small amounts in many foods but only a smali proportion is absorbed. Aluminium salts are found in the abnormal nerve tangles in the brain in Alzheimer's disease, and it has been suggested that aluminium poisoning may be a factor in the development of the disease, although there is little evidence. Aluminium is used in cooking vessels and as foil for wrapping food, as well as in cans and tubes; it is a soft flexible metal, resistant to oxidation and deterioration, although it is dissolved by alkalis. The 'silver' beads used to decorate confectionery are coated with either silver foil or an alloy of aluminium and copper. Baking powders containing sodium aluminium sulphate as the acid agent were used at one time (alum baking powders), and aluminium hydroxide and silicates are commonly used in antacid medications.

Alveographe A device for measuring the stretching quality of dough as an index of its protein quality for baking. A standard disc of dough is blown into a bubble and the pressure curve and bursting pressure are measured to give the stability, extensibility, and strength of the dough.

Alzheimer's disease This disease causes progressive memory loss and dementia in its victims as it kills brain cells (neurons). It is named after Alois Alzheimer who in 1906 first described the Amyloid ί Protein (AίP) plaques in the human brain that are caused by this disease. The drug Tacrine appears to slow the progression of Alzheimer's disease, but there is currently no way to stop the disease.

Amabile Italian; wines intermediate between medium sweet (abboccato) and sweet (dulce).

Amaranth Amaranth is from the Greek for "never-fading flower" or "everlasting." It is an annual herb, and therefore not a true grain. It has broad leaves and large flower heads that produce thousands of tiny, protein-rich seeds. There are hundreds of varieties of amaranth. It is grown for its leaves-some varieties are good in salad, some are delicious steamed or stir-fried-and its somewhat peppery seeds. Amaranth can be cooked as a cereal. The seeds are very tiny-looking, a bit like caviar when cooked, and their lack of substance makes them rather unsatisfactory as the base of pilaf-type dishes. Amaranth is most often ground into flour, which has a fairly strong malt-like vegetable taste and is beige in colour. It is the only known food that contains between 75% and 87% of total human nutritional requirements. Amaranth is used in several cultures in very interesting ways, In Mexico, it is popped and mixed with a sugar solution to make a candy called alegria and the roasted seed is used to create a traditional Mexican drink called atole. People from Peru use fermented amaranth seeds to make chichi (beer). During the carnival festival, women dancers often use the red amaranth flower as rouge, painting their cheeks, and then dancing while carrying bundles of amaranth on their backs.

Amaranthus A genus of plants cultivated for their leaves and sometimes for their seeds also. The leaves are promoted in South East Asia as a good source of carotene.

Amaretti Meaning 'little bitter things' in Italian, amaretti are small almond biscuits similar to macaroons. Some are made using ground sweet and bitter almonds, baked with egg and sugar, others from ground apricot kernels. They're light and airy, crunchy on the outside and chewy in the middle. Serve them as an after-dinner treat with sweet wine or liqueurs - Italians like to dip them in red wine. They can be used instead of sponge fingers in trifles and tiramisu, or ground up and used in cakes and desserts. Amarettini are the mini version. For an easy dessert, sandwich them together with buttercream, or serve a large plateful alongside your favourite ice cream so guests can just dip in.

Amaretto An Italian almond flavored liqueur (or cordial) that is made from apricot pits and flavored with almonds and aromatic extracts.

Amazone French garnish for meat; lentil fritters, hollowed out and stuffed with morel mushrooms and chestnut purie.

Ambergris A waxy concretion obtained from the intestine of the sperm whale, containing cholesterol, ambrein, and benzoic acid. Used in drugs and perfumery.

Amberlite Group of polystyrene resins (ion-exchange resins) used to absorb specific ions in water softening and purification in general.

Ambrosia 1. The name is sometimes applied to certain beverages.

2. A traditional Christmas dish in many Southern homes, where the dessert is served in the best cut-glass bowl from the sideboard. It usually consists of chilled fruit (usually oranges and bananas) mixed with coconut.

Amenorrhoea Cessation of menstruation, normally occurring between the ages of 40 and 55 (the menopause), but sometimes at an early age, especially as a result of severe under-nutrition (as in anorexia nervosa) when body weight falls below about 45 kg.

Amer Picon Trade name; pungent bitters invented in 1830 by Gaston Picon; contains quinine, gentian, and orange.

American Breakfast It is an restaurant term that usually consists of eggs, juice, bacon or sausage, toast or hashbrowns.

Ames test An in vitro test for the ability of chemicals, including potential food additives, to cause mutation in bacteria (the mutagenic potential). Commonly used as a preliminary screening method to detect substances likely to be carcinogenic.

Aminapaptidase An enzyme secreted in the pancreatic juice which removes amino acids sequentially from the free amino terminal of a peptide or protein (i.e. the end which has a free amino group exposed), until the final product is a dipeptide. Since it works at the end of the peptide chain, it is an exopeptidase.

Amincaciduria Excretion of abnormal amounts of one or more amino acids in the urine, usually as a result of a genetic disease. See also amino acid disorders.

AmInctransferase Any enzyme that catalyses the reaction of transamination.

Amine Amines are organic compounds and a type of functional group that contain nitrogen as the key atom. Structurally amines resemble ammonia, wherein one or more hydrogen atoms are replaced by organic substituents such as alkyl and aryl groups. An important exception to this rule is that compounds of the type RC(O)NR2, where the C(O) refers to a carbonyl group, are called amides rather than amines. Amides and amines have different structures and properties, so the distinction is chemically important. Somewhat confusing is the fact that amines in which an N-H group has been replaced by an N-M group (M = metal) are also called amides. Thus $(CH_3)2NLi$ is lithium dimethylamide.

Amino acids The basic units from which proteins are made. Chemically compounds with an amino group ($-NH_2$) and a carboxyl group (-COOH) attached to the same carbon atom.

Thirteen of the amino acids involved in proteins can be synthesized in the body, and so are called non-essential or dispensable amino acids, since they do not have to be provided in the diet. They are alanine, arginine, aspartic acid, asparagine, cysteine, cystine, glutamic acid, glutamine, glycine, hydroxyproline, proline, serine, and tyrosine.

Eight amino acids cannot be synthesized in the body at all and so must be provided in the diet; they are called the essential or indispensable amino acids - isoleucine, leucine, lysine, methionine, phenylalanine, threonine, tryptophan, and valine. In addition, histidine is partially essential, since it cannot be synthesized in adequate amounts to meet requirements without some dietary intake, and arginine may be essential for infants, since their requirement is greater than their ability to synthesize this amino acid. Two of the non-essential amino acids are made in the body from essential amino acids: cysteine (and cystine) from methionine, and tyrosine from phenylalanine.

The limiting amino acid of a protein is that essential amino acid present in least amount relative to the requirement for that amino acid. The ratio between the amount of the limiting amino acid in a protein and the requirement for that amino acid provides a chemical estimation of the nutritional value (protein quality) of that protein, termed chemical score. Most cereal proteins are limited by lysine, and most animal and other vegetable proteins by the sum of methionine + cysteine (the sulphur amino acids). In whole diets it is usually the sulphur amino acids that are limiting.

A number of other amino acids also occur in proteins, including hydroxyproline, hydroxylysine, -carboxyglutamate and methylhistidine, but are nutritionally unimportant since they cannot be re-utilized for protein synthesis. Other amino acids occur as intermediates in metabolic pathways, but are not required for protein synthesis, and are nutritionally unimportant, although they may occur in foods. These include homocysteine, citrulline, and ornithine. Some of the non-protein amino acids that occur in plants are toxic in excess.

The amino acids are sometimes classified by the chemical nature of the side-chain. Two are acidic: glutamic acid (glutamate) and aspartic acid (aspartate) and have a carboxylic acid (-COOH) group in the sidechain. Three, lysine, arginine and histidine, have basic groups in the side-chain. Three, phenylalanine, tyrosine, and tryptophan, have an aromatic group in the side-chain. Three, leucine, isoleucine, and valine, have a branched chain structure. These three have very similar metabolism, and a rare genetic disease affecting their metabolism results in maple syrup urine disease. Two, methionine and cysteine, contain sulphur in the side-chain; although cysteine is not an essential amino acid, it can only be synthesized from methionine, and it is conventional to consider the sum of methionine plus cysteine (the sulphur amino acids) in consideration of protein quality.

An alternative classification of the amino acids is by their metabolic fate; whether they can be utilized for glucose synthesis or not. Those that can give rise to glucose are termed glucogenic (or sometimes antiketogenic); those that give rise to ketones or acetate when they are metabolized are termed ketogenic. Only leucine and lysine are purely ketogenic; isoleucine, phenylalanine, tyrosine, and tryptophan give rise to both ketogenic and glucogenic fragments; the remainder are purely glucogenic.

Amino acid chelate A term used to describe a mineral that has been bonded to an amino acid, i.e Magnesium Aspartate. The body can absorb amino acid chelated minerals more easily than standard forms i.e Magnesium Oxide.

Amino acid disorders A number of extremely rare genetic diseases, occurring in 1-80 per million live births which affect the metabolism of individual amino acids; if untreated many result in mental retardation. Screening for those conditions that can be treated is carried out shortly after birth in most countries. Treatment is generally by feeding specially formulated diets providing minimal amounts of the amino acid involved. See also argininaemia; argininosuccinic aciduria; citrullinaemia, cystinuria; cystathioninuria; Hartnup disease; homocystinuria; hyperammonaemia; maple syrup urine disease; phenylketonuria.

Aminogram A diagrammatic representation of the amino acid composition of a peptide or protein. A plasma aminogram is the composition of the free amino acid pool in blood plasma.

Amla Indian gooseberry, Emblica officinalis Gaertn, important in Ayurvedic medicine and reported to reduce hypercholesterolaemia. An extremely rich source of vitamin C (600 mg/100 g).

Amoebiasis Infection of the intestinal tract with pathogenic amoeba (commonly Entamoeba histolytica) from contaminated food or water, causing profuse diarrhoea, intestinal bleeding, pain, jaundice, anorexia, and weight loss.

Amomum A group of tropical plants including cardamom and melegueta pepper, which have pungent and aromatic seeds.

Amour Purple-coloured liqueur, flavoured with citrus fruits and violets.

Amourettes French; marrow from calves' bones, normally cooked as a garnish.

AMP Adenosine monophosphate.

Amphetamine A chemical at one time used as an appetite suppressant; addictive, and a common drug of abuse ('speed'), its use is strictly controlled by law.

Amtlicher Prufungsnummer (AP) German; batch number on labels of quality wines. See wine classification, Germany.

Amuse-bouche Also known as amuse-gueule, amusee, petite amuse, and lagniappe are used interchangeably to describe these tasty morsels. A French term that literally means "mouth amusement." These are tiny bites of food served before a meal to whet the palate and invigorate the appetite. They're more whimsical than hors d'oeuvres, and smaller than appetizers. The best restaurants offer a tiny serving of something interesting (also known as palate teasers) soon after you sit down, which ideally previews the cooking style of the restaurant. In some restaurants, it's also a way to present something luxurious to favoured customers. In the United States we think of them as 'hors-d'oeuvre'. Customers regard them as tokens of appreciation. In this age of frequently getting less than what is expected, gestures like this make diners feel welcome and can promote customer loyalty.

Amydon A traditional starchy material made by steeping wheat flour in water, then drying the starch sediment in the sun, used for thickening broths, etc.

Amygdalin 1. A glycoside in almonds and apricot and cherry stones which is hydrolysed by the enzyme emulsin to yield glucose, hydrocyanic acid, and benzaldehyde. It is therefore highly poisonous, although it has been promoted, with no evidence, as a nutrient, laetrile or so-called vitamin B 17. Unfounded claims have been made for its value in treating cancer.

2. French name for cakes and sweets made with almonds.

Amylases Enzymes that hydrolyse starch and glycogen. a-Amylase (dextrinogenic amylase or diastase) acts to produce small dextrin fragments from starch, while ι-amylase (maltogenic amylase) liberates maltose, some free glucose, and isomaltose from the branch points in amylopectin.

Salivary amylase (sometimes called by its obsolete name of ptyalin) and pancreatic amylase are both a-amylases.

Amyli Dried tamarind.

Amyloamylose Old name for amylose, as distinct from erythroamylose, the old name for amylopectin.

Amylodyspepsia An inability to digest starch.

Amylograph A device to measure the viscosity of flour paste as it is heated from 25°C to 90°C (the same increase in temperature as occurs in baking), which serves as a measure of the diastatic activity of the flour.

Amyloins Carbohydrates that are complexes of dextrins with varying proportions of maltose.

Amylopectin The branched chain form of starch. About 75-80% of starch is in this form, the remainder is amylose.

Amylopeptic A general description of enzymes that are able to split starch to give soluble products.

Amylopsi Alternative name for pancreatic amylase.

Amylose The straight chain form of starch. About 20-25% of starch is in this form, the remainder is amylopectin.

Anabolic Pertaining to the putting together of complex substances from simples ones, especially to the building of muscle protein from amino acids.

Anabolism The process of building up or synthesizing. See metabolism.

Anacard Brazilian; vinegar made by fermentation of the pulp surrounding the cashew nut.

Anadama bread It is a specialty yeast bread of the New England States that is made with flour, cornmeal, and molasses.

Anaemia 1. A shortage of red blood cells, leading to pallor and shortness of breath, especially on exertion. Most commonly due to a dietary deficiency of iron, or excessive blood losses resulting in iron losses greater than can be met from the diet. Other dietary deficiencies can also result in anaemia, including deficiency of vitamin B 12 or folic acid (megaloblastic anaemia), vitamin E (haemolytic anaemia), and rarely vitamin C or vitamin B 6. 2. Haemolytic Anaemia caused by premature and excessive destruction of red blood cells; not normally due to nutritional deficiency, but can occur as a result of vitamin E deficiency in premature infants.

Anaemia, megaloblastic Release into the circulation of immature precursors of red blood cells, due to deficiency of either folic acid or vitamin B 12. See also anaemia, pernicious.

Anaemia, pernicious Anaemia due to deficiency of vitamin B 12, most commonly as a result of failure to absorb the vitamin from the diet. There is release into the circulation of immature precursors of red blood cells, the same type of megaloblastic anaemia as is seen in folic acid deficiency. There is also progressive damage to the spinal cord (sub-acute combined degeneration), which is not reversed on restoring the vitamin. The underlying cause of the condition may be the production of antibodies against either the intrinsic factor that is required for absorption of the vitamin, or the cells of the gastric mucosa that secrete intrinsic factor. Atrophy of the gastric mucosa with ageing also impairs vitamin B 12 absorption, and causes pernicious anaemia. Dietary deficiency of vitamin B 12, leading to a similar anaemia with spinal cord degeneration, may occur in strict vegetarians.

Anaerobes Micro-organisms that grow in the absence of oxygen. Obligate anaerobes cannot survive in the presence of oxygen, facultative anaerobes normally grow in the presence of oxygen but can also grow in its absence.

Anaerobic literally "without oxygen". A high-intensity energy system where the muscles lack sufficient oxygen to successfully burn fuel, resulting in the production of lactic acid. Anaerobic exercise is very intense and can only be sustained for short periods of time.

Anaheim chile Mild, long green chile peppers that are named after the area near Los Angeles where they were first cultivated. Also known as Chile Verde (green), Chile Colourado (red) or the California Long Green, the Anaheim Chile is light green in colour and slightly bent. It is the most commonly found variety in the United States. Mild, sweet, and slightly bitter in flavor, this chile pepper can be used fresh or roasted and is often available canned. If you buy them fresh, Anaheim Chile peppers can be stored in the refrigerator for one week.

Anal fissure Crack in the skin in or adjacent to the anal canal.

Anal stenosis A condition in which the anus is narrowed

Analgesic Pain relieving.

Analytical epidemiology Epidemiological investigations specifically aimed at studying the determinants of diseases in study populations.

Anaphylaxis 1. In medicine, anaphylaxis is a severe and rapid multi-system allergic reaction. Anaphylaxis occurs when a person is exposed to a trigger substance, called an allergen, to which they have become sensitized. Minute amounts of allergens may cause a life-threatening anaphylactic reaction. Anaphylaxis may occur after ingestion, inhalation, skin contact or injection of an allergen. The most severe type of anaphylaxis—anaphylactic shock—will usually lead to death in minutes if left untreated.

2. A generalised inflammatory immune reaction to a foreign protein in a sensitised individual which may be severe enough to be life-threatening.

Anchovy Anchovies vary in size and can be bought either fresh or cured. Fresh anchovies look and taste similar to sardines. They're not easy to find in the UK because there isn't a great demand for them, but try Italian or Spanish delis. Cured anchovies were originally left whole and packed in salt, but now they tend to be boned, cleaned and preserved in salt or oil and sold in tins or jars. The type packed in oil need to be drained before use. You may want to soak the salted variety in milk for a while to get rid of any excess saltiness. Supermarkets have a limited range but delis tend to sell a wider range.

Use anchovies to make anchovy butter to serve with fish, anchovy toast, tapenade or the Italian bagna cauda - a mixture of butter or olive oil, garlic, basil and anchovy fillets mashed into a sauce and served hot with vegetables as a type of fondue. Anchovies have an affinity with red meat and also form the basis of condiments such as anchovy essence, Worcestershire sauce, Asian fish sauce and Patum Peperium.

Anchovy essence A natural juice concentrate from anchovies, this is the British equivalent of Asian fish sauce and is a good substitute for it. Used sparingly it can add an extra kick to soups, stews and sauces.

Anchovy paste A paste of pureed anchovies with oil and salt. Available in tubes at most supermarkets and specialty food stores. You can also make your own using a can of anchovy fillets. First wash them in cold water, then mash them with a fork, and add just enough olive oil to make a smooth paste.more

Anchoyade French (Provennale); anchovies purıed with garlic and olive oil.

Andalouse 1. Dishes with rice and tomatoes.

2. French sauce based on mayonnaise with tomato purıe and diced peppers.

3. Garnish of tomatoes stuffed with rice, aubergine, and tomatoes.

4. Clear chicken soup garnished with tomatoes, rice, ham, and beaten egg.

Andouille 1. Traditionally, the andouilles from France were made from the large intestines and stomach of the pig (seasoned heavily and smoked).

2. Andouille is also the Cajun smoked sausage so famous nationally today. Made with pork butt, shank, and a small amount of pork fat. This sausage is seasoned with salt, cracked black pepper, and garlic. The andouille is then slowly smoked over pecan wood and sugar cane. True andouille is stuffed into the beef middle casing, which makes the sausage approximately one and a half inches in diameter. When smoked, it becomes very dark to almost black in colour. It is not uncommon for the Cajuns to smoke andouille for seven to eight hours at approximately 175 degrees.

Anemia Anemia is a condition in which a deficiency in the size or number of erythrocytes (red blood cells) or the amount of hemoglobin they contain limits the exchange of oxygen and carbon dioxide between the blood and the tissue cells. Most anemias are caused by a lack of nutrients required for normal erythrocyte synthesis, principally iron, vitamin B-12, and folic acid. Others result from a variety of conditions, such as hemorrhage, genetic abnormalities, chronic disease states or drug toxicity.

Aneurine Obsolete name for vitamin B_1.

Aneurysm Local dilatation (swelling and weakening) of the wall of a blood vessel, usually the result of atherosclerosis and hypertension; especially serious when occurring in the aorta, when rupture may prove fatal.

Angel Food Cake Angel Food Cake is also known as foam-style cake. They are made with a large quantity of egg whites and no shortening or leavening. Angel Food or "angel cake" is thought to be a takeoff of the cornstarch cake and the sponge cake.

Angel's hair Jam made from the fibrous part of mature pumpkin or squash, preferably kept from the previous year's harvest.

Angelica Angelica may be familiar as the acid green crystallised or candied strips used as a decoration on cakes and desserts, but angelica itself is a herb. It's known as 'herb of the angels' (hence the name) because it was believed to have medicinal properties. This tall plant, which has a long firm stem and bright green leaves, is a member of the parsley family.

Candied angelica is made by boiling the stems in sugar syrup. If you can find the fresh herb (almost impossible) the stems can be cooked with rhubarb or apple for pies or crumbles. They're also used in jams and preserves, and the leaves go well with fish or in salads.

Angelman syndrome A genetic disorder characterized by mental retardation, hyperactivity, and unprovoked laughter

Angel's hair Jam made from the fibrous part of mature pumpkin or squash, preferably kept from the previous year's harvest.

Angels on horseback Oysters wrapped in bacon, skewered, and grilled.

Anghiti Indian; charcoal brazier used for grilling kebabs.

Angina Paroxysmal thoracic pain and choking sensation, especially during exercise or stress, due to partial blockage of the coronary artery (the blood vessel supplying the heart), as a result of atherosclerosis.

Angioedema, hereditary A genetic form of angioedema. (Angioedema is also referred to as Quinke's disease.) Persons with it are born lacking an inhibitor protein (called C1 esterase inhibitor) that normally prevents activation of a cascade of proteins leading to the swelling of angioedema. Patients can develop recurrent attacks of swollen tissues, pain in the abdomen, and swelling of the voice box (larynx) which can compromise breathing. The diagnosis is suspected with a history of recurrent angioedema. It is confirmed by finding abnormally low levels of C1 esterase inhibitor in the blood. Treatment options include antihistamines and male steroids (androgens) that can also prevent the recurrent attacks. Also called hereditary angioneurotic edema.

Anglaise 1. Plainly cooked in stock or water;

2. coating of eggs on foods that are then dipped in breadcrumbs and fried;

3. garnish for boiled salt beef consisting of boiled vegetables.

Angostura The best known of the bitters, widely used in cocktails; a secret blend of herbs and spices, including the bitter aromatic bark of either of two trees of the orange family (Galipea officinalis, Cusparia felorifuga). Invented in 1824 by Dr Siegert in the town of Angostura in Bolivia, originally as a medicine, and now made in Trinidad. A few drops of Angostura in gin makes a 'pink gin'.

Angostura bitters Named after a town in Venezuela and made in Trinidad from roots, bark, leaves, and alcohol. It is used in small amounts to lend an aromatic and slightly bitter element to mixed drinks. It is best known as the essential ingredient of the popular cocktail called the "Manhattan."

Engstrom A unit of length equal to 10-8 cm (10-10 m) and hence = 10 nm; not an official SI unit, but still commonly used in structural chemistry and crystallography. See Appendix I.

Angular stomatitis A characteristic cracking and fissuring of the skin at the angles of the mouth, a symptom of vitamin B 2 deficiency, but also seen in other conditions.

Animal and Plant Health Inspection Service (APHIS) A government agency which resides in the United States Department of Agriculture and governs the field-testing of agricultural biotechnology crops.

Animal protein factor A name given to a growth factor or factors which were found to be present in animal but not vegetable proteins. Vitamin B 12 was identified as one of these.

Anion A negatively charged ion.

Anise (anis) Liqueur made by infusion of aniseed berries (not star anise) in spirit; may be sweet or dry. French sweet anise liqueur is anisette. Pastis is prepared by distillation of anise and liquorice rather than infusion.

Anise pepper A pungent spice from the Sichuan region of China (the fruit of Zanthoxylum piperitum); the flavour develops gradually after biting into the pepper.

Anise, star A spice, the seeds of Illicium verum, widely used in Chinese cooking. Distinct from aniseed.

Aniseed The dried fruit of Pimpinella anisum, a member of the parsley family, which is used to flavour baked goods, meat dishes, and drinks, including anise, anisette, and ouzo. See also anise, star.

Aniseed milk Dutch (anijs melk); hot milk drink flavoured with aniseed, traditionally drunk when one is ice skating.

Anisette A sweet liqueur flavoured with aniseed.

Annata Year of vintage on Italian wine labels. See wine classification, Italy.

Annatto A paste produced from achiote seeds, which are ground and used as a spice in parts of Latin America. Annatto is more important as a colouring agent than as a spice. It's used to make a bright orange-yellow dye that's produced commercially and used to colour butter, margarine, cheese (such as Cheshire and

Lancashire) and smoked fish such as mackerel and kippers.

Anorectal manometry A test that can be used to measure resting and squeezing anal sphincter pressures, rectal sensation and compliance, and sphincter response.

Anorectic drugs Drugs that depress the appetite, used as an aid to weight reduction. The most commonly used are diethylpropion, fenfluramine (and dexfenfluramine), phenmetrazine hydrochloride, and mazindol. Amphetamines were used at one time, but are addictive and subject to special control.

Anorexia Lack of appetite. anorexia nervosa A psychological disturbance resulting in a refusal to eat, possibly with restriction to a very limited range of foods, and often accompanied by a rigid programme of vigorous physical exercise, to the point of exhaustion. Anorectic subjects generally do not feel sensations of hunger. The result is a very considerable loss of weight, with tissue atrophy and a fall in basal metabolic rate. It is especially prevalent among adolescent girls; when body weight falls below about 45 kg there is a cessation of menstruation.

Anosmia Lack or impairment of the sense of smell.

Anserine A dipeptide found in muscle, of unknown function. It consists of ß-alanine and methylhistidine.

Antabuse Trade name for the drug disulfiram, used in the treatment of alcoholism. It inhibits the further metabolism of acetaldehyde arising from the metabolism of alcohol, and so causes headache, nausea, vomiting, and palpitations if alcohol is consumed.

Antacids Bases or buffers that neutralize acids, used generally to counteract excessive gastric acidity and to treat indigestion. Antacid preparations generally contain such compounds as sodium bicarbonate, aluminium hydroxide, magnesium carbonate, or magnesium hydroxide.

Anthocyanidins A type of flavonoid found in various fruits which provides the health benefits of neutralizing free radicals and possibly reducing the risk of cancer.

Anthropometer An instrument for measuring dimensions of the human body; arm span measurements are made with an anthropometer, a stainless steel detachable rod, approximately seven feet long with etched gradations to 0.1 cm or 1/8 inch and one movable sleeve.

Anthropometric deficit Growth delays in the ratios of weight/age, weight/height and height/ age, using as a reference conventionally recommended charts of averages. Can also refer to other indices of body measurements.

Anthropometry Body measurements used as an index of physiological development and nutritional status; a non-invasive way of assessing body composition. Weight for age provides information about the overall nutritional status of children; weight for height is used to detect acute malnutrition (wasting); height for age to detect chronic malnutrition (stunting). Mid-upper arm circumference provides an index of muscle wastage in undernutrition. Skinfold thickness is related to the amount of subcutaneous fat as an index of over- or under-nutrition.

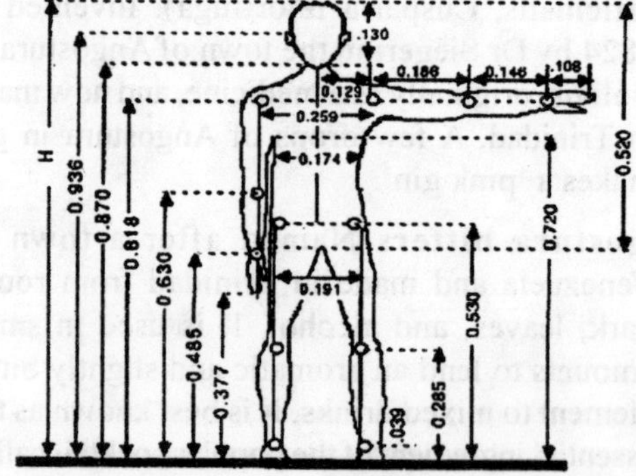

Fig. Anthropometry (Body Measurement)

Antibiotic resistance The ability of a bacterium to synthesize a protein that neutralizes an antibiotic.

Antibiotics Antibiotics are used in animal agriculture for two reasons. First, to improve the rate of growth and the feed efficiency of animals so they produce more meat or milk on less feed. The second reason is to prevent and treat diseases, just as in humans.

Antibodies A class of proteins formed in the body in response to the presence of antigens (foreign proteins and other compounds), which bind to the antigen, so inactivating it. Immunity to infection is due to the production of antibodies against specific proteins of bacteria, viruses, or other disease-causing organisms, and immunization is the process of giving these marker proteins, generally in an inactivated form, to stimulate the production of antibodies. Adverse reactions to foods (food allergies) may be due to the production of antibodies against specific food proteins. Chemically the antibodies form a class of proteins known as the ?-globulins or immunoglobulins; there are five types, classified as IgA, IgD, IgE, IgG, and IgM.

Antibody 1. An antibody or immunoglobulin is a large Y-shaped protein used by the immune system to identify and neutralize foreign objects like bacteria and viruses. Each antibody recognizes a specific antigen unique to its target. This is because at the two tips of its "Y", it has structures akin to locks. Every lock only has one key, in this case, its own antigen. When the key is inserted into the lock, the antibody attaches, tagging the microbe or an infected cell for attack by other parts of the immune system or by directly neutralizing its target (i.e. blocking a part of the microbe that is essential for its invasion and survival). The production of antibodies is the main function of the humoral immune system.

2. A type of protein made by plasma cells (a type of white blood cell) in response to an antigen (foreign substance). Each antibody can bind to only one specific antigen. The purpose of this binding is to help destroy the antigen. Antibodies can work in several ways, depending on the nature of the antigen. Some antibodies destroy antigens directly. Others make it easier for white blood cells to destroy the antigen.

Antibody therapy Treatment with an antibody, a substance that can directly kill specific tumor cells or stimulate the immune system to kill tumor cells.

Anti-caking agents Compounds added in small amounts to powdered foodstuffs to prevent clumping or caking - e.g. anhydrous disodium hydrogen phosphate is added to salt and icing sugar, aluminium calcium silicate or calcium or magnesium carbonate to table salt, calcium silicate to baking powder.

Anticarcinogens Substances which inhibit the formation of cancers or the growth of tumors. More than 600 chemicals are claimed to be anti-cancer agents. These range from natural chemical constituent present in garlic, broccoli, cabbage and green tea to manmade antioxidants, such as butylated hydroxyanisole (BHA) and derivatives of retinoic acid.

Anticoagulants Compounds that prevent or slow the process of blood clotting or coagulation, either in samples of blood taken for analysis or in the body. One of the most commonly used such substances is heparin, which is formed in the body (especially the lungs and liver).

People at risk of thrombosis are often treated with Warfarin and similar compounds as an anticoagulant, to reduce the risk of intravenous blood clot formation. These act by antagonizing the action of vitamin K in the synthesis of blood clotting proteins, and people taking anticoagulants should be careful not to take supplements containing large amounts of vitamin K. It is most unlikely that the vitamin K in foods would be enough to have any such adverse effect.

Anticonvulsant An agent used to prevent or minimize the occurrence or severity of seizures; medication-nutrient interactions can include interference with metabolism of folic acid, carnitine and vitamins B6, B12, and D

Antidiarrhoeal Drug used to treat diarrhoea by absorbing water from the intestine, altering intestinal motility, or adsorbing (bacterial) toxins.

Antidiuretic Drug used to reduce the formation of urine and so conserve fluid in the body. See also water balance.

Antiemetic Drug used to prevent or alleviate nausea and vomiting. antigalactic Drug that reduces or prevents the secretion of milk in women after parturition.

Antigen 1. An antigen is a substance that stimulates an immune response, especially the production of antibodies. Antigens are usually proteins or polysaccharides, but can be any type of molecule, including small molecules (haptens) coupled to a carrier-protein.

2. Something potentially capable of inducing an immune response. Antibodies are elicited by antigens.

3. A substance that causes the immune system to make a specific immune response.

Anti-grey-hair factor Deficiency of the vitamin pantothenic acid causes loss of hair colour in black and brown rats, and at one time the vitamin was known as the anti-grey-hair factor. It is not related to the loss of hair pigment in human beings.

Antihistamine Drug that antagonizes the actions of histamine; those that block histamine H 1 receptors are used to treat allergic reactions; those that block H 2 receptors are used to treat peptic ulcers.

Antihypertensive Drug, diet, or other treatment used to treat hypertension by lowering blood pressure.

Antilipidaemic Drug, diet, or other treatment used to treat hyperlipidaemia by lowering blood lipids.

Antimetabolite Compound that inhibits a normal metabolic process, acting as an analogue of a normal metabolite. Some are useful in chemotherapy of cancer, others are naturally occurring toxins in foods, frequently causing vitamin deficiency diseases by inhibiting the normal metabolism of the vitamin.

Antimony Toxic metal of no known metabolic function, and therefore not a dietary essential. Antimony compounds are used in treatment of some parasitic diseases.

Antimycotics Substances that inhibit the growth of moulds and fungi, such as sodium and calcium propionates, methyl hydroxybenzoate, quaternary ammonium chloride, sodium benzoate, sorbic acid.

Antinociception Increased tolerance to pain.

Antioxidant An antioxidant is a chemical that reduces the rate of particular oxidation reactions in a specific context, where oxidation reactions are chemical reactions that involve the transfer of electrons from a substance to an oxidising agent.Antioxidants are particularly important in the context of organic chemistry and biology: all living cells contain complex systems of antioxidant chemicals and enzymes to prevent chemical damage to the cells' components by oxidation.A diet containing polyphenol antioxidants from plants is required for the health of most mammals, since plants are an important source of organic antioxidant chemicals. Antioxidants are widely used as ingredients in dietary supplements that are used for health purposes such as preventing cancer and heart disease. However, while many studies have suggested benefits for antioxidant supplements in laboratory experiments, several large clinical trials have failed to clearly demonstrate a benefit for the formulations tested, and excess supplementation may be harmful. It is logical to assume that a one dimensional approach to dietary supplementation with one specific antioxidant is not a panacea, since a broad diet rich in phytonutrients will yield thousands of different polyphenol antioxidants available for metabolism.

Antioxidant nutrients Highly reactive oxygen radicals are formed both during normal oxidative metabolism and in response to infection and some chemicals. They cause damage to fatty acids in cell membranes, and the products of this damage can then cause damage to proteins and DNA. The most widely accepted theory of the biochemical basis of much cancer, and also of atherosclerosis and possibly kwashiorkor, is that the key.factor in precipitating the condition is tissue damage by such radicals. A number of different mechanisms are involved in protection against, or repair after, oxygen radical damage, including a number of nutrients, especially vitamin E, carotene, vitamin C, and selenium. Collectively these are known as antioxidant nutrients.

Antipasto The term antipasto, usually translated as "appetizer" in English. It literally means "before the meal" and denotes a relatively light dish designed to stimulate the palate before the service of more substantial courses. Antipasti are not essential to the Italian kitchen; a formal Italian dinner without antipasti would not betray the traditions of Italian gastronomy. Today, however, it is difficult to imagine a formal dinner that would not include some dishes classified as antipasto. In the regional Italian kitchen, antipasti are an important element, not on a daily basis, but certainly on holidays and special occasions. Many dishes, served as accompaniments to main courses, are today considered too rich for such use. So, through the years, many of these dishes have been adapted to serve as antipasto. Antipasto takes full advantage of all kinds of different foods not generally regarded as being substantial enough to be served as main courses. The ingredients may be varied, but generally they must all be eaten with a fork.

Antisense A piece of DNA that produces the mirror image, or antisense messenger RNA, that is exactly opposite in sequence to one that directs the cells to produce a specific protein. Since the antisense RNA binds tightly to its image, it prevents the protein from being made.

Anti-spattering agents Compounds such as lecithin, sucrose esters of fatty acids, and sodium sulpho-acetate derivatives of mono- and diglycerides, which are added to oils and fats used for frying to prevent potentially dangerous spattering. They function by preventing the coalescence of water droplets.

Anti-staling agents Substances that retard the staling of baked products, and soften the crumb, e.g. sucrose stearate, polyoxyethylene monostearate, glyceryl monostearate, stearoyl tartrate.

Antivitamins Substances that interfere with the normal metabolism or function of vitamins, or destroy them. Dicoumarol in spoiled sweet clover antagonizes the function of vitamin K, thiaminase in raw fish destroys vitamin B1, the drug methotrexate antagonizes folic acid action (this is part of its mechanism of action in treating cancer), the drug isoniazid antagonizes the action of vitamin B6.

Anus The opening of the rectum.

AOC Appellation d'origine contrтlиe; see wine classification, France.

AP Amtlicher Prófangsnummer, German; batch number on labels of quality wines. See wine classification, Germany.

Apastia Refusal to take food, as an expression of a psychiatric disturbance. See also anorexia nervosa.

Aperitif A French term referring to a light alcoholic drink taken before a meal. Ideally an aperitif should stimulate the appetite and tantalise the palate, preparing it for greater things to come. The French often enjoy a glass of pastis before a meal.

Other popular aperitifs include drinks based on wine (for example, vermouth) or alcohol (for example, anise, bitters) and certain spirits and liqueurs. Arak (an aniseed-flavoured clear spirit) is drunk as an aperitif in some Arabic countries, ouzo in Greece and a glass of fino or manzanilla sherry in Spain.

Aphagia Inability to swallow. Difficulty in swallowing is dysphagia.

Aphagosis Inability to eat.

Apoenzyme The protein part of an enzyme which requires a coenzyme for activity, and is therefore inactive if the coenzyme is absent. See also coenzyme; enzyme activation; prosthetic group.

Apokreo Greek: literally 'fast from meat'; the three weeks of abstinence from meat ordained by the Greek Orthodox Church during Lent.

Apolipoprotein The protein part of lipoproteins without the associated lipid. See also lipids, plasma.

Apollinaris water An alkaline, highly aerated, mineral water containing sodium chloride and calcium, sodium, and magnesium carbonates, from a spring in the valley of Ahr (in Germany).

Aporrhegma Ptomaine or other toxic substance formed from an amino acid during the bacterial decomposition of a protein.

Aposia Absence of sensation of thirst.

Apositia Aversion to food.

Appellation controlee (AC) Or appellation d'origine controlee (AOC); see wine classification, France.

Appendix A residual part of the intestinal tract, a small sac-like process extending from the caecum, some 4-8 cm long. Acute inflammation, caused by an obstruction (appendicitis) can lead to perforation and peritonitis if surgery is not performed in time. See also gastro-intestinal tract.

Appertization French term for the process of destroying all the micro-organisms of significance in food, i.e. 'commercial sterility'; a few organisms remain alive but quiescent. Named after Nicholas Appert (1752-1841), a Paris confectioner who invented the process of canning.

Appetizer It is a small portion of bite-size food which is served before a main meal as the first course in order to stimulate the appetite. If served before a meal it should be small. They may be hot or cold, plated, or served as finger food. If served at a cocktail party, it is usually called hors d' oeuvres.

Apple Fruit of the tree Malus sylvestris and its many cultivars and hybrids; there are more than 2000 varieties in the British National Fruit Collection. Crab apples are grown mainly for decoration, and for pollination of fruit-bearing trees, although the sour fruit can be used for making jelly. Cooking apples are generally sourer varieties than dessert apples, and normally have flesh which crumbles on cooking; cider apples are sour varieties especially suited to the making of cider. One apple (110 g) provides 2.2 g of dietary fibre and supplies 40 kcal.

Apple brandy Spirit made by distillation of cider, known in France as Calvados. See also apple jack.

Apple butter Apple butter is a kind of jam made of tart apples, boiled in cider until reduced to a very thick smooth paste, to which is added a flavoring of allspice, while cooking. It is then placed in jars and covered tightly.

Apple Charlotte It is a golden-crusted dessert made by baking a thick apple compote in a mold lined with buttered bread.

Apple cider Most cider is made from fermented apple juice. Natural cider has nothing added and relies, for fermentation, upon the wild yeast present in the apples. For mass-produced ciders, a yeast culture is added in order to achieve consistency. Although much of today's cider is produced from apple concentrate, many traditional cider-makers use only cider apples, cultivated specifically for the purpose. When the Romans arrived in England in 55 B.C., they were reported to have found the local Kentish villagers drinking a delicious cider-like beverage made from apples. It has been recorded that the Romans and in particular their leader, Julius Caesar, embraced the pleasant pursuit with enthusiasm! How long the locals had been making this apple drink, prior to the arrival of the Romans, is anybody's guess. In America, cider was an everyday drink up until the middle of the 19th century. Anytime was considered a good time for drinking in the New England Colonies, and upon rising in the morning, the downing of a mug of cider was considered customary. Most of the early apple crops were made into cider since the apples had not yet been perfected into the sweet, juicy, eating apples of today. By the 1670s, cider was the most abundant and least expensive drink in New England. It quickly took the place of water, which was considered unsafe. During the colonial period, hard cider was the most popular beverage in America and often the measure of a town's wealth was measured by how many barrels of cider were stored for the winter.

Apple jack American name for apple brandy, normally distilled, but traditionally prepared by leaving cider outside in winter, when the water froze out as ice crystals, leaving the alcoholic spirit.

Apple juice It is the juice squeezed from apples. As long as apple juice (fresh cider) remains in its natural state and is not sweetened, preserved, clarified, or otherwise altered, it is apple juice. In sweet cider, fermentation is not permitted at all. See apple cider.

Apple nuggets Crisp granules of apple of low moisture content, used commercially for manufacture of apple sauce.

Apple sauce Pulped stewed apple; in the UK it is made from sour apples, as an accompaniment to pork and goose; in the USA also used for stewed apple as a dessert.

Apple, liquid American preparation of apple juice with pulverized apple pulp in suspension.

Applejack A brandy made by distilling apple cider. The name is also given to a beverage produced by freezing hard cider. As early as 1698, William Laird began it distill cider for himself and neighbors, producing apple brandy or applejack. Applejack, because of its power, was also know as "jersey Lighting." In 1780, a descendant of laird began commercial production of applejack and the company still distills it today.

Apple-pear Not a cross between apple and pear but a distinctive varietal type of pear-shaped fruit with apple texture. Also called Japanese pear, pear-apple, and shalea or chalea.

Apricot The apricot derives its name from the Latin world "praecox" meaning "precocious." The apricot has a long history of cultivation, starting in China some 4,000 years ago and traveling along the trade routes to the shores of the Mediterranean. In Iraq and Iran, apricots are served with lamb, and a regional specialty is "kamraddin" (a kind of apricot leather). A drink is made from it to mark the end of a period of religious fasting. The Spanish missionaries introduced the apricot trees to the Santa Clara Valley in California.

Aquaculture It is the cultivation of the sea. The term refers specifically to the intensive production of fish and shellfish in a controlled environment for human food. It is an ancient practice in Asia but it has only began approximately 20 years ago in the U.S., but in virtually no time has become one of the fastest growing segments of the United States economy.

Aquavit Scandinavian; spirit flavoured with herbs (commonly caraway, cumin, dill, or fennel). Also known as snaps, and in Germany as schnapps.

Arachidonic acid A fatty acid with twenty carbon atoms and four double bonds (20:4 ?6). Not strictly an essential fatty acid, since it can be formed from linoleic acid, but three times more potent than linoleic acid in curing the signs of essential fatty acid deficiency. Found in animal tissues, especially fish, eggs, liver, and brain.

Arachin One of the globulin proteins from the peanut.

Arachis oil Oil extracted from the groundnut or peanut, Arachis hypogea, 20% saturated, 50% mono-unsaturated (oleic acid), 30% polyunsaturated (linolenic acid), less than 1% linolenic acid.

Arak Arabic; anise- and liquorice- flavoured spirit. Also used generally in the Middle and Far East to mean any one of a variety of spirits, often distilled from fermented dates or palm wine.

Arborio rice An Italian short grain rice that was virtually synonymous with risotto for many years. It is the best known of the top-grade varieties of Italian rice. When purchasing arborio rice, the only precaution is to check the label to be sure it is not precooked.

Arbroath smokie 'Smokies' are whole wood-smoked haddock with the backbone still intact. They're still produced in small family smokehouses in the east coast fishing town of Arbroath in Scotland. Good for poaching, grilling, making fishcakes and pies, and used in kedgeree and soups.

The Arbroath smokie joined a select band of European speciality products when it was awarded Protected Geographical Indication (PGI) status by the European Commission on 2 March 2004, joining names such as Roquefort cheese, Stilton and Jambon d'Ardenne in achieving protection against imitators.

Arbute Fruit of the southern European strawberry tree (Arbutus unedo); resemble strawberries in appearance but have a grainy texture and little taste.

Architectural cuisine Menu items that are stacked for height. Also called Vertical Cuisine.

Area-eligibility A process within the child nutrition programs that allows all program participants in a low-income area to be eligible for free meals (for children in schools and child care settings) or the highest reimbursement level (for child care providers in the CACFP). Area eligibility is based on the percentage of children in families with income at or below 185 percent of the Federal Poverty Level in an area. Census data or school data showing the percentage of children qualifying for free or reduced price lunch at the neighborhood elementary school is used to determine area eligibility.

Arepas Similar to an English muffins but made from precooked corn flour, it is a cornmeal patty or pancake that is considered like bread in other countries. Arepas are popular throughout South America, but especially popular in Colombian and Venezuelan. It is considered the national dish of Venezuela (the local equivalent of an American hamburger). You can find arepas in small restaurants called Areperas. The most famous arepa is La reina pepiada, made with chopped meat, avocado and cheese. The favourite way to serve them in Venezuela is to split them open, remove some of the steaming moist corn meal, and then stuff them with your favourite ingredients. The arepa is wrapped in a square of slick paper (like butcher paper), and handed to the purchaser to eat standing up. Very few people make arepas at home, choosing to buy them at the store or have them delivered directly to their homes. You can also find them all over Miami, Florida (the traditional arepa served in Miami has two cornmeal pancakes with a layer of cheese inside).

Argan oil Believed to be one of the rarest oils in the world, argan oil comes from the nuts of the argan tree which is indigenous to Morocco. Argan trees used to cover much of North Africa but they're now greatly reduced in numbers, hence the high price of argan oil. It's related to the olive but has a distinct flavour of its own.

Argan oil can be drizzled over food before serving or stirred into soups, couscous and tagines. It has numerous health benefits and is also used as a skincare product. You should be able to buy it from specialist food shops or delis.

Argininaemia A genetic disease affecting the metabolism of the amino acid arginine, and hence the normal formation of urea and elimination of end-products of protein metabolism. Depending on the severity of the condition, affected infants may become comatose and die after a moderately high intake of protein. Treatment is by severe restriction of protein intake. Sodium benzoate may be given to increase the excretion of nitrogenous waste as hippuric acid.

Arginine A basic amino acid. Not a dietary essential for adult human beings, but infants may not be able to synthesize enough to meet the high demands of growth so some may be required in infant diets.

Argininosuccinic aciduria A genetic disease affecting the formation of urea, and hence the elimination of end-products of protein metabolism. Depending on the severity of the condition, affected infants may become comatose and die after a moderately high intake of protein. Treatment is by restriction of protein intake and feeding supplements of the amino acid arginine, which permits elimination of nitrogenous waste as argininosuccinic acid. Sodium benzoate may be given to increase the excretion of nitrogenous waste as hippuric acid. See also benzoic acid.

Argol Crust of crude cream of tartar (potassium acid tartrate) which forms on the sides of wine vats, also called wine stone. It consists of 50-85% potassium hydrogen tartrate and 6-12% calcium tartrate, and will be coloured by the grapes, so white argol comes from white grapes and red argol from red grapes. Used in vinegar fermentation, in the manufacture of tartaric acid and as a mordant in dyeing.

Ariboflavinosis Deficiency of riboflavin (vitamin B2) characterized by swollen, cracked, bright red lips (cheilosis), an enlarged, tender, magenta-red tongue (glossitis), cracking at the corners of the mouth (angular stomatitis), congestion of the blood vessels of the conjunctiva and a characteristic dermatitis with filiform (wire-like) excrescences.

Arm span The distance between a child's extended right and left middle fingers, measured across the back; sometimes used as an estimator of stature (length or height)

Armagnac Brandy made from white wine from one of three defined areas of France: Bas-Armagnac, Haut-Armagnac, or Tinartze. See also cognac.

Armenian bole Ferric oxide (iron oxide), either occurring naturally as haematite or prepared by heating ferrous sulphate and other iron salts. Used in metallurgy, polishing compounds, paint pigment, and as a food colour.

Arnold Chiari malformation A malformation that can accompany myelomeningocele and other neural tube disorders where the cerebellum and medulla oblongata protrude into the spinal cord

Arogel Trade name for a potato starch preparation which is stable to heating and is used as a thickener in gravies, sauces, and canned foods.

Aros See P-4000.

Aromatic 1. A vegetable, herb, or spice used to enhance the flavor and fragrance of food and drinks. In classic cooking, a reference to "aromatics" most often means onions, carrot, and celery.

2. It also means spicy, pungent, or having a fragrant aroma.

Arrack Also called arak. It is an anise-flavored liqueur, often homemade. It's a popular aperitif in the Middle East. It is a distilled from grapes, dates, and other fruits. In its countries of origin, it's included in cooking in some recipes for fish stews.

Arrowroot A starch extract of the root of a tropical plant native to the Americas called maranta. Arrowroot is used for thickening sauces, juices and syrups; when heated the starch turns to jelly and so thickens the liquid. Its great advantage over cornflour is that it's completely tasteless (whereas cornflour can need cooking to get rid of its 'raw' taste) and gives a clear finish when used to thicken certain soups, fruit syrups or sauces.

Arroz con pollo It is a popular chicken and rice Spanish and Mexican dish that is actually a paella without any shellfish or meat.

Arroz Spanish word for long-grain white rice. This is a main staple in Mexican cooking.

Arsenic A toxic metal, with no known metabolic function. Organic arsenic derivatives (arsenicals) have been used as pesticides and in treatment of diseases such as syphilis, leprosy, and yaws. Arsenic can accumulate in crops treated with arsenical pesticides, and in fish and shellfish living in arsenic-polluted water.

Arteriosclerosis Thickening and calcification of the arterial walls, leading to loss of elasticity, occurring with ageing and especially in hypertension.

Artesian-well water Water obtained from an underground source; the water rises to the surface under pressure.

Artichoke Confusingly, three different, unrelated plants are all known by this name. The globe artichoke is related to the thistle. Its leaves are edible, as is the bottom part of the flower, called the heart (which you can also buy tinned or frozen). Globe artichokes make a delicious starter simply boiled whole and served with melted butter, mayonnaise, hollandaise or vinaigrette for dipping the leaves. Break off each leaf and draw the soft fleshy base through your teeth. Once you've removed all the leaves, you can pull or slice off the hairy 'choke' and then eat the heart and the meaty bottom with the remaining sauce.

The Jerusalem artichoke belongs to the sunflower family and it's the plant's underground tubers that are eaten. They're rather knobbly and irregular in shape, with a pale brown or purple-red skin. Scrub them and boil or steam until tender and then peel. If a recipe calls for peeled Jerusalem artichokes, peel them and drop into acidulated water until ready to use to stop them from discolouring.

The Chinese artichoke is a perennial herb of the mint family, grown for its edible tuberous underground stems. It has a sweet, nutty taste, similar to the Jerusalem artichoke. It's much more difficult to find in shops than globe or Jerusalem artichokes.

Arugula It is also known as rocket, rulola, Italian cress, and roquette. It is a delicate salad green that is related to mustard. When the leaves are young, they are tender and nutty, with a subtle peppery flavor. The leaves look like radish leaves. The white blossoms are also edible. It is used as a salad green, as a garnish, and in combination with other ingredients in sandwiches.

Asafetida This pungent resinous gum is used widely in Indian vegetarian cooking. Also called stinking gum and devil's dung because of its unpleasant smell, this seasoning is obtained from the gum of a plant native to Afghanistan, Iran, and northern India. A perennial of the carrot family that grows wild to 12 feet high in natural forests. The whole plant exudes a characteristic smell, described by some as stink. The milky resin comes from both the thick stems and the root and it dries into asafoetida. A popular ingredient in Indian vegetarian dishes, it imparts a subtle flavor if used sparingly (the odor does not transmit to cooked food). In the raw state, the resin or the powder has an unpleasant smell. This completely disappears when the spice is added to a variety of fish, vegetable pulse, and pickle ingredients. Also used in the curries and pickles of West and South India. The powdered version is easier to handle. Buy asafoetida in small quantities. The powder resin is usually mixed with flour to provide bulk and is sold in bright yellow plastic tubs.

Ascorbic acid Vitamin C, chemically L-xyloascorbic acid, to distinguish it from the isomer D-araboascorbic acid (isoascorbic acid or erythorbic acid), which has only slight vitamin C activity. Both ascorbic acid and erythorbic acid have strong chemical-reducing properties, and are used as antioxidants in foods and to preserve the red colour of fresh and preserved meats, and in the curing of hams.

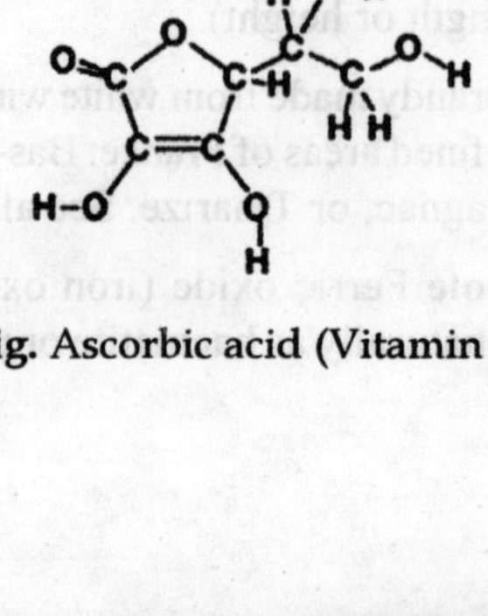

Fig. Ascorbic acid (Vitamin C)

Ascorbic acid oxidase An enzyme in plant tissues that oxidizes ascorbic acid to dehydro-ascorbic acid. In the intact fresh plant the enzyme is separated from the ascorbic acid, and is only released when the plant wilts or is cut. To preserve the vitamin in cooked vegetables, it is generally recommended that they be plunged into boiling water, to denature and therefore inactivate the enzyme, as soon as possible after cutting.

Ascorbin stearate An ester of ascorbic acid and stearic acid; a fatsoluble form of the vitamin which is used as an antioxidant.

Ascorbyl palmitate An ester of ascorbic acid and palmitic acid which is used as an anti-staling compound in bakery goods (E-304).

Aseptic filling The filling of cans or other containers with food that has already been sterilized, the process thus having to be carried out under aseptic conditions. Continuous sterilization as the food passes along narrow pipes (followed by aseptic filling) allows more rapid heating, with less effect on the quality of the food, than sterilization by heating after canning.

Ash The residue left behind after all organic matter has been burnt off, a measure of the total content of mineral salts in a food.

Asiago cheese Asiago cheese is a semi-firm Cheese from Italy. Also known as "poor man's Parmesan cheese." It is made from whole or part-skim cow's milk. It comes in small wheels with glossy rinds and is yellow inside with many small holes called "eyes." Asiago is rich and nutty in flavor and used as a table cheese when young; when matured for 6 months or more it hardens and may be grated.

Asparagine A non-essential amino acid, chemically the í-amide of aspartic acid.

Asparagus The name asparagus comes from the Greek language meaning "sprout" or "shoot," and it is a member of the lily family. Plants in the lily family are also related to various grasses. In the dialects of 18th and 19th century cookbooks, asparagus was referred to as sparagrass or sparrowgrass. People throughout Europe, Asia, and the United States use fresh Asparagus in their favourite cuisine. In China, Asparagus spears are candied and served as special treats. It is widely popular today as a scrumptious, fresh, healthy vegetable.

Aspartame Aspartame is a low calorie sweetener used in a variety of foods and beverages and as a tabletop sweetener. It is about 200 times sweeter than sugar. Aspartame is made by joining two protein components, aspartic acid and phenylalanine.

Aspic In Greek it is called aspis and means a "shield." A clear jelly made from meat stock (or occasionally from fruit or vegetable juices) thickened with gelatin. Used to coat foods or it is cubed and used as a garnish. It also refers to a molded, usually tomato-based, gelatin salad. It is basically the same as jellied consommı, except that more gelatin is added.

Aspic jelly A clear jelly made from fish, chicken, or meat stock, sometimes with added gelatine, flavoured with lemon, tarragon, vinegar, sherry, peppercorns, and vegetables, used to glaze foods such as meat, fish, and game. The name may be derived from the herb espic or spikenard.

Aspiration Inspiratory sucking into the lungs of foreign material, including food and liquid

Assiette anglaise French; plate of cold assorted meats (literally 'English plate').

Astaxanthin Astaxanthin belongs to a group of compounds called carotenoids. In nature, there are more than 700 different carotenoids, which are responsible for the dazzling array of colours to plants and the animal kingdom.

Astaxanthin is present as a vibrant red pigment in birds, fish, crustaceans, and shellfish. Even certain plants and bacteria produce it. The antioxidative properties of astaxanthin are very powerful, as shown in trials comparing it with other fat-soluble antioxidants such as Vitamin E and í-carotene.

Astaxanthin One of the carotenoids, the pink colour of salmon and trout muscle; has no vitamin A activity.

Asthma The difficulty experienced in breathing due to excessive contraction of the involuntary muscle in the walls of bronchial tubes leading into the lungs, with consequent narrowing of the tubes. The muscle reacts excessively to a wide range of stimuli such as infections, exertion, and, most importantly, allergens, the substances that cause allergies. If the attack is prolonged it is complicated by plugging of the small airways by abnormal secretion, and it is this that can make asthma a threat to life. Asthma commonly starts in childhood, and about half those affected improve or recover around puberty. The condition can be alleviated by drug treatment.

Astringency The action of unripe fruits and cider apples, among other foods, to cause a contraction of the epithelial tissues of the tongue (literally astringency means 'a drawing together'). It is believed to result from a destruction of the lubricant properties of saliva by precipitation by tannins.

Atheroma The fatty deposit composed of various lipids, complex carbohydrates, and fibrous tissue which forms on the inner wall of blood vessels in atherosclerosis.

Atherosclerosis A condition that exists when too much cholesterol builds up in the blood and accumulates in the walls of the blood vessels.

Atherosclerosis Atherosclerosis is a disease affecting the arterial blood vessel. It is commonly referred to as a "hardening" or "furring" of the arteries. It is caused by the formation of multiple plaques within the arteries.Pathologically, the atheromatous plaque is divided into three distinct components:The atheroma ("lump of porridge", from Athera, porridge in Greek,) is the nodular accumulation of a soft, flaky, yellowish material at the centre of large plaques, composed of macrophages nearest the lumen of the artery, sometimes with Underlying areas of cholesterol crystals, and possibly also Calcification at the outer base of older/more advanced lesions.

2. A disease characterized by the deposition of lipids and platelets at the innermost coat of certain arteries, which causes progressive narrowing of their lumen and a decrease in their elasticity.

3. One of many diseases in which fat builds up in the large- and medium-sized arteries. This buildup of fat may slow down or stop blood flow. This disease can happen to people who have had diabetes for a long time.

Athetosis or diskinesis A condition characterized by involuntary, slow, writhing continuous movements; seen in some neurological disorders, e.g., cerebral palsy

ATP Adenosine triphosphate, the coenzyme that acts as an intermediate between energy-yielding (catabolic) metabolism (the oxidation of metabolic fuels) and energy expenditure as physical work and in synthetic (anabolic) reactions. ADP (adenosine diphosphate) is phosphorylated to ATP linked to oxidations; in energy expenditure ATP is hydrolysed to ADP and phosphate ions.

Attention deficit hyperactivity disorder (ADHD) Commonly called "hyperactivity," Attention Deficit Hyperactivity Disorder is a clinical diagnosis based on specific criteria. These include excessive motor activity, impulsiveness, short attention span, low tolerance to frustration and onset before 7 years of age.

Attention The ability to focus selectively on a selected stimulus, sustaining that focus and shifting it at will. The ability to concentrate.

Au bleu The French term for the method of preparing fish the instant after it is killed. Used especially for trout, as in "truite au blue," when the freshly killed fish is plunged into a boiling court bouillon, which turns the skin a metallic blue colour.

Au gratin To dress up vegetables, meats, and fish with a layer of bread crumbs and/or grated cheese on top. It is then broiled or baked until a thin brown crust forms.

Au jus 1. French and has the same meaning as a la and be translated as "in" or "with."

2. It also describes meat served in its own natural juices, not with gravy.

Aubergine Aubergines are an essential Mediterranean vegetable, featuring in classic dishes such as ratatouille, moussaka and imam bayildi (stuffed aubergines). They're also an important ingredient in many Indian vegetable-based dishes and are the basis of the Arabic mezze dish baba ganoush.

Use them in vegetable curries and summer vegetable stews or just sliced and fried or grilled. With the skin left on they hold their shape quite well, but remove the skin and the flesh can be cooked down to a thick pulp. Also known as eggplant, after the egg-shaped, white-skinned variety, aubergines should be firm and heavy with a taut, shiny skin and a bright green calyx, or stalk end.

As well as the deep purple variety, there are white, mauve, green and striped varieties, although the purple and white are most widely available. Home-grown aubergines are available from April to October in the UK.

They store we'l in the fridge or cool larder for about four to six days. In the past, many recipes recommended salting aubergines to reduce their bitter flavour. This isn't really necessary now, although salting does make them absorb less oil when they're fried. To prepare, wash the skin and trim off the stalk. Slice or cut the flesh into chunks just before cooking because it discolours quickly.

Aurantiamarin A glucoside present in the albedo of the bitter orange which is partly responsible for its flavour.

Autism spectrum disorders A group of pervasive developmental disorders; diagnostic criteria include communication problems, ritualistic behaviours and inappropriate social interaction

Autoclave A vessel in which high temperatures can be achieved by using high pressure; the domestic pressure cooker is an example. At atmospheric pressure water boils at 100 °C; at 5 lb (35 kPa) above atmospheric pressure the boiling point is 109 °C; at 10 lb (70 kPa), 115 °C; at 15 lb (105 kPa), 121 °C, and at 20 lb (140 kPa), 126 °C. Autoclaves have two major uses. In cooking, the higher temperature reduces the time needed. At these higher temperatures, and under moist conditions, bacteria are destroyed more rapidly, so permitting sterilization of foods, surgical dressing and instruments, etc.

Autolysis The process of self-digestion by the enzymes naturally present in tissues. For example, the tenderizing of game while hanging is due to autolysis of connective tissue. Yeast extract is produced by autolysis of yeast.

Autonomic dysreflexia A condition resulting from the blocked function of the autonomic nervous system that occurs in individuals with paralysis; caused by simultaneous sympathetic and parasympathetic activity; symptoms include hypertension and bradycardia

Autonomic nervous system The part of the nervous system that controls involuntary actions of internal organs such as the bowel.

Autotrophes Organisms that can synthesize all the compounds required for growth from simple inorganic salts, as distinct from heterotrophes, which must be supplied with complex organic compounds. Plants are autotrophes, whereas animals are heterotrophes. Bacteria may be of either type; heterotrophic bacteria are responsible for food spoilage and disease.

Availability Also known as bioavailabitity or biological availability. In some foodstuffs, nutrients that can be demonstrated to be present chemically may not be available, or only partially so, when they are eaten. This is because the nutrients are chemically bound in a form that is not susceptible to enzymic digestion, although it is susceptible to the strong acid or alkali hydrolysis used in chemical analysis. For example, the niacin in cereal grains, calcium bound to phytate, and lysine combined with sugars in the Maillard complex, are all biologically unavailable. See also available lysine.

Available lysine Not all of the lysine in proteins is biologically available, since some is linked through its side-chain amino group, either to sugars in the Maillard complex, or to other amino acids. These linkages are not hydrolysed by digestive enzymes, and so the lysine cannot be absorbed. Available lysine is that proportion of the protein-bound lysine in which the side-chain amino group is free, so that it can be absorbed after digestion of the protein.

Avicel Trade name for microcrystalline a-cellulose. It is natural cellulose which has been partially hydrolysed with acid, and reduced to a fine powder. It disperses in water and has the properties of a gum. it is used in oily foods such as cheese and peanut butter, as well as in syrups and honey, sauces and dressings.

Avidin A protein in egg white which binds the vitamin biotin, so rendering it unavailable to the body. Cooking denatures proteins, and denatured avidin in cooked eggs does not bind biotin.

Avitaminosis The absence of a vitamin; may be used specifically, as, for example, avitaminosis A, or generally, to mean a vitamin deficiency disease.

Avocado Sometimes called an avocado pear, the avocado is the fruit of the Persea Americana tree, which is native to the subtropical regions of the American continent. It has green, buttery flesh and a large central stone. It's very high in both protein and oil. In Britain, two main varieties are available Hass and Fuerte. The Hass variety has a knobbly purple-black exterior and a creamy-textured, richly flavoured interior; the Fuerte variety has a smooth green skin.

Mexican guacamole is probably the best known avocado dish, but avocados are very versatile. Look for ones that have unblemished skins with no soft spots, which suggest bruising. They're ready to eat when the flesh yields slightly when pressed with the thumb. The flesh discolours once cut, but lemon juice helps to minimise the effect.

Azo dyes Synthetic chemicals used as dye-stuffs and food colours, made by reacting a diazonium salt (which has two nitrogen atoms linked to each other) with a phenol or aromatic amine. Also known as diazo or diazonium compounds.

B

B and B Mixture of equal parts of brandy and Benedictine; also an abbreviation for accommodation offering bed and breakfast.

Baba Baba is called babka in Poland and Babas Au Rhum in France. In French, the word baba meaning, "falling over or dizzy." These are small cakes made from yeast dough containing raisins or currants. They are baked in cylindrical molds and then soaked with sugar syrup usually flavored with rum (originally they were soaked in a sweet fortified wine). After these cakes were soaked in the wine sauce for a day, the dried fruits would fall out of them.

Baba Au Rhum In the 18th century, French chef, Jean Anthelme Brillat-Savarin (1755-1826), created a cake that he served with a rum sauce that he called Baba Au Savarin. The dessert became very popular in France, but the people called it Baba Au Rhum and soon dropped the name Savarin.

Baba ganoush When aubergine is roasted, peeled, puried and mixed with lemon juice, garlic, tahini (sesame paste) and salt, it's transformed into the heavenly baba ganoush (or moutabal as it's known in Lebanon) - a smooth, smoky-flavoured spread or dip that's a favourite Middle Eastern meze dish.

Babaco The seedless fruit of the tree Carica pentagona, related to the pawpaw, discovered in Ecuador in the 1920s, introduced into New Zealand in 1973, and more recently into the Channel Islands. A 100-g portion is a rich source of vitamin C.

Babassu oil Edible oil from the Brazilian palm nut, similar in fatty acid composition to coconut oil, and used for food and in soaps and cosmetics.

Babcock test A test for the fat content of milk.

Babka 1. Russian; yeast cake with grated carrot or potato and flour.

2. Polish; a cake similar to baba, but baked without yeast.

Baby foods General term to include infant formula milk and weaning foods.

Baby-Friendly Hospital Initiative Maternity and other hospitals that fulfil the "Ten Steps to Breastfeeding Sucess" endorsed by WHO/ Unicef.

Bacalao Spanish and South American name for dried salted cod; Portuguese is bacalhau. See klipfish.

Backerbsen German; garnish for soup, batter mixture poured through a colander into hot oil and fried to resemble dried peas.

Backerei German for baked goods; Austrian name for a variety of different types of biscuit made with baking powder.

Bacon Cured (and usually smoked) meat from the back, sides, and belly of a pig; variety of cuts with differing fat contents. A 100-g portion of boiled collar joint is a rich source of protein, niacin, and vitamin B1, a source of vitamin B2 and iron; contains 30 g of fat of which 40% is saturated; supplies 320 kcal (1345 kJ). A 100-g grilled gammon rasher is exceptionally rich in vitamin B1 (0.9 mg); a rich source of protein and niacin; a good source of iron; a source of vitamin B2; contains 12 g of fat of which 40% is saturated; supplies 230 kcal (970 kJ). A 100-g portion of fried, streaky bacon is a rich source of protein, niacin, and vitamin B1; a source of vitamin B2 and iron; contains 45 g of fat of which 40% is saturated; supplies 500 kcal (2100 kJ). Also a source of zinc, copper, and selenium. Gammon is bacon made from the top of the hind legs; green bacon has been cured but not smoked.

Bacteria Unicellular micro-organisms, ranging between 0.5 and 5 [mu]m in size. They may be classified on the basis of their shape: spherical (coccus), rodlike (bacilli), spiral (spirillum), comma-shaped (vibrio), corkscrew-shaped (spirochaetes), or filamentous. Other classifications are based on whether or not they are stained by Gram's stain, aerobic(need oxygen to grow) or anaerobic(grows without oxygen), and autotrophic or heterotrophic. Some bacteria form spores which are relatively resistant to heat and sterilizing agents.

Bacteria are responsible for much food spoilage, and for disease (pathogenic bacteria which produce toxins), but they are also made use of, for example in the pickling process and fermentation of milk, as well as in the manufacture of vitamins and amino acids and a variety of enzymes and hormones. Between 45 and 85% of the dry matter of bacteria is protein, and some can be grown on petroleum residues, methane, or methanol for use in animal feed.

Bacterial filter A filter fine enough to prevent the passage of bacteria (0.5-5 μm in diameter), which permits removal of bacteria from solutions. Viruses are considerably smaller, and will pass through a bacterial filter.

Bacteriophage Viruses which attack bacteria, commonly known as phages. They pass through bacterial filters, and can be a cause of considerable trouble in bacterial cultures (for example milk starter cultures).

Badminton A drink prepared with claret, sugar, and soda water.

Bagasse The residues from sugar-cane milling, consisting of the crushed stalks from which the juice has been expressed; it consists of 50% cellulose, 25% hemicelluloses, and 25% lignin. It is used as a fuel, for cattle feed, and in the manufacture of paper and fibre board. The name is sometimes also applied to the residues of other plants, such as beet, which is sometimes incorporated into foods as a source of dietary fibre.

Bagel Bagel derives from the Yiddish word beygl, which comes from the German word beugel meaning a "bracelet." Bagels are bread rolls in the shape of a doughnut or an old-fashioned curtain ring. The brown crust is obtained on the rolls by first boiling them in water and then baking them in an oven. Over time, its shape evolved into a circle with a hole in the centre and its named was converted to its modern form, bagel. In the 1880s, hundreds of thousands of Eastern European Jews immigrated to America, bringing with them a love for bagels. In 1927, Polish baker Harry Lender opened the first bagel plant outside New York City in New Haven, Conn. The bagel's popularity began to spread in the United States.

Bagna cauda An Italian term that means "hot Bath." It is like a Swiss fondue except that it has a much more boisterous flavor. The original recipe called for walnut oil, but olive oil is now used and is considered the key to a successful sauce. The sauce is made up of anchovy fillets, olive oil, garlic, cream, butter, and vinegar. It always includes one or more members of the cabbage family along with such other ingredients as steak, shrimp, and cheese.

Baguette French for a "rod," "wand," or "stick." Baguette is the name for anything long and skinny, including drumsticks, strips of wood, etc. The baguette is generally known as a French white bread due to its popularity in that country. Baguettes are formed into a long, narrow, cylindrical loaf. It usually has a thin, crisp brown crust and an open-holed, chewy interior.

Bain-marie 1. A hot water bath that is used to keep food warm on the top of a stove. It is also to cook custards and baked eggs in the oven without curdling or cracking and also used to hold sauces and to clarify butter.

2. The term is also used for a cooking utensil, which is a fairly large pan (or tray) which is partly filled with water. The food to be cooked is placed in another container in order that the food is not cooked too quickly or harshly. Most authorities think that it was named after Maria Prophetissa. Maria Prophetissa was also known as "Miriam," "Maria the Jewess" or simply "Maria" and lived during the first century A.D. She is called The Jewess because Zosimos, Egyptian alchemist and historian, called her a Sister of Moses. It is held that Mary Magdalene and the noted first century alchemical author known as Mary the Jewess was one and the same individual. Whoever she was, Mary the Jewess was an accomplished practical alchemist and the inventor of a series of technical devices still in use today, such as the hot ash box for steady heat, the dung box for prolonged heat and the double boiler, still called the "bain-marie" in French and Marienbad in German. Although no complete works by her have been found, enough fragments exist to establish her as a historical fact. Yet her personal information, even her birthplace, remains a mystery.

Bake blind It is the technique used for baking an unfilled pastry shell. The pastry shell is first pricked with a fork to prevent puffing, covered with aluminum foil or parchment paper, and then weighted with rice or beans. It is then baked for a short period of time, about 10 to 15 minutes.

Bake stone A bake stone is a flat, round iron plate, usually with an attached semicircular iron loop, which allows it to be hung over a fire from a crane. It can also be set down directly on hot embers. Before baking ovens, and even after them, this was a common utensil for baking simple quick breads.

Baked alaska A dessert that consists of a sponge cake that is covered with ice cream, then with a layer of stiffly beaten egg whites, and lastly put in a hot oven to be browned. Also known as omelette α la norvigienne, Norwegian omelette, omelette surprise, and glace au four.

Baked Apple a la Josephine - The soaked, pruned apples are boiled for 15 minutes. Boiled milk is mixed with rice, salt and sugar are added, and then it is cooled down and divided into four portions. The cores of the apples are removed and are covered with butter and sprinkled with sugar. They are placed in a pre-warmed oven and baked for 20 minutes. The apples are served in the middle of the rice pudding, sprinkled with sugar, and toppled with raspberry syrup.

Bakers' ammonia (Ammonium carbonate) It is also called hartshorn. It is an ammonia compound and not harmful after baking. However, don't eat the raw dough. Your kitchen will stink of ammonia while the cookies bake - but once baked, the cookies will not taste of it. Can be substituted for equal amount of baking powder in any cookies recipe. It is an old-time leavening favoured for cookies, such as German Springerle. It is said to give a "fluffiness" of texture baking powder can't. Its leavening is only activated by heat, not moisture (such as baking powder).

Bakewell tart An open pastry tart with an almond-flavoured cake filling, originally made in Bakewell in Derbyshire, England.

Baking additives Materials added to flour products for a variety of purposes, including bleaching the flour, ageing, slowing the rate of staling, and improving the texture of the finished product.

Baking blind Making a pastry case for a tart or flan, which is baked empty and then filled.

Baking Cooking in an oven by dry heat.

Baking powder A raising agent used in cakes, biscuits and breads. Commercial baking powder contains bicarbonate of soda and tartaric acid (with a dried starch or flour to absorb any moisture during storage). When these chemicals become moist and warm they react and give off carbon dioxide, which causes food to rise. It has a limited shelf life so check the sell-by date when using it; otherwise your cakes might literally be a flop! Make your own baking powder by combining 15ml/1tbsp bicarbonate of soda with 30ml/2tbsp cream of tartar. Measure carefully because too much or too little can upset a recipe's balance.

Baking soda Baking soda, which is the alkaline element bicarbonate of soda, is used solely as a chemical leavener in baking. Because it is not premixed with an acid, as is baking powder, it is used alone in baked goods where other ingredients, which also contain acid, are present (yogurt, buttermilk, lemon juice, or sour cream). When the baking soda and acid are combined, they neutralize each other, causing carbon dioxide gas bubbles to form. The bubbles make the dough or batter grow bigger, or rise. Baking soda is more volatile than baking powder because it begins to act the minute you moisten it with the wet ingredients. You must put whatever you are baking right in the oven once the baking soda has been activated. See also bicarbonate of soda. Baking soda was previously known as saleratus, a combination of the Latin "sal" (salt) and "aeratus" (aerated.) John Dwight of Massachusetts and his brother-in-law, Dr. James A. Church of Connecticut, started the manufacture of bicarbonate of soda in this country in 1846. The first factory was in the kitchen of his home with baking soda put in paper bags by hand. A year later, in 1847, the firm of John Dwight and Company was formed, and subsequently Cow Brand was adopted as a trademark for Dwight's Saleratus (aerated salt) as it was called. The standard package at that time weighed one pound. The cow was adopted as a trademark because of the use of sour milk with saleratus in baking. In 1867, James A. Church began marketing sodium bicarbonate as baking soda under the Arm & Hammer label. He formed a partnership known as Church & Company, doing business under that firm name with his sons James A. Church and E. Dwight Church.

Baking stone Also referred to as a pizza stone. Unglazed ceramic, clay, or stone tiles that allows for high temperature and dry heat, which is necessary for crisp crusts when making breads and pizzas. A stone can be placed in the oven (and kept there when not in use) where it retains heat and makes an ideal surface for baking breads. A baking stone is invaluable for getting the "perfect" crust and it can also help your oven to run more efficiently because of its heat retaining properties. They should only be washed with clear, plain water, as these stones are actually molded sand, which is tightly compacted under high pressure. Like sand on the beach, they will suck in any liquid exposed to the surface.

Baklava A popular middle eastern (especially Greece and Turkey) pastry that is made with buttered layers of phyllo dough. How it is traditionally made depends on the region. In some areas, it is made with walnuts; in other areas, it is made with pistachios or almonds. Sometimes dried fruit is added between the layers. Baklava consists of 30 or more sheets of phyllo dough brushed with lots of butter, and layered with finely chopped nuts. After baking, a syrup of honey, rose water and lemon juice (sometimes spiced with cinnamon, cardamom, cloves, etc) is poured over the pastry and allowed to soak in. This dessert is known as baglawa in Syrian and Lebanese. Most historians agree that the first people, the Assyrians, in the 8th century B.C. were the first to put together thin layers of bread dough, with chopped nuts in between those layers, added some honey and baked it in their primitive wood burning ovens. This earliest known version of baklava was baked only on special occasions. Baklava was considered a food for the rich until mid-19th century. In Turkey the sheets of pastry for baklava are rolled out so thinly that when held up the person standing behind can be seen as if through a net curtain. In Turkey, to this day one can hear a common expression often used by the poor, or even by the middle class, saying: "I am not rich enough to eat baklava and boerek every day". The Greek seamen and merchants traveling east to Mesopotamia soon discovered the delights of Baklava and brought the recipe to Athens. The Greeks' major contribution to the development of this pastry is the creation of a dough technique that made it possible to roll it as thin as a leaf, compared to the rough, bread-like texture of the Assyrian dough. Phyllo means "layer" or "leaf" in the Greek language. The Armenians, located on ancient Spice and Silk Routes, integrated for the cinnamon and cloves into the baklava. The Arabs introduced the rose water and cardamom. The taste changed in subtle nuances as the recipe started crossing borders.

Balance 1. With reference to diet, positive balance is a net gain to the body and negative balance a net loss from the body. When intake equals excretion the body is in equilibrium or balance with respect to the nutrient in question. Used in reference to nitrogen (protein), mineral salts, and energy.

2. A balanced diet is one containing all nutrients in appropriate amounts.

3. A weighing device.

Balka Polish; conical yeast cake traditionally eaten for festivals, similar to Italian panettone.

Ball mill A vessel in which material is ground by rolling with heavy balls, used especially for hard materials.

Balling A table of specific gravity of sugar solutions published by von Balling in 1843, giving the weight of cane sugar in 100 g of a solution for the specific gravity determined at 17.5 'C. It is used to calculate the percentage extract in beer wort. The original table was corrected for slight inaccuracies by Plato in 1900, and extracts are referred to as percent Plato.

Ballottine A kind of galantine of meat, poultry, game, or fish, boned, stuffed, and rolled into a bundle; also small balls of meat or poultry.

Balm A herb with hairy leaves and a lemon scent, therefore often known as lemon balm. Used for its flavour in fruit salads, sweet or savoury sauces, etc., as well as for preparation of herb teas. Claimed to have calming medicinal properties, and promoted at one time as an elixir of life and a cure for impotence; it is rich in tannins.

Balsamic vinegar A dark-brown syrupy vinegar with a smooth sweet-sour flavour, produced in the Modena region of Italy. It's made from reduced grape juice that's aged in wooden casks. The best quality balsamic vinegar can be more than 100 years old but is more commonly sold at three to four years of age.

True balsamic vinegars are very expensive but have an exceptional flavour. Balsamic vinegars made on a commercial basis are less pricey (although still fairly expensive) but luckily a little goes along way. Use with a dash of olive oil for a subtle salad dressing or add a few drops to meaty stews, when frying steak or chops or in marinades. Alternatively, lightly sprinkle sliced strawberries with it. It really brings out the flavour of the fruit.

Balti Balti is an Indian dish, which may have originated in Northwest Pakistan. It is a form of a meat curry, but one that's cooked quickly (like a stir-fry). The spice mix used to flavor the dish is a combination of seeds (coriander, cardamom, cumin, black mustard, fennel, wild onion, and fenugreek). It can be made as either a masala paste or used dry. The name comes from the cast-iron pot "balti," in which it was originally both made and served. Now the term "balti" seems to refer to the food, and the pot is called a "karahi." In some parts of the world, the dish is also called karai, or karah.

Bambarra groundnut Also known as the Madagascar peanut or earth pea, Voandseia subterranea. It resembles the true groundnut, but the seeds are low in oil. They are hard and require soaking or pounding before cooking.

Bamboo shoot Young shoots of the bamboo plant. The shoots grown from an underground stock, and they are cut soon after their appearance above the ground. The outer sheaths are removed and the shoots are prepared for the table much in the same manner as asparagus. They are used a lot in Chinese and Japanese cooking.

Bami Indonesian, Dutch; noodles with fried shredded vegetables, served with diced pork, chicken or prawns, topped with strips of omelette.

Banana Bananas aren't grown on trees. They're part of the lily family, a cousin of the orchid, and a member of the herb family. With stalks 25 feet high, they're the largest plant on earth without a woody stem. The banana is harvested green, even for local consumption. It is the one fruit, which if left to ripen on the plant, never develops its best flavor. After they are picked, the sugar content increases from 2% to 20%. The banana was probably one of the first plants to be cultivated. The earliest historical reference to the fruit was 327 B.C., when Alexander the Great found them flourishing in India. Traders in the Indian Ocean carried the banana to the eastern coast of Africa, and Chinese traders introduced the banana to the Polynesians before the second century A.D. During Alexander the Great's life, bananas were called pala in Athens. North America got its first taste of the tropical fruit in 1876 at the Philadelphia Centennial Exhibition. Each banana was wrapped in foil and sold for 10 cents.

Banana figs Bananas that have been split longitudinally and sun-dried without treating with sulphur dioxide. The product is dark in colour and sticky.

Banana, false The fruit of Ensete ventricosum, related to the banana. The fruits are small and, unlike bananas, contain seeds. The rhizome and inner tissue of the stem are eaten after cooking, and form a major part of the diet in southern Ethiopia.

Bananas foster A dish made of bananas and rum, flamed and served over vanilla ice cream. The original Banana Foster was created in the New Orleans restaurant called Brennan's in the old French Quarter. In the 1950's, New Orleans was the major port of entry for bananas shipped from Central and South America. Owen Edward Brennan challenged his talented chef, Paul Blangi, to include bananas in a new culinary creation - Owen's way of promoting the imported fruit. Simultaneously, Holiday Magazine had asked Owen to provide a new recipe to appear in a feature article on Brennan's. In 1951, Chef Paul created Bananas Foster. The scrumptious dessert was named for Richard Foster, who, as chairman, served with Owen on the New Orleans Crime Commission, a civic effort to clean up the French Quarter. Richard Foster, owner of the Foster Awning Company, was a frequent customer of Brennan's and a very good friend of Owen. Source:

Banbury cake Flat oval cake of flaky pastry filled with dried fruit; originated in Banbury, Oxfordshire, England.

Bangers Colloquial English term for sausages. When served with mashed potatoes, the dish is known as bangers and mash.

Banian days Days on which no meat was served; named after Banian (Hindu) merchants who abstained from eating meat. An obsolete term for 'days of short commons'.

Banitsa bulgarian Tarts made from phyllo pastry, filled with nuts and cream, cheese, or spinach.

Bannock A flat round cake made from oat, rye, or barley meal and baked on a hearth or griddle. Pitcaithly bannock is a type of almond shortbread containing caraway seeds and chopped peel.

Bap Traditionally a soft, white, flat, flour-coated Scottish breakfast roll. Now also used for any relatively large soft-crusted roll, made from white, brown, or wholemeal flour.

Bara brith A Welsh yeast- or baking soda-raised sweet bread, quite dense and cake-like in texture, containing spices and tea-soaked dried fruit. Delicious served warm, sliced and spread with salty Welsh butter.

Barbary duck Bred in large quantities in France, Barbary ducks are intensively reared for ten to 12 weeks. You should be able to find Barbary duck breasts and leg portions, as well as whole, oven-ready ducks, in supermarkets.

Barbary ducks are less fatty than many other breeds, with a thin skin and no layer of fat underneath. It needs careful basting when cooking so that it doesn't dry out. A six to seven-pound duck is enough to feed four to six people.

Barbecue There are several theories on where or how the word "barbecue" originated. 1. One is that it is a derivative of the West Indian term barbacoa, which denotes a method of slow-cooking meat over hot coals.

2. It is also thought that the word barbecue comes from the French phrase "barbe a queue," meaning "from heat to tail."

3. Another theory is that the word comes from a 19th century advertisement for a combination whiskey bar, beer, hall, pool establishment and purveyor of roast pig, known as the "Bar-Beer-Cue-Pig.)

4. The final explanation is that the method of roasting meat over powdery coals was picked up from indigenous peoples in the colonial period, and the word barbacoa became barbecue in the lexicon of early settlers. Barbecuing is a long, slow, indirect, low-heat method that uses smoldering logs, charcoal, or wood chunks to smoke-cook the food (usually some kind of meat). "Indirect" meant that the heat source is located away from the food to be cooked. "Barbecuing" and "grilling" are two different techniques. The earliest example of barbecue is in 1661, when it is used as a verb meaning 'to cook on a barbecue'. Other early senses include 'the wooden framework for supporting food'; 'a whole animal, or a piece of an animal, roasted on a barbecue'; and 'a social gathering at which food is cooked on a barbecue'. Barbecuing is primarily a New World phenomenon, originating in the Caribbean and then spreading to the United Sates (the American South in particular).

In the Southern United States, barbecue is considered a cherished cultural icon. In other areas of America, the word barbecue is a verb (Northerners barbecue food on the backyard grill). In the South, barbecue is most definitely a noun (a barbecue is a gathering of food aficionados who appreciate the aroma of roasted meant that has been painstakingly smoked for several hours) During the colonial period, the practice of holding a neighborhood barbecue was well established, but it was in the fifty years before the Civil War that the traditions associated with large barbecues became entrenched. Plantation owners regularly held large and festive barbecues, including "pig pickin's" for slaves. In the 19th century, barbecue was a feature at church picnic and political rallies as well as at private parties. A barbecue was a popular and relatively inexpensive way to lobby for votes, and the organizers of political rallies would provide barbecue, lemonade, and usually a bit of whiskey. Unlike most food preparation in the South, which is dominated by women, barbecue is a male preserve. In 1951, George Stephen of Palatine, Illinois invented the kettle grill and revolutionized the art of outdoor cookery throughout the US.

Barbecue sauce Chopped onions fried in butter, made into a sauce with tomato paste and seasoned with sugar, vinegar, mustard, and Worcestershire sauce, served with barbecued meat and sausages.

Barbera A grape variety widely used for wine making, although not one of the classic varieties;

makes the dark fruity and often sharp red wines of northern Italy.

Barcelona nut Spanish variety of hazel nut. A 30-g portion is a rich source of copper; contains 19 g of fat of which 7% is saturated; provides 3 g of dietary fibre; supplies 190 kcal.

Barding To cover the breast of a bird with slices of fat before roasting, to prevent the flesh from drying.

Bariatric surgery Surgery on the stomach and/or intestines to help the patient with extreme obesity lose weight. Bariatric surgery is a weight-loss method used for people who have a body mass index (BMI) above 40. Surgery may also be an option for people with a BMI between 35 and 40 who have health problems like heart disease or type 2 diabetes.

Barium A metal of no known metabolic function, and hence not a dietary essential. Barium sulphate is opaque to X-rays and a suspension is used (a barium meal) to allow examination of the shape and movements of the stomach for diagnostic purposes, and as a barium enema for X-ray investigation of the lower intestinal tract.

Barley Barley, as a food, is most commonly identified as pearl barley, which is traditionally used in soups and stews. In the last few years, we've become more creative with barley and have used it in summer salads, casseroles, and side dishes. Barley is also used as a commercial ingredient in prepared foods such as breakfast cereals, soups, pilaf mixes, breads, cookies, crackers, and snack bars. Today it is the world's fourth largest cereal crop. Barley has held a prominent and long-standing place in the history of food, being the world's oldest grain, and has been cultivated for about 8,000 years. Babylonians brewed beer from barley around 2500 B.C. Both the ancient Greeks and Hebrews made use of barley in porridge and bread. Barley remained an important bread grain in Europe until the 1500s when wheat breads became popular.

Barley sugar Sugar confectionery made by melting and cooling sugar, originally made by boiling with a decoction of barley.

Barley water A drink made by boiling pearl barley with water, commonly flavoured with orange or lemon.

Barley wine Fermented malted barley, stronger than beer (8-10% alcohol by volume), bottled under pressure, so sparkling.

Barleycorn An obsolete measure of length; the size of a single grain of barley; 1/3 inch (0.85 cm).

Barlow's disease Infantile scurvy, also known as Moeller's disease and Cheadle's disease.

Barm An alternative name for yeast or leaven, or the froth on fermenting malt liquor. Sport (short for spontaneous) or virgin barm is made by allowing wild yeast to fall into sugar medium and multiply.

Barm brack Irish; yeast cake made with butter, egg, buttermilk, and dried fruit, flavoured with caraway seed. Similar Welsh cake is bara brith.

Barmene Trade name for yeast extract, prepared from autolysed brewer's yeast, plus vegetable juices, used for flavouring.

Baron of beef The pair of sirloins of beef, left uncut at the bone.

Barrel A standard barrel contains 36 gallons. (36 imperial gallons (UK)= 163.6 L; 36 US gallons = 113.7 L.)

Bartlett pear The Bartlett pear variety originated in Berkshire, England, in the 17th century, by a schoolmaster named John Stair. Stair sold some of his pear tree cuttings to a horticulturist named Williams, who further developed the variety and renamed it after himself. After pear seedlings crossed the Atlantic with the early colonists, the Williams pear found fame and fortune in 1812 under the tutelage of nurseryman, Enoch Bartlett, of Dorchester, Massachusetts. Bartlett, unaware of the pear's true name, distributed it under his own name. Ever since, the pear has been known as the Bartlett in the United States, but is still referred to as the Williams pear in other parts of the world. Bartlett pear trees eventually came out West in the covered wagons of the 49ers heading for the Great California Gold Rush.

Basal metabolic rate (BMR) The energy cost of maintaining the metabolic integrity of the body, nerve and muscle tone, respiration and circulation. It depends on the amount of metabolically active body tissue, and hence can be calculated from body weight, using different factors for males and females, and at different ages. For children the. BMR also includes the energy cost of growth. Experimentally, BMR is measured as the heat output from the body, or the rate of oxygen consumption, under strictly standardized conditions, 12-14 hours after the last meal, completely at rest (but not asleep) and at an environmental temperature of 26-30 °C, to ensure thermal neutrality. Measurement of metabolic rate under less rigorously controlled conditions gives the resting metabolic rate (RMR).

For people with a sedentary lifestyle and relatively low physical activity, BMR accounts for about 70% of total energy expenditure. The energy costs of different activities are generally expressed as the physical activity ratio, the ratio of energy expenditure in the activity to BMR.

Basal metabolism Basal metabolism is the energy (calories) a body burns when completely at rest. Basal metabolism rate (BMR) is the level of energy needed to keep involuntary body processes going. These processes include heartbeat, breathing, generating body heat, perspiring to keep cool, and transmitting messages to the brain. For a sedentary person, BMR accounts for about 60-70 percent of daily energy expenditure; the remaining 30-40 percent is from physical activity and from body heat produced after a meal. Physical activity is responsible for as much as 50-60 percent of the total energy expenditure in people who include frequent aerobic activity into their lifestyles

Base Base is a soup reduction paste similar to bouillon, but richer, more flavorful, and less salty. You can find it in the soup section of the super market. It comes in a jar and must be refrigerated after opening.

Basic science The fundamental approach to understanding how systems work. Basic research takes place in the laboratory and often involves the study of molecules and cells.

Basil A versatile and widely used aromatic herb. There are numerous species of basil; some have scents reminiscent of pineapple, lemon, cinnamon or cloves; others have beautiful purple leaves. The plant grows well in warm climates and is widely used throughout southern Europe, particularly the Mediterranean, and in many parts of Asia.

The variety called holy basil (tulsi) is an essential part of an authentic Thai curry. In Mediterranean regions, basil and tomato are a classic combination. Pesto, made from basil leaves and pine nuts, with parmesan or pecorino cheese and olive oil (traditionally pounded together in a mortar and pestle) is another classic dish.

Basil, an annual plant, is very easy to grow from seed but is sensitive to cold. Basil is widely available in supermarkets; look for bright green leaves with no hint of wilting or black spotting. Dried basil retains little of the aroma and flavour of fresh basil, so is of limited use in the kitchen.

Basmati Long-grain Indian variety of rice; much prized for its delicate flavour (the name means 'fragrant' in Hindi).

Basmati rice Basmati is a long-grain rice from India, considered to be one of the best-quality white rices. It has a distinctive aroma and, when cooked, each grain should remain separate, giving a light, fluffy result. Basmati should be rinsed thoroughly in a few changes of water before cooking, in order to remove the starch. It's the perfect accompaniment to Indian curries or used in biryani and pilaf dishes.

Basophils Blood cells which when connected to immunoglobulin E antibodies release histamine or other substances causing allergic symptoms.

Baste To spoon, brush or pour drippings or liquid over a food before or during cooking in order to prevent drying, to add flavor, or to glaze it.

Basting The process of spooning stock or fat over meat at intervals to prevent it from drying out during roasting. You can buy a bulb baster - a kind of large pipette - for the job. They're made of glass or plastic; although delicate, the glass one tends to be better because the plastic ones can melt if the liquid is very hot.

Bath bun A small English cake made from milk-based yeast dough, with dried fruit and a topping of sugar crystals, attributed to Dr W. Oliver of Bath (18th century).

Bath chap The cheek and jawbones of the pig, salted and smoked. Originated in Bath.

Bath cheese A small English cheese, made from cow's milk with the subsequent addition of cream.

Bath oliver A biscuit made with yeast, attributed to Dr W. Oliver of Bath (18th century).

Baton In culinary terms, a baton means something - usually a vegetable, such as a carrot, courgette or piece of celery - cut into a long, thin rectangle shape. Vegetables cut into this shape are often steamed or sautéed, or served raw, as in a classic French cruditı selection. If you're making a cruditı selection, the recipe below would make a good dip.

Battenberg cake A two-coloured sponge cake, baked in an oblong tin, usually covered with almond paste; named in honour of the marriage of Queen Victoria's granddaughter to Prince Louis of Battenberg, 1884.

Batter The name of many semi-liquid, floury mixtures of flour, water or milk (or both) or some other liquid. It also usually includes sugar and eggs. Batters may be thin or thick (but even when thick, they must be fluid enough to drop from a spoon). When thin, they should pour out like creamy milk.

Batterie de cuisine An expression commonly used by chefs to describe the essential equipment that every good cook needs for the preparation of food in the kitchen, from saucepans to knives.

Bauernschmaus Austrian; pork loin chops, bacon, and sausages cooked in beer with sauerkraut, grated raw potato, and seasoning.

Bavarian cream It is a molded cream that is made from custard sauce or sweetened fruit puree that is bound with gelatin and lightened with whipped cream. Bavarian cream can be served on its own or used as a filling for cold charlottes or molded cakes.

Bavarois(e) 1. A hot drink made from eggs, milk, and tea, sweetened and flavoured with a liqueur; seventeenth-century Bavarian.

2. French; (crome bavarois) a cold dessert made from egg custard with gelatine and cream.

3. Hollandaise sauce with crayfish garnish.

Bay (bay leaf) A herb, the leaf of the Mediterranean sweet bay tree (Lauris nobilis) with a strong characteristic flavour. Rarely used alone, but an important component of bouquet garni, and used with other herbs in marinades, pickles, stews, and stuffing.

Bay boletes or boletus A robust and meaty wild mushroom, often found in areas where conifers grow. Use in risottos or omelettes or simply fry with a little garlic. Bay boletes are also good for pickling and drying.

Bay leaves The aromatic leaf from the bay laurel tree, it is an essential component of the classic bouquet garni parsley, thyme and a bay leaf. It's one of the few herbs that doesn't lose its flavour when dried. Although fresh leaves are becoming more widely available, they're usually sold dried.

The dried bay leaves are more strongly flavoured than fresh ones, but the uses for both are the same. The bittersweet, spicy leaves impart their pungent flavour to a variety of dishes and ingredients, making bay a versatile store-cupboard ingredient. Bay leaves can be used to flavour vinegars, in pickling and in marinades or to flavour pates.

Long cooking draws out the aroma of this herb and most braised, poached and stewed dishes benefit from its flavour. A leaf dropped into soups and stocks is particularly good. Add a bay leaf when braising red or pickled cabbage, to poaching liquid for fish, or to infuse the milk for custard or rice pudding. Bean soups and stews are enhanced by a bay leaf, as are rice dishes such as risotto or pilaf.

Bay lobster Or Moreton Bay bug, a variety of sand lobster found in Australia.

B-Carotene The most abundant of the carotenoids. b-Carotene has strong provitamin A activity. Unlike vitamin A itself, b-carotene is a strong antioxidant.

Basophil granulocyte Basophils are the least common of the granulocytes, representing about 0.5% to 1% of circulating leukocytes. They contain large cytoplasmic granules which obscure the cell nucleus under the microscope. However, when unstained, the nucleus is visible and it usually has 2 lobes. A cell in tissues, the mast cell, has many similar characteristics. For example, both cell types store histamine, a chemical that is secreted by the cells when stimulated in certain ways (histamine causes some of the symptoms of an allergic reaction). Like all circulating granulocytes, basophils can be recruited out of the blood into a tissue when needed.

Bdelygmia An extreme loathing for food.

Bean curd Of all the vegetarian products, bean curd is the most versatile and important in the Chinese cuisine. Bean curds are made of soybean powder and come in square cakes measuring 2 1/2 or 3 inches to a side. They are white and have the consistency of firm custard. They are bland but absorbent, soft-textured but strong, and are conducive to all types of cooking. Because they are inexpensive, there is an eastern Chinese expression for taking advantage of a person that is "eating bean curd."

Bean sauce After soy sauce is brewed, the soybean pulp is removed from the vats and made into several types of condiments. The first is bean sauce, sometimes called brown bean sauce or soybean condiment. Use this rich condiment to replace soy sauce where thicker gravy is desired. Especially good used as a marinade for roasted meats.

Bean sprouts Any of a number of peas, beans, and seeds which can be germinated and the sprouts eaten raw or cooked. The sprouting causes the synthesis of vitamin C. One of the commonest sprouts is that of the mung bean, but alfalfa and adzuki beans are also used. An 80-g portion is a good source of folate; provides 2.4 g of dietary fibre; supplies 7 kcal.

Bean, black-eyed Also known as black-eyed pea or cow pea, Vigna sinensis; creamy white bean with a black mark on one edge.

Bean, borlotti Italian variety of Phaseolus vulgaris, haricot or common bean.

Bean, broad Also known as fava or horse bean, Vicia faba. A 75-g portion is a good source of copper; a source of niacin, folate, and vitamin C; contains 0.5 g of fat of which 16% is saturated; provides 3 g of dietary fibre; supplies 35 kcal.

Bean, butter Several large varieties of Phaseolus vulgaris, also known as Lima, curry, Madagascar, and sugar bean. A 100-g cooked portion is a source of protein, copper, iron; provides 5 g of dietary fibre; supplies 80 kcal.

Bean, French Unripe seeds and pods of Phaseolus vulgaris; ripe seeds are haricot beans. A 100-g portion is a rich source of folate; a source of vitamin A (as carotene) and copper; provides 3 g of dietary fibre:; supplies 7 kcal.

Bean, haricot Ripe seed of Phaseolus vulgaris (the unripe seed is the French bean). Also known as navy, string, pinto, or snap bean. A 100-g portion of dried haricot beans is a good source of copper; a source of protein, vitamin B1, and iron; contains 0.5 g of fat of which 20% is saturated; provides 7 g of dietary fibre; supplies 100 kcal.

Bean, mung Whole or split seed of Vigna radiata (Phaseolus aureuis, P. radiatus), green gram. A 150-g portion is a rich source of folate, copper, and selenium; a good source of vitamin B6, iron, and zinc; a source of protein and vitamin B 1,; provides 3 g of dietary fibre; supplies 90 kcal.

Bean, red kidney Ripe seed of Phaseolus vulgaris. A 100-g portion of dried raw beans is a rich source of protein, vitamin B 1, folate, iron, copper, and selenium; a good source of vitamin B6 and zinc; a source of vitamin B 2, niacin, and calcium; contains 1.7 g of fat of which 11% is saturated; provides 25 g of dietary fibre; supplies 280 kcal (1180 kJ). Like all pulses contains toxic lectins; uncooked or partially cooked beans cause vomiting, diarrhoea, and serious damage to the intestinal mucosa. The lectins are inactivated by boiling for about 10 min., but not by cooking below boiling point.

Bean, runner A 100-g portion is a rich source of folate; contains 0.2 g of fat of which 50% is saturated; provides 3 g of dietary fibre; supplies 20 kcal (85 kJ).

Bean, string Either runner beans or French beans which have a climbing habit rather than growing as small bushes. The name derives from the method of growing them up strings.

Beans Beans can be divided into two main groups those with edible pods (green beans) and those with edible seeds. The former group includes French beans, runner beans and yellow 'wax' beans; the latter includes the likes of cannellini or borlotti beans and a myriad of similar varieties. Dried beans need to be soaked, preferably overnight, before using.

Dried beans shouldn't be kept more than a year because they tend to toughen with age. Tinned beans are already cooked and only need rinsing and draining before using. The flavour of each variety of bean is distinct, but they all share a wholesome, earthy taste. Beans can be served on their own, but they combine well with other flavourings and food.

Many cuisines have their own classic bean dishes the French cassoulet, the Spanish cocido or the smoked bacon or pork and bean stews of Romania, Hungary and throughout the Balkans. Beans can also be used to thicken wintry soups and stews, cooked whole and then mashed or purıed. They can also be mixed with pasta or rice in soup to make a hearty, warming dish.

Beans are a good substitute for meat in vegetarian 'burgers' because they're high in protein. Mexican fajitas wouldn't't be the same without refried beans - purıed beans that are fried and spread on a tortilla. Cold, cooked beans are also excellent mixed with garlic vinaigrette for a salad to accompany fish or cold meats.

Bearnaise sauce A classic French sauce made with a reduction of vinegar, white wine, tarragon, black peppercorns and shallots. It's finished with egg yolks and butter. Delicious served with any plain meat or fish. The Food Standards Agency recommends that pasteurised egg should be used in any dish in which the egg will not be completely cooked, such as Bıarnaise sauce. Pasteurised egg is available in frozen, liquid or powder form and eggs pasteurised in their shells are also available.

Beat 1. To agitate an ingredient or a mixture by vigorously turning it over and over with an upward motion, in order to introduce air, using a spoon, fork, whisk, or electric mixer.

2. Raw meat is beaten by hitting it briskly all over the surface to break down the fibres and make it more tender when cooked.

Beaten biscuit Southerners describe beaten biscuits as a cross between a soda cracker and a baking powder biscuit. To achieve the right texture and lightness, the dough had to be beaten hard (usually with a mallet) for at least half an hours. The purpose of the beating was to incorporate air into the mixture (this was a time in history before the invention of baking powder). They were a very heavy biscuit, not like our present day baking powder biscuits. Beaten biscuits originated in Virginia and traveled across the mountains to Kentucky and then south to Maryland. Chuck wagon cooks also made them, recruiting a gullible new cowhand for help. They were considered the pride of the South, and in earlier days no Southern hostess would fail to offer these at any and all times of the day They are one of the delicious hot breads that have made Southern cooks famous They were basically considered an upper-class status symbol dish that depended on a lot of labor. Making the beaten biscuits was the daily duty of the plantation cook.

Beau monde seasoning salt Beau Monde is a seasoning salt containing ground dried onion and celery seed. It can be found in the spice section of your grocery store. Check out the web page on Beau Monde Seasoning Salt.

Beaujolais red wine from the Beaujolais region of France, made from Gamay grapes. Beaujolais nouveau (primeur in French) is the new season's wine, drunk young. It is 'officially' available on 18 November.

Bechamel sauce A white sauce given extra flavour by infusing the milk with carrot, onion, celery, black peppercorns, mace and bay leaf for 30 minutes.

Like hollandaise, mayonnaise and crıme anglaise, bıchamel forms the basis of numerous other sauces. It was named after its inventor, Louis XIV's steward Louis de Bıchamel. It's a versatile sauce for all sorts of dishes including macaroni cheese, lasagne and croque-monsieur.

Bıchamel sauce In France, it is one of the four basic sauces called "meres" or "mother sauces" from which all other sauces derive. It is also know as "white sauce." It is a smooth, white sauce made from a roux made with flour, boiled milk, and butter. It is usually served with white meats, eggs, and vegetables. It forms the basis of many other sauces.

Bee wine Wine produced by the usual fermentation of sugar, but using yeast in the form of a clump of yeast and lactic bacteria; the clump rises and falls with the bubbles of carbon dioxide formed, during fermentation, hence the name 'bee'.

Beef Flesh of the ox (Bos taurus); flesh from young calves is veal. A 150-g portion of most cuts is a rich source of protein, niacin, iron, copper, and vitamin B12; a good source of vitamin B 2 and copper; a source of vitamins B 1, B 6, and selenium; contains 20-30 g of fat of which half is saturated (lean part is 5% fat); supplies 350-500 kcal.

Beef olives Thin strips of beef filled with savoury stuffing, braised in stock.

Beef on Weck Sandwich Also called Beef On Wick, an alternative spelling usually used by older people from Buffalo and eastern suburbanites. It is a roast beef sandwich on a salty kummelweck roll. This sandwich is a unique staple of Buffalo, New York's bars and taverns. Few, if any, restaurants outside of the Buffalo area serve this sandwich or even know what it is. The important ingredient to these sandwiches is the German roll, called kummelweck. These rolls are large, hard rolls with chunks of salt and caraway seeds on the top. Kummelweck is simply shortened to "weck."

Beef stroganoff A dish that consists of thin slices of tender beef (usually tenderloin or top loin), onions, and sliced mushrooms. The ingredients are quickly sautued in butter and combined with a sour-cream sauce. It is usually accompanied by rice pilaf. The recipe did not appear in English cookbooks until 1932, and it was not until the 1950s, after World War II, that beef stroganoff became popular for elegant dinner parties in America. There is more than one story on who first created this elegant dish: Beef Stroganoff was created in the 1890s by chef Charles Briere for Count Paul Stroganoff, a 19th century Russian diplomat, who was in a friendly competition with the chefs of other families in St. Petersburg, the cultural centre of Russian society.< The Stroganoff's chef won the prize with his recipe. Another version is that Count

Pavel Stroganov, a celebrity in turn-of-the-century St. Petersburg, was a noted gourmet as well as a friend of Alexander III. He is frequently credited with creating Beef Stroganoff or having a chef who did so. The name of this dish comes from Russian Count Grigory Stroganove (1770-1857) who was one of the richest noblemen and held the highest diplomatic posts. Great gourmet, he loved delicious dishes and always had the best cooks. One of them invented an original dish from scraped meat and it was on the Count's taste. The dish took the name Stroganoff, but, as to the cook, his name was unfairly forgotten but some people told ("bitter tongues") that the dish was made especially for the Count when he, being old, lost all his teeth and couldn't chew a simple beef stake.

Beef tea An extract of stewing beef, formerly used for invalids, since the extractives stimulate the appetite. See also meat extract.

Beef Wellington It is a choice fillet of beef (often flambіed in brandy) that is covered with liver pate and sliced mushrooms. The meat is then placed in a case of puff pastry and baked in a hot oven. It was named in the mid 19th century in honour of Arthur Wellesley (1769-1852), British soldier and statesman. He is best known for his military victory over Napoleon at the battle of Waterloo in 1815. He was a national hero and was made the first Duke of Wellington to honour him. Because of his love of a dish of beef, truffles, mushrooms, Maderia wine, and pate cooked in pastry, this dish was name Beef Wellington in his honour. He was also Prime Minister of Britain and Ireland. According to Queen Victoria, the Duke was The pride of this country. He was the GREATEST man this country ever produced. To think that all of this is gone; and that this great and immortal man belongs now to History."

Beef, pressed (Salt beef); boned brisket beef that has been salted, cooked, and pressed. Known as corned beef in USA.

Beefalo A cross between the domestic cow (Bos taurus) and the buffalo (Bubalus spp.) which can be fattened on range grass rather than requiring cereal and protein supplements.

Beefsteak fungus Large edible fungus (Fistulina hepatica) with a stringy, meat-like texture and deep red juice.

Beer Alcoholic beverage made by the fermentation of cereals; traditionally barley, but also maize, rice, and sorghum. The first step is the malting of barley: it is allowed to sprout, when the enzyme amylase hydrolyses some of the starch to dextrins and maltose. The sprouted (malted) barley is dried, then extracted with hot water (the process of mashing) to produce wort. After the addition of hops for flavour, the wort is allowed to ferment. Two types of yeast are used in brewing: top fermenting yeasts which float on the surface of the wort and bottom or deep fermenters. Most traditional British beers (ale, bitter, stout, and porter) are brewed with top fermenting yeasts.

UK beers, brown ale, and stout: around 3% alcohol by volume, 2-4 % carbohydrate, 75-110 kcal (315-460 kj) per 300 mL (half pint). Strong ale is 6.6% alcohol, 6% carbohydrate, 210 kcal (880 kJ) per 300 mL, (half pint). Ale is a light-coloured beer, relatively high in alcohol content, and moderately heavily hopped. Bitter beers are darker and contain more hops. Porter and stout are almost black in colour; they are made from wort containing some partly charred malt; milk stout is made from wort containing added lactose.

Lager is the traditional mainland European type of beer, sometimes called Pilsner lager or Pils, since the original lager was brewed in Pilsen in Bohemia. It is brewed by deep fermentation.

Lite beer is beer which has been allowed to ferment until virtually all the carbohydrate has been converted to alcohol and so it is low in carbohydrate and high in alcohol.

Low alcohol beer may be made either by fermentation of a low carbohydrate wort, or by removal of much of the alcohol after fermentation (de-alcoholized beer).

Sorghum beer (African, made also from millet, maize, or plantain) is a thick sour beverage consumed while still fermenting. Also known by numerous local names, kaffir beer, bouza, pombı, bantu beer. 3-8% alcohol, 3-10% carbohydrate, a rich source of vitamin B1 per 300 mL portion.

Beestings The first milk given by the cow after calving, the colostrum, rich in immunoglobulins.

Beet Scientific name is Beta vulgaris. Among its numerous varieties are the red, or garden, beet, the sugar beet, and Swiss chard. In the United States, sugar beets are grown extensively from Michigan to Idaho and in California, accounting for :nore than half of United States sugar production. Greens are used, as you would cook spinach. The beet has been cultivated since pre-Christian times. The beet comes from the Mediterranean area where the people in Babylonia, Egypt, and Greece grew them. Then as now were used not only to eat but for their red dye.

Beetroot The root of Beta vulgaris, eaten cooked or pickled. Known simply as beet in North America. The violet-red pigment, betanin, is used as a food colour (E-162). One small beetroot (40 g) is a good source of folate; provides 1.6 g of dietary fibre; supplies 18 kcal.

Beeturia Excretion of red-coloured urine after eating beetroot, due to excretion of the pigment betanin. It occurs, not consistently, in about one person in eight.

Beignets Puffy squares of deep-fried dough dusted with powdered sugar. The word beignet comes from the early Celtic word "bigne" meaning "to raise." Beignet is also French for "fritter." It is a New Orleans specialty that is a fried, raised piece of yeast dough, usually about two inches in diameter or two inches square. After being fried, they are sprinkled with sugar or coated with various icings. It is like a sweet doughnut, which is square-shaped, and minus the hole. Traditional fare at New Orleans coffee houses, most notably Cafe du Monde in the French Quarter.

Beluga The Russian name for a sturgeon found in the Black and Caspian Seas (they can grow up to 2,000 pounds). It is the largest of the sturgeon family and is considered the finest caviar. The eggs are light to dark gray in colour.

Bemax Trade name for a wheat germ preparation. A 30-g portion is a rich source of vitamins B 1 and E, folate, copper, and zinc; a good source of iron; a source of protein, vitamins B 2, B 6, and niacin; provides 5 g of dietary fibre; contains 2.4 g of fat; supplies 120 kcal (500 kJ).

Benedictine A French liqueur invented in about 1510 by the monks of the Benedictine Abbey of Fıcamp in France. The Abbey was closed, and the recipe lost after the French Revolution, then rediscovered about 1863. It is based on double-distilled brandy, flavoured with some 75 herbs and spices; it contains 40% (by volume) alcohol and 30% sugar; 300 kcal (1.3 MJ)/100 mL. See also B and B.

Benzoic acid A preservative normally used as the sodium, potassium, or calcium salts and their derivatives (E-210-E-219), especially in acid foods such as pickles and sauces. It occurs naturally in a number of fruits, including cranberries, prunes, greengages, and cloudberries, and in cinnamon. Cloudberries contain so much benzoic acid that they can be stored for long periods of time without any precautions being taken against bacterial or fungal spoilage. Benzoic acid and its derivatives are excreted from the body conjugated with the amino acids glycine (hippuric acid) and alanine. Because of this, benzoic acid is sometimes used in the treatment of argininaemia, argininosuccinic aciduria, and citrullinaemia, permitting excretion of nitrogenous waste from the body as these conjugates.

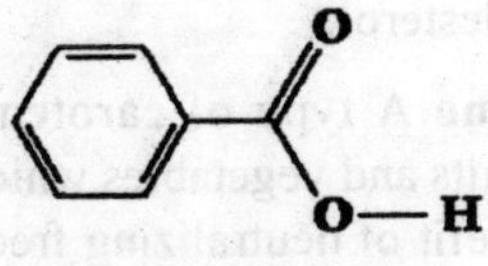

Fig. Benzoic acid

Bergamot 1. A pear-shaped orange, Citrus bergamia, grown mainly in Calabria, Italy, for its peel oil;

2. An ornamental herb, Monarda didyma, the dried leaves of which were used to make Oswego tea;

3. A type of pear, Pyrus persica.

Beriberi The result of severe and prolonged deficiency of vitamin B 1, still a problem in parts of South East Asia where the diet is high in carbohydrate (polished rice) and poor in vitamin B 1. In developed countries vitamin B1 deficiency is associated with alcohol abuse; while it may result in beriberi, more commonly the result is central nervous system damage, the Wernicke-Korsakoff syndrome. In beriberi there is degeneration of peripheral nerves, starting in the hands and feet and ascending the arms and legs, with a loss of sensation and deep muscle pain. There is also enlargement of the heart, which may lead to oedema (wet beriberi), and death results from heart failure. Fatal heart failure may develop without the nerve damage being apparent (Shoshin or sudden beriberi). The name is derived from the BahasaMalay word for sheep, to describe the curious sheep-like gait adopted by sufferers.

Berry Botanical term for fleshy juicy fruits with one or more seeds not having a stone e.g. grape, gooseberry, tomato, banana, blackcurrant, cranberry.

Beta carotene A type of carotenoid found in various fruits and vegetables which provide the health benefit of neutralizing free radicals that may cause damage to cells.

Beta glucan A soluble fiber in oats which provides the health benefit of reducing the risk of cardiovascular disease by decreasing circulating blood cholesterol.

Beta-carotene A type of carotenoid found in various fruits and vegetables which provide the health benefit of neutralizing free radicals that may cause damage to cells.

Betel Leaf of the creeper Piper betel, which is chewed in some parts of the world for its stimulating effect, due to the presence of the alkaloids arecoline and guvacoline. The leaves are chewed with the nuts of the areca palm, Arecha catechu, which is therefore often called the betel palm, and the nut is called betel nut. The Indian delicacy pan is based on betel leaf and areca nut, together with aromatic spices and herbs.

Betty or Brown Betty A Betty is a baked dessert dating back to Colonial America, It is a baked pudding made with layers of spiced sweetened fruit (usually apples) and buttered breadcrumbs.

Beurre manie This is a French term for a kneaded mixture of butter and flour.

Beurre This is the French word for "butter."

Bezoar A hard ball of undigested food, sometimes together with hair, which forms in the stomach or intestine and can cause obstruction. Foods with a high content of indigestible pectin, such as orange pith, can form bezoars if swallowed without chewing. The name is derived from the Arabic meaning 'protection against poison', since bezoars were formerly believed to have protective properties.

Bhaji 1 Chinese spinach (Amaranthus gangeticus), also known as callaloo.

2 Also bhajia, Indian; vegetable fritters, normally made with gram (lentil) flour.

Bharak palinka Hungarian; dry apricot brandy.

Bhoona Indian term for frying. Sukha bhoona is a simple sauti. Dumned bhoona is a pot roast, or steam-fried dish; marinated meat is seared, moistened, and cooked in a tightly closed vessel in the oven. Ard bhoona is a dry pot roast; the meat is seared then cooked in a tightly closed vessel in the oven with butter but no water.

Bhujia Indian; vegetable dishes, highly spiced. In the final stage of cooking they are fried in ghee which has been heated with onions, chillies, garlic, and ginger.

Bialy A bialy is similar to a bagel, in that it is a round, chewy roll. But it is unlike a bagel in two important ways: One, it does not have a hole in the middle, but a depression; and two, it never became popular outside of New York City. The indentation in the middle of the dough is can be filled with onion, garlic, or poppy seeds. As the bialy has a very short shelf life, about six hours, they do not lend to being shipped around the country. They can be modest in size, three to four inches, or the size of a small pizza.

Bias 1. A bias is a prejudice in a general or specific sense, usually in the sense for having a preference to one particular point of view or ideological perspective. However, one is generally only said to be biased if one's powers of judgment are influenced by the biases one holds, to the extent that one's views could not be taken as being neutral or objective, but instead as subjective. A bias could, for example, lead one to accept or deny the truth of a claim, not on the basis of the strength of the arguments in support of the claim themselves, but because of the extent of the claim's correspondence with one's own preconceived ideas. This is called confirmation bias.

2. In a clinical trial, bias refers to effects that a conclusion that may be incorrect as, for example, when a researcher or patient knows what treatment is being given. To avoid bias, a blinded study may be done.

BIBRA The British Industrial Biological Research Association.

Bicarbonate of soda Another common name for baking soda is bicarb which is short for bicarbonate of soda or sodium bicarbonate. Baking soda, is a naturally occurring substance that is present in all living things. It helps living things maintain the pH balance necessary for life. Baking Soda is made from soda ash, also known as sodium carbonate. It is found in all grocery stores in the baking section.

Bierplinse German; batter made with dark beer, used for sweet or savoury fritters.

Biersuppe German soup made from light beer, thickened with potato flour and flavoured with cinnamon and lemon peel.

Biffins Apples that have been peeled, partly baked, then pressed and dried.

Bifidus factor A carbohydrate in human milk which contains nitrogen and stimulates the growth of Lactobacillus bifidus in the intestine. In turn, this organism lowers the pH of the intestinal contents and suppresses the growth of E. coli and other pathogenic bacteria. See also lactulose.

Bigos Polish; casserole of sauerkraut, cooked meat, game, sausages, ham, etc., with vodka and wine.

Bilberry The berry of wild shrubs of the genus Vaccinium, not generally cultivated. Variously known as whortleberry, blaeberry, whinberry, huckleberry. A 110-g portion is a rich source of vitamin C; a source of copper; provides 7.7 g of dietary fibre; supplies 60 kcal.

Bile Fluid produced by the liver and stored in the gall bladder before secretion into the small intestine (duodenum) via the bile duct. It contains the bile salts, which function in the emulsification and hence digestion of fats, bile pigments (bilirubin and biliverdin, which are the result of breakdown of the haemoglobin of red blood cells) and cholesterol. It is alkaline, and hence neutralizes the acid from the stomach as the food reaches the small intestine. Relatively large amounts of vitamin B 12 and folic acid are secreted in the bile and then reabsorbed from the small intestine. Most of the cholesterol and bile salts are also reabsorbed from the small intestine.

Bile salts Salts of cholic and deoxycholic acid and their glycine and taurine conjugates, secreted in the bile; they assist the digestion of fats by emulsifying them.

Bile Secretions of the liver that aid in digestion and absorption, and stimulate peristalsis.

Biltong South African; strips of dried meat, salted, spiced, and dried in air for 10-14 days.

Bind To add liquid, fat, or egg to a mixture to hold it together. See also panada.

Binge-purge syndrome A feature of the eating disorder bulimia nervosa, characterized by the ingestion of excessive amounts of food and the excessive use of laxatives.

Bioassay Biological assay; measurement of biologically active compounds (e.g. vitamins and essential amino acids) by their ability to support growth of micro-organisms or animals.

Bioavailability The extent to which the body can utilise a particular nutrient.

Biocides Chemicals used to kill unwanted organisms: herbicides, insecticides, fungicides.

Biocytin The main form of the vitamin biotin in most foods, bound to the amino acid lysine.

Biodegradable Describes any material that can be broken down by biological action (e.g., dissimilation, digestion, denitrification). The breakdown of material (chemicals) by microorganisms (bacteria, fungus, etc.).

Bio-electrical impedance (BIE) A method of measuring the proportion of fat in the body by the difference in the resistance to passage of an electric current between fat and lean tissue.

Bioelectrical impedance analysis (BIA) A way to estimate the amount of body weight that is fat and nonfat. Nonfat weight comes from bone, muscle, body water, organs, and other body tissues. BIA works by measuring how difficult it is for a harmless electrical current to move through the body. The more fat a person has, the harder it is for electricity to flow through the body. The less fat a person has, the easier it is for electricity to flow through the body. By measuring the flow of electricity, one can estimate body fat percent.

Biological activity The effect (change in metabolic activity upon living cells) caused by specific compounds or agents. For example, the drug aspirin causes the blood to thin, that is to clot less easily.

Biological controls An integrated pest management method which includes the use of living organisms to reduce the extent of pest problems. This includes the use of beneficial or predatory insects such as ladybugs and parasitic wasps to control crop destroying bugs.

Biological group See nutritional supervision, supervision of siblings and contacts, and vulnerability. Designates risks induced by biological factors.

Biological oxygen demand (BOD) A way of assessing bacterial contamination of water, milk, etc. by micro-organisms which take up oxygen for their metabolism.

Biological utilization of food Process that involves the continuum digestion / absorption / metabolism / excretion, or partial resynthesis of foods in living organisms. Can be adversely altered by the occurrence of diseases at any one or more of the steps in the process.

Biomarker 1. For other meanings, see the disambiguation page Marker Biomarker is a substance used as an indicator of a biologic state. It may mean the following:It can be any kind of molecule indicating the existence (past or present) of living organisms. In particular, in the fields of geology and astrobiology biomarkers are also know as biosignatures. The term is also used to describe biological involvement in the generation of petroleum (see Biomarker (petroleum)). In medicine, a biomarker can be a substance that is introduced in an organism as a means to examine organ function or other aspects of health. For example, rubidium chloride is used as a radioactive isotope to evaluate perfusion of heart muscle.In biology and medicine, a biomarker can be a substance whose detection indicates a particular disease state (for example, the presence of an antibody may indicate an infection).In cell biology, a biomarker is a molecule that allows for the detection and isolation of a particular cell type (for example, the protein Oct-4 is used as a biomarker to identify embryonic stem cells).

A biomarker can also be used to indicate exposure to various environmental substances in epidemiology and toxicology. In these cases, the biomarker may be the external substance itself (e.g. asbestos particles or NNK from tobacco), or a variant of the external substance processed by the body (a metabolite). In genetics, a biomarker (identified as genetic marker) is a fragment of DNA sequence that causes disease or is associated with susceptibility to disease.

2. A substance sometimes found in the blood, other body fluids, or tissues. A high level of biomarker may mean that a certain type of cancer is in the body. Examples of biomarkers include CA 125 (ovarian cancer), CA 15-3 (breast cancer), CEA (ovarian, lung, breast, pancreas, and gastrointestinal tract cancers), and PSA (prostate cancer). Also called tumor marker.

3. An effect in a biological system. Measurements in the human body or its products. Some biomarkers, such as the levels of certain vitamins in blood serum, are used as indices of nutritional status. Others are used as indices of the risk or progression of disease.

Biomedical model The model of illness and disease in Western medical education and research. It has two assumptions 1. reductionism - that all conditions can be linearly reduced to a single cause, and

2. dualism - where illness and disease are divided either to an "organic" disorder having an objectively defined cause, or a "functional" disorder, with no specific cause or pathophysiology. The biomedical model is not sufficient to explain the functional GI disorders.

Bioperine Bioperine is a standardized piperine extract obtained from the fruits of the Piper nigrum L. (black pepper) and/or Piper longum L. (long pepper) plants that are cultivated in the damp, nutrient-rich soil regions of south India. The delicate pepper berries are hand harvested just prior to ripening and then sun dried to assure optimum maturity and quality.

The extract of piperine, developed by Sabinsa Corporation in its patented form of Bioperine, has been clinically tested in the United States and shown to significantly enhance the bioavailability of supplemented nutrients through increased absorption.

Biopesticide A biopesticide is any material of natural origin used in pest control derived from living organisms, such as bacteria, plant cells or animal cells.

Biopsychosocial model A model that proposes that illness and disease result from simultaneously interacting systems at the cellular, tissue, organismal, interpersonal, and environmental level. It incorporates the biologic aspects of the disorder with the unique psychosocial features of the individual, and helps explain the variability in symptom expression among individuals having the same biologic condition.

Biopterin The coenzyme for a number of enzymes, including phenylalanine, tyrosine, and tryptophan hydroxylases. Not a dietary requirement, since it can readily be synthesized in the body. Rare patients with a variant form of phenylketonuria cannot synthesize biopterin, and have to receive supplements.

Bios A name given to a factor in cell-free extract of yeast which was essential for the growth of yeast, by Wildiers in 1901. Three components were subsequently identified: inositol, ί-alanine and biotin. Of these, only biotin is a vitamin and essential for human beings.

Biotechnology The simplest definition of biotechnology is "applied biology." The application of biological knowledge and techniques to develop products. It may be further defined as the use of living organisms to make a product or run a process. By this definition, the classic techniques used for plant and animal breeding, fermentation and enzyme purification would be considered biotechnology. Some people use the term only to refer to newer tools of genetic science. In this context, biotechnology may be defined as the use of biotechnical methods to modify the genetic materials of living cells so they will produce new substances or perform new functions. Examples include recombinant DNA technology, in which a copy of a piece of DNA containing one or a few genes is transferred between organisms or "recombined" within an organism.

Biotin A vitamin, sometimes known as vitamin H, required for the synthesis of fatty acids and glucose, among other reactions. Biotin is widely distributed in foods such as liver, kidney, egg yolk, yeast, vegetables, grains, and nuts; dietary deficiency is unknown. There is no evidence on which to base reference intakes other than to state that current average intakes (between 15-70 μg/day) are obviously more than adequate to prevent deficiency.

The protein, avidin, in raw egg-white binds biotin strongly, preventing its absorption, and individuals who consume abnormally large amounts of uncooked egg (several dozen eggs per week) have been reported to show biotin deficiency. Avidin is denatured on cooking, and does not combine with biotin; indeed cooked egg is a rich source of available biotin.

Biovailability The degree of utilization of specifc nutients contained in foods, using as a reference the total content 100% - of the nutritive factor being considered.

Birch beer A non-alcoholic carbonated beverage flavoured with oil of wintergreen or oils of sweet birch and sassafras.

Bird's nest pudding A pudding containing apples whose cores have been replaced by sugar. The apples are nestled in a bowl created by the crust. Also called Crow's Nest Pudding.

Bird's nest soup A classic Chinese soup, called yin waw, is made using the nests of the swiftlet (a sea swallow), a tiny bird found throughout Southeast Asia and especially high in the caves of Thailand's southern islands. These small birds live on high cliffs in the isolated islands of Indonesia and in parts of Western China bird. Instead of twigs and straw, it makes its nest from strands of gummy saliva, which harden when exposed to air. When dried, these nests are translucent and grayish in colour and have the texture of soft plastic. They are about the size and shape of a human ear. Once the nests are harvested, they are cleaned and sold to restaurants, where they are served simmered in chicken broth. Both the Indonesian and the Chinese governments have limited harvesting of swallow's nests to twice a year, because of the fear of causing extinction to these cliff swallows.

This is when the swallows have left their nest and migrated elsewhere (before the eggs are laid and after the swallows have left their nests). The soup has the reputation of being an aphrodisiac. The soup is popular because it is believed to help growth, skin complexion and sex drive, prevent lung disease and stave off aging. All through the ages in China, swallow's nest soup is fed to very old people and to sick people that could not eat anything in order to sustain themselves. It is also quite costly (a bowl of bird's nest soup at a good Hong Kong restaurant can go for as much as $60), many western restaurants serve a less expensive version consisting of soup with noodles shaped to resemble a bird's nest. Chinese began eating the nests of edible-nest swiftlets in soup or in jelly mixed with spices or sweets about 1,500 years ago. It was during times of famine that the imaginative Chinese discovered that not only were sharks' fins and car's tongues edible, but that swallows' nests were as well. According to legends, Empress Dowager of the Qing Dynasty was able to keep her youthful looks because of her daily intake of swallow nests.

Biriani Indian; highly spiced rice dish flavoured with saffron and layered with meat. See also pilau.

Biscotti In Italian, biscotti means, "twice cooked." The word biscotto is derived from bis (twice) and cotto (cooked). Biscotti is also the generic term for cookies in Italian. The dough is formed into logs and baked until golden brown. The logs are then sliced, and the individual biscotti are baked again to give them their characteristic dryness. The shelf life of biscotti are three to four months without preservatives or additives. Other countries have their version of this cookie - Dutch rusk, French biscotte, and the German zwieback. Early Seaman's biscuits, also known as hard tack, probably were the first version of biscotti. They were the perfect food for sailors who were at sea for months at a time on long ocean voyages. The biscuits were thoroughly baked to draw out the moisture, becoming a cracker-like food that that was resistant to mold. Biscotti were a favourite of Christopher Columbus who relied on them on his long sea voyage in the 15th century. Historians believe that the first Italian biscotti were first baked in 13th century Tuscany in the in a city called Prato.

Biscuit A baked flour confectionery dried down to low moisture content. The name is derived from the Latin bis coctus, meaning cooked twice. A 100-g portion provides 400-500 kcal. Known as cookie in the USA, where 'biscuit' means a small cake-like bun.

Five chocolate fingers (30 g) provide 0.6 g of dietary fibre and 8 g of fat of which 60% is saturated; supplies 160 kcal. Four cream crackers (30 g) provide 1.2 g of dietary fibre and 5 g of fat; supplies 135 kcal (570 kJ). Two plain digestive biscuits (30 g) provide 1.5 g of dietary fibre and are a source of copper; provide 6 g of fat of which 45% is saturated; supply 145 kcal. Four semi-sweet biscuits (30 g) provide I g of dietary fibre and 5 g of fat of-which 50% is saturated; supply 140 kcal. One piece of shortbread (30 g) provides 1 g of dietary fibre and 8 g of fat of which two-thirds is saturated; supplies 155 kcal. Four filled wafer biscuits (30 g) provide 0.6 g of dietary fibre and 9 g of fat of which 40% is saturated; supplies 165 kcal (695 kJ). Four water biscuits (30 g) provide 1 g of dietary fibre and 4 g of fat of which 20% is saturated; supplies 140 kcal.

Biscuit check The development of splitting and cracking in biscuits immediately after baking.

Biscuit In England, it is the equivalent of U.S. cookies (small, sweet cakes). In the U.S., a type of non-yeast bread made of flour, milk, and shortening, usually served with breakfast - small, and similar to what much of the world refers to as "scones."

Bishop A medieval beverage of hot spiced and sweetened wine (commonly port).

Biskoids Trade name for saccharin.

Bismarck herring Pickled and spiced whole herring.

Bisque A bisque is a thick, rich, creamy sauce in the form of a puree. Bisque in French means a "shellfish soup." The word is a corruption of "biscuit," as the soup was cooked twice to thicken it. Bisques in the 18th century were made of poultry and game, not with shellfish as they usually are today.

Bistro 1. In France, a bistro used to be a bar that also sold wine. Sometimes, they would have one or two tables and the wife of the owner would have made a dish she would sell. Today a bistro is a small neighborhood restaurant with a comforting, predictable menu and reliable daily specials. It functions as a home away from home for many people, drawn by the familiar atmosphere, honest food and consistent prices.

2. Bistro also means a style of cooing (simple home cooking - it's similar to old-fashioned American food). It's a return to the era before fast food, before speed and convenience became more important than flavor and quality, but not quite to the complexity of old school French cooking.

Bitki Polish, Russian; meatballs made from raw minced beef with fried onions, grilled or fried.

Bitot's spots Irregularly shaped foam-like plaques on the conjunctiva of the eye, characteristically seen in vitamin A deficiency, but not considered to be a diagnostic sign without other evidence of deficiency.

Bitter Traditional British beer with a bitter flavour due to its content of hops.

Bitterballen Dutch; fried meatballs flavoured with Worcestershire sauce and nutmeg.

Bitterness One of the five senses of taste.

Bitters Extracts of herbs, spices, roots, and bark, steeped in, or distilled with, spirits. Originally prepared for medicinal use (tinctures or alcoholic extracts of the natural products); now used mainly to flavour spirits and cocktails, or as aperitifs. See also Angostura; wine, aperitif.

Biuret test A chemical test for proteins (actually for the presence of peptide bonds) which depends on the formation of a violet colour when copper sulphate reacts with a peptide bond in alkaline solution.

Bixin A carotenoid pigment found in the seeds of the tropical plant Bixa orellana; the crude extract is the colouring agent annatto (E-160).

Blachan A pungent, dark-brown dried shrimp paste. It's an essential ingredient in South-east Asian cooking, particularly Thailand, and is used in very small amounts in soups and curries. It's sold in tins or jars, or as hard slabs or cakes. Available in Asian shops and markets.

Black bream The black bream is a dark grey sea fish with tough scales that need to be removed before cooking. It isn't a hugely popular fish so is relatively inexpensive, but it has sweet firm flesh and is delicious eaten whole after being stuffed and baked, or as fillets.

Black butter This is a classic accompaniment to fish, particularly skate and plaice. It is made by browning butter in a pan and adding lemon juice and parsley. In French it is known as 'beurre noir'.

Black cumin Seeds of Nigella sativa, used as a spice; unrelated to cumin.

Black forest gateau Chocolate sponge with whipped cream and cherries, decorated with chocolate curlicues.

Black forest mushroom Or shiitake, Lentinula (Lentinus) edodes, see mushrooms.

Black fungus Or wood-ears, edible wild fungus, Auricularia polytricha.

Black pepper Black pepper comes from a climbing vine, the fruits of which - small round berries - ripen from green to red and finally to brown. Black peppercorns are actually berries that are picked when they're just turning red. They're then dried whole before being sold. Peppercorns can be green, white or black, depending on when they're harvested. Pink 'peppercorns', however, aren't true pepper.

Peppercorns can be used whole, or crushed or ground to add heat and flavour to cooking. Used whole, they can be added loose to stews and soups or used as part of a bouquet garni. You'll often find whole peppercorns spicing up salamis or sausages.

Freshly ground peppercorns have much more flavour than ready-ground pepper, so buy fresh whole peppercorns and invest in a pepper grinder. Freshly ground or crushed black pepper adds a flavour of its own to dishes, as well as enhancing the taste of other ingredients. Lightly crushed or cracked peppercorns can be used to spice up creamy sauces or to coat fillet steaks or chicken breasts.

The light crushing releases the fragrant spiciness; using ground pepper in this way would just release too much heat. Try grinding fresh black pepper over a bowl of strawberries and see how it enhances the flavour of the fruit, releasing a very subtle pepper flavour.

Black PN A black food colour (E-151), also known as brilliant black BN.

Black pudding Called "Marag" (Blood Pudding) in Gaelic (it also means a fat, shapeless person!), this is one of the famous blood dishes that Scottish people love. It usually accompanies other fried dishes, such as bacon and eggs. While it might seem shocking to eat blood, don't forget that all meat dishes contain blood and it's the basis, with fat, of gravy. Blood dishes are popular all over Europe, especially in Transylvania.

Black tongue disease A sign of niacin deficiency in dogs, the canine equivalent of pellagra, historically important in the isolation of the vitamin.

Black velvet Mixture of equal parts of sparkling wine and stout (traditionally Guinness stout).

Blackberry Berry of the bramble, Rubus fruticosus. A 100-g portion is a good source of vitamin C (a source when stewed); a source of folate and copper; provides 7.5 g of dietary fibre; supplies 25 kcal (105 kJ).

Blackcurrant Fruit of the bush Ribes nigra, of special interest because of its high vitamin C content (150-230 mg/100g). The British National Fruit Collection has 120 varieties. A 100-g portion is a rich source of vitamin C; a source of iron and copper; provides 9 g of dietary fibre; supplies 35 kcal (145 kJ).

Blackened A cooking technique where meat or fish is usually seasoned with a Cajun spice mixture and then cooked in a cast-iron skillet that has been heated almost red-hot. This technique gives the food an extra crispy crust and sears in the juices. It is also guaranteed to set off your smoke detector—unless the battery is dead!

Blackened Redfish A dish made by searing seasoned redfish fillets in a smoking hot skillet (usually a cast-iron skillet). This cooking technique and popular fish dish was introduced by Louisiana chef Paul Prudhomme, causing a worldwide culinary phenomenon in the early to mid-1980s. As the dish's fame grew in the late 1980s, stiff limits had to be placed on redfish catches to prevent the disappearance of the species from Gulf Coast waters. Chef Paul Prudhomme's non-traditional "blackened redfish" dish sparked a worldwide Cajun food craze which inspired creative chefs to start "blackening" everything from chicken to veal in order to continue to cash in on the craze.

Blanc de blancs White wine made from white grapes. By contrast, blanc de noirs is white wine made from black grapes; but the skin is removed before fermentation begins.

Blanch The process of plunging food, frequently vegetables, into and out of boiling water for just a few seconds or minutes. Blanching preserves the colour and texture of food, and can be used to get rid of strong flavours (such as older garlic cloves). Blanching can also be used to par-cook food. For example, potatoes can be blanched before roasting or sautiing. The process can also help to loosen the skins of nuts, tomatoes or other fruits before skinning them.

Blanch, blanching 1. To briefly plunge food into boiling water and then into cold water to stop cooking.

2. Blanching allows you to cook vegetables completely, then cool them quickly for use in dishes like salad, soup, stew, and pasta. Blanching is used to loosen skins of fruits and vegetables or to prepare them for more cooking by another method.

3. To scald shelled nuts until the thin outer skins are sufficiently loosened to remove easily.

Blanching A partial precooking by plunging the food into hot water (82-95°C) for 1/2-5 min. Fruits and vegetables are blanched before canning, dehydrating, or freezing, to soften the texture, shrink the food or remove air, destroy enzymes that may cause spoilage when frozen, and remove undesirable flavours. Blanching is also performed to remove excess salt from preserved meat, and to aid the removal of skin, e.g. from almonds and tomatoes. There can be a loss of 10-20% of the sugars, salts, and protein, as well as some of the vitamins B 1, B 2 and niacin, and up to one third of the vitamin C.

Blancmange powder Usually a cornflour base with added flavour and colour, mixed with hot milk to make a dessert.

Bland diet A diet that is non-irritating, does not over-stimulate the digestive tract and is soothing to the intestines; generally avoiding alcohol, strong tea or coffee, pickles, spices, and high intake of dietary fibre.

Blanquette A stew of white meat (veal, lamb or poultry) cooked in white stock or water with aromatic flavourings. The cooking liquor is thickened to make a sauce after the meat is cooked and finished with egg yolks and cream. Blanquettes are also made with fish and vegetables.

Blawn fish Scottish (Orkney); fresh fish, rubbed with salt and hung in a windy passage for a day, then grilled.

Bleach figure A measure of the extent of bleaching of the flour from the relative paleness of the extracted (yellow) pigments.

Bleaching The removal or destruction of colour. In the context of food it usually refers to the bleaching of flour. It also refers to the bleaching of oils, a stage in the purification by which dispersed impurities and natural colouring materials are removed by activated or fuller's earth. See also ageing.

Bleeding bread A bacterial infection with Bacillus prodigiosus, which stains the bread bright red. Under warm and damp conditions the infection can appear overnight, and contamination of the shewbread in churches has led to accusations and riots against religious minorities over the centuries.

Blend To mix ingredients together thoroughly (either by hand or mixer).

Bleu cheese Also called fromage bleu. It is the French name for a group of Roquefort-type (blue-veined) cheeses made in the Roquefort area in southeastern France. Roquefort-type cheeses made in the United States are called blue cheese.

Bleu D'Ambert The name comes from the mold or form traditionally used to shape the cheese in its tall, cylindrical shape. Originally, the cow's milk used for this ancient cheese came from the pastures around the town of Ambert in the heart of France. Fourme was made long before the English Stilton that it resembles visually and in terms of recipe and flavor, but is not as crumbly as Stilton. This liberally veined blue cheese has a pronounced but not evenly sharp flavor.

Bleu des Causses This is always unpasteurized. The texture is creamer than Bleu d'Auvergne though the recipe is the same. The difference is in the quality of the milk. They are made in 5 to 5 1/2 pound wheels. It is made by only a few small producers and is quite rare.

Blind experiment In a single blind experiment, the subjects do not know whether they are receiving an experimental treatment or a placebo. In a double blind experiment, neither the researchers nor the participants are aware of which subjects receive the treatment until after the study is completed.

Blind baking A method of preparing a pastry case before adding the filling, in order to prevent the bottom becoming soggy and undercooked. The pastry is first baked with a lining weighted with beans. You can use dried beans (haricot beans are good) or you can buy ceramic or glass baking beans from good cook shops specifically made for the purpose. Crumpled up tin foil also does the job if you haven't got any beans in your cupboard.

Blind staggers Acute vitamin B 1 deficiency in horses and other animals, caused by eating bracken, which contains thiaminase, which destroys the vitamin.

Blinding A process in a clinical study that conceals a treatment from the patient.

Blini They are Russian pancakes made with yeast and buckwheat flour, and have been made in Russia for hundreds of years. They are used in place of puff pastry for canapıs to serve caviar, smoked salmon, and a number of other savory foods.

Blinis Russian; small yeast pancakes made from buckwheat flour, served with salt herring, smoked salmon, or caviar, and sour cream.

Blintz This is the Yiddish word, derived from blini for a small pan-fried battercake that is rolled with meat, potato, cheese, or fruit filling.

Blintzes Middle European (and especially Jewish); pancakes, stuffed with either curd cheese (and then served with soured cream) or minced meat.

Blood The familiar red fluid in the body that contains white and red blood cells, platelets, proteins, and other elements. The blood is transported throughout the body by the circulatory system. Blood functions in two directions arterial and venous. Arterial blood is the means by which oxygen and nutrients are transported to tissues while venous blood is the means by which carbon dioxide and metabolic by-products are transported to the lungs and kidneys, respectively, for removal from the body.

Blood cells Three main types of cell are present in blood: erythrocytes or red cells, leucocytes or white cells, and platelets. Red blood cells carry the red colouring matter of the blood, the protein haemoglobin, which is responsible for the transport of oxygen from the lungs to tissues, and of carbon dioxide from tissues to the lungs. White blood cells are generally concerned with protection against invading microorganisms, and platelets with the ability of the blood to coagulate, and so prevent excessive blood loss through bleeding. Platelets are also involved in the inappropriate formation of blood clots in the blood vessels, thrombosis.

Blood clotting The process by which the soluble protein fibrinogen in blood plasma is converted to insoluble fibrin, thus preventing blood loss through cuts, etc. Vitamin K is required and deficiency is characterized by excessive bleeding.

Thrombosis is the inappropriate formation of blood clots in the blood vessels, and can be a cause of serious illness and death when blood vessels are blocked. Antagonists of vitamin K, including Warfarin, are commonly used to reduce the ability of blood to clot in patients at risk of thrombosis.

Blood orange The blood orange generally is sweeter than its orange cousins, with a slight raspberry aftertaste. It can be enjoyed as any other orange, for its juice, or in fruit salads, or as a garnish for desserts, but its high price dictates that it should be reserved for special occasions. The blood orange is generally about the same size as a Florida juice orange (about the size of a tennis ball), though it has none of the green streaks common to juice oranges. Blood oranges are generally seedless, or close to it, and may outwardly range from bright orange to orange with red areas.

Blood plasma The liquid component of blood, accounting for about half the total volume of the blood, Plasma is a solution of nutrients and various proteins, mainly albumin and various globulins, including the immunoglobulins which are responsible for much of the body's defence against infection, as well as some adverse reactions to foods. When blood has clotted (see blood clotting), the resultant fluid is known as serum. See also lipids, plasma.

Blood pressure 1. The blood pressure is the pressure of the blood within the arteries. It is produced primarily by the contraction of the heart muscle. It's measurement is recorded by two numbers. The first (systolic pressure) is measured after the heart contracts and is highest. The second (diastolic pressure) is measured before the heart contracts and lowest. A blood pressure cuff is used to measure the pressure. Elevation of blood pressure is called "hypertension."

2. The force of the blood on the walls of arteries. Two levels of blood pressure are measured-the higher, or systolic, pressure, which occurs each time the heart pushes blood into the vessels, and the lower, or diastolic, pressure, which occurs when the heart rests. In a blood pressure reading of 120/80, for example, 120 is the systolic pressure and 80 is the diastolic pressure. A reading of 120/80 is said to be the normal range. Blood pressure that is too high can cause health problems such as heart attacks and strokes.

3. The pressure exerted by the circulating blood on the walls of arteries and veins and in the heart

chambers. When the heart contracts, the maximum pressure exerted is the systolic pressure; during relaxation, the minimum pressure is the diastolic.

Blood sugar Glucose; normal concentration is about 5 mmol (90 mg)/L, and is maintained in the fasting state by mobilization of tissue reserves of glycogen and synthesis from amino acids. Only in prolonged starvation does it fall below about 3.5 mmol (60 mg)/L. If it falls to 2 mmol (35 mg)/L there is loss of consciousness (hypoglycaemic coma). See also hypoglycaemia.

After a meal the concentration of glucose rises, but this rise is limited by the hormone insulin, which is secreted by the pancreas to stimulate the uptake of glucose into tissues. Diabetes mellitus is the result of failure of the insulin mechanism.

Blood volume The average blood volume is 5.3 L (78 mL/kg body weight, 9 pints) in males and 3.8 L (56 mL/kg body weight, 6.5 pints) in females.

Bloom Fat bloom is the whitish appearance on the surface of chocolate which sometimes occurs in storage. It is due either to a change in the form of the fat at the surface or to fat diffusing outwards and being deposited as crystals on the surface. Sugar bloom is due to the deposition of sugar crystals on the surface, but is less common than fat bloom.

Bloom gelometer An instrument for measuring the strength of jellies, and also for any test of firmness, e.g. the staleness of bread.

Blue cheese Blue, blue-mold, or blue-veined cheese is the name for cheese of the Roquefort type that is made in the United States and Canada. It was not until about 1918 that attempt to make Roquefort-type cheese in the United States met with success. See bleu cheese.

Blueberry The blueberry of the genus "Vaccinium," is a Native American species. One of only three berries native to North America; Wild Blueberries were well known to the earliest inhabitants. To settle the question about blueberries and huckleberries being the same berry, they are not. Huckleberries have ten large hard bony seeds, which do not disappear when the berries are baked, boiled, or eaten fresh. Wild blueberries have many tiny seeds that are so soft they literally melt in your mouth. Low bush blueberries (often referred to as "wild blueberries") were the first to be cultivated commercially (the first attempts were made by the Indians who practiced burning as a pruning technique). When the explorers and settlers arrived on the North American Continent, they found the native Indians using berries as an integral part.

Bluefin tuna Regarded as the highest grade tuna, bluefin tuna is used in top-class restaurants for sashimi and sushi. However, the southern bluefin tuna is endangered, so be very choosy about what exactly you're buying.

Blush wine Californian term for rose wines.

BMI (Body Mass Index) A number that shows body weight adjusted for height that can be calculated with simple math using inches and pounds. For adults, BMI falls into one of these categories: underweight, normal, overweight and obese. For children and teens, BMI is used to assess underweight, risk for overweight and overweight. In addition, BMI for children and teens takes into account age and gender.

Boar, wild Meat of Sus scrofa. Hunted in parts of Europe, farmed on small scale in UK. A 150-g portion is a rich source of protein; contains 4.5 g of fat of which one third is saturated; and supplies 160 kcal (670 kJ).

Bocadillo Spanish; a sandwich made by slicing a long crusty loaf or roll lengthways.

Bocal French; wide-mouthed glass jar used for bottling or pickling fruit and vegetables.

Bocconcini 1. Bocconcini means "a mouthful" and refers to small nuggets (about 1-inch in diameter) of fresh mozzarella. They are usually sold packed in whey or water.

2. It can also describe tempting Italian dishes.

Body surface area Heat loss from the body is related to surface area and basal metabolic rate and energy expenditure are sometimes expressed per unit body surface area. It is commonly calculated according to the formulae of: Du Bois: area (cm2) = 71.84 x weight0.425(kg) x height0.725(cm) Meeh: area (cm2) = 11.9 x weight?kg).

The surface area of adults is about 18,000 cm2 (men) or 16,000 cm2 (women).

Body-building food A term used indiscriminately, but generally referring to proteins. The Code of Practice in advertising suggests that no claim should be made for the body-building properties of a food unless a reasonable (unspecified) amount of protein is present in a normal portion.

Bog butter Norsemen, Finns, Scots and Irish used to bury firkins of butter in bogs to ripen and develop a strong flavour.

Bog myrtle A wild plant (Myrica gale) with a strong resinous flavour. The leaves and seeds are used to flavour soups and stews.

Boil To cook submerged in a boiling liquid.

Boiled peanuts These are green or raw peanuts that are boiled in salty water for hours over open flames. Green peanuts must be obtained at just the right time to ensure their high quality. One of the drawbacks of boiled peanuts is that they are a low-acid food and highly perishable. Because of this, they have a very short shelf life unless refrigerated or frozen. Boiled peanuts are considered a traditional southern snack in the states of South Carolina, Georgia, northern Florida, Alabama, and Mississippi. They are an acquired taste, but according to Southerners, they are totally addictive. In the months of May through November, you will see roadside stands that can range from woodsheds to shiny trailers offering fresh boiled peanuts. A traditional way that old-timers like to eat boiled peanuts is to drop the shelled peanuts into a bottle of cold RC Cola and gulp the combo down. The origin of who first boiled peanuts remains a mystery. It is known that boiled peanuts have been a southern institution since the Civil War (1861-1865) when General Sherman led his troops through Georgia. When troops of the Southern Confederacy were almost with food, peanuts suddenly became very important. Soldiers roasted the peanuts in a campfire and boiled them.

Boiled sweets Sugar and water boiled at such a high temperature (150-166°C) that practically no water remains and a vitreous mass is formed on cooling.

Boiler Danish, Norwegian; dumplings.

Boiling point The temperature at which the saturated vapour pressure of a liquid equals the external atmospheric pressure. As a consequence, bubbles form in the liquid and the temperature remains constant until all the liquid has evaporated. As the boiling point of a liquid depends on the external atmospheric pressure, boiling points are usually quoted for standard atmospheric pressure (760 mmHg = 101 325 Pa).

Bok choi Closely related to the pak choi, this leafy green Chinese vegetable belongs to the cabbage family (although it tastes nothing like cabbage!). It has fleshy, white, slightly ribbed leaf stalks and soft, oval green leaves. The leaves and stems are best suited to brief stir-frying or steaming so they retain their mild flavour. Occasionally you may be able to find baby bok choi, which can be cooked whole.

Bolete, boletus The name of a large group of (mostly edible) fungi, which includes the cep (cepe). Boletes are characterised by the sponge-like texture of the bottom side of the cap. Boletes are found in most parts of the world from Europe to China and Africa. Despite popular belief, not all boletes/boletus are edible, so be very careful if picking wild mushrooms.

Boletus Edible wild mushroom, Boletus edulis or B. granulatus, also known as the yellow mushroom or cep.

Bollito misto An Italian dish of various kinds of meat - usually chicken, ox tongue and pigs' trotters - boiled in stock. It's served with sauces that vary from region to region, but salsa verde and mostarda di frutta (a whole fruit preserve with hot mustard in sweet syrup) are common accompaniments. Bollito misto is traditionally served on New Year's Eve in northern Italy, with lentils and preserved, candied fruit. The meat represents good health, the lentils wealth and the fruit good spirits.

Bologna Italian smoked pork and veal sausage, also known as polony.

Bolognese sauce Ragω Bolognese, often known simply as ragω, is the all-purpose thick Italian sauce made from minced beef and tomatoes. It can form the basis of lasagne or be served with spaghetti. Slow cooking is the key, until the sauce has reduced to a thick, mahogany richness.

Bombay duck Also called bummalo, this isn't a duck at all, but a small dried fish from India and Bangladesh. The fish are landed, then hung on racks on the beach to dry in the sun. In cooking, Bombay duck is usually heated in the oven or fried until it is crisp enough to be crumbled over stews and curries. It was once banned by the EU, but can now be imported to the UK; you can find it in tins or packets in Asian supermarkets.

Bombe Bombe is French for a "bomb" which was used in a cannon. In France, they had at one time, a spherical mold for food shaped like a round bomb. Originally it was made of copper and had a tight lid so that it could be buried with its contents in salted ice to keep the contents frozen. It is a dessert made with two different ice cream mixtures. The first is a simple plain ice cream, which is used to line a mold. The second is a more elaborate ice cream mixture (usually with a strong flavoring), which, is used as a filling. The bombe is usually decorated when it is complete with crystallized fruit. It is then frozen and served cold as a dessert.

Bon Appeti Seasoning Salt Bon Appetit Seasoning is a spice, put out by McCormick Company. Bon Appetite is a very mild blend of Celery, Onion, Salt, and MSG. Its light colour makes it ideal for chicken, fish, white sauces and vegetables, tossed salads and baked potatoes. Check out the web page on Bon Appetit Seasoning.

Bon appetit A French phrase that literally means "good appetite" or "enjoy your meal."

Bondon French (Normandy); soft cheese shaped in the form of a bun.

Bone Bones consist of an organic matrix composed of collagen and other proteins and crystalline mineral, mainly hydroxyapatite (calcium phosphate and calcium hydroxide), together with magnesium phosphate, fluorides, and sulphates. See also calcium.

Bone broth Prepared by prolonged boiling of bones to break down the collagen and extract it as gelatine. Of little nutritive value, since it consists of 2-4% gelatine, with little calcium. See also stock.

Bone charcoal Charcoal produced by heating pieces of bone sufficiently to burn off the organic matter, leaving the carbon deposited on a framework of calcium carbonate. It is used to purify solutions because it will absorb colouring matter and other impurities. Also known as animal charcoal.

Bone-meal Prepared from degreased bones and used as a supplement in both animal and human foods as a source of calcium and phosphate. Also used as a plant fertilizer as a slowly released source of phosphate.

Bonito Large fish from the same family as tuna and mackerel. Bonito is an oily fish and is prepared in the same way as tuna. It's labelled as skipjack tuna when tinned.

Bonk depletion of glycogen and blood sugar while exercising. Symptoms include a dramatic reduction in performance and feeling disoriented and weak.

Bonne femme Cooked in a simple or 'housewifely' style, with a garnish of fresh vegetables or herbs, usually including mushrooms. Applied especially to fish dishes and cream soups.

Bontrae Trade name for textured vegetable protein prepared by spinning or extrusion.

Boonchi Caribbean name for yard-long beans or asparagus beans, Vigna sesquipedalis.

Boquerones Spanish; fresh anchovies, floured and joined together by making a small incision at the tail of one and slipping the tails of 3 or 4 others through. Fried in the shape of a fan.

Borborygmi Audible rumbling abdominal sounds due to gas gurgling with liquid as it passes through the intestines.

Bordeaux Red and white wines produced in the Bordeaux region of France; red Bordeaux wines are called claret in the UK.

Boric acid Chemically H_3BO_4, derived from the element boron, boric acid has been used in the past as a preservative in bacon and margarine, but boron accumulates in the body. It was formerly used as an anti-infective agent and eyewash (boracic acid) but there was a high incidence of toxic reactions.

Borlotti beans A variety of kidney bean, this is a large, plump bean, pinkish brown in colour with reddish brown streaks, widely used in Italian cooking. You can buy borlotti beans dried or tinned - cannellini beans make a good replacement if you can't find them. They have a sweetish flavour with a smooth creamy texture. Good for using in salads and casseroles. The dried variety needs to be soaked in cold water before cooking.

Boron An element, known to be essential for plant growth, but not known to have any function in human beings or animals. Suggested to modify the actions and metabolism of oestrogens, and sometimes used in preparations to alleviate the pre-menstrual syndrome, although there is little evidence of efficacy; toxic in excess. Occurs mainly as salts of boric acid.

Borsch or borscht Eastern European soup usually made with beetroot and served with a good dollop of soured cream and, sometimes, dumplings.

Borscht Also known as borsch and borsch. A beef soup that originated in Ukraine and is considered their national soup. This delicious soup is served in many variations with up to 25 different ingredients, which usually contain either beef, cabbage, or chicken with dumplings stuffed with meat, mushrooms, or vegetables. The best known of these soups is a cold version based on beets and served with sour cream, but hot versions are also very common. Ukrainian cuisine stems from peasant dishes based on grains and staple vegetables like potatoes, cabbage, beets and mushrooms. Meat is typically boiled, fried or stewed. This soup was so popular with the American Jewish people in the 1930s to 1950s, that the popular resorts in the Catskill Mountains of upper New York State became know as the "Borscht Belt," due to their largely Jewish clientele.

Boston baked beans Beans baked slowly over a long period of time. When the first colonist arrived, the local Indians were cultivating several types of beans that they baked in small holes in the ground lined with stones. The colonist called the holes "ban holes." This was the first way of baking beans and every colonial family had a bean hole until fireplaces with brick ovens were built in their homes. The Pilgrims baked their beans on Saturday because of the religious mandate that dictated Sunday as a day of rest. The beans were baked overnight in brick ovens.

Boston Cream Pie It is really a cake, not a pie. Two layers of sponge cake are filled with thick vanilla custard and topped with a chocolate glaze or a sprinkling of confectioners' sugar. It is cut in wedges like a pie. The Boston Cream Pie was proclaimed the official Massachusetts State Dessert on December 12, 1996. A civics class from Norton High School sponsored the bill.

Botargo A relish or dip prepared from fish roe (usually mullet or tuna); see also taramasalata.

Boti kabab Indian; small pieces of meat, marinated and cooked rapidly under intense heat, basted with butter or ghee.

Bottarga Also known as bottarga di muggine. It is salted Mediterranean salted tuna or mullet roe. Bottarga is made with gray mullet in Sardinia and tuna in Sicily. The term Bottarga, from the Arabic bot-ah-rik, means "raw fish eggs." This delicacy is a specialty of the islands of Sardinia and Sicily. The mullet's eggs, after being extracted, in their protective sacs, are washed and purified, put under salt, rinsed and laid to dry. The aging process takes four to five months. The dried eggs are then pressed and vacuum packed. The colour of the roe goes from yellow-gold to dark amber; the change of colour does not affect the quality or taste. The Sardinians serve it simply, with spaghetti, extra-virgin olive oil, and chopped garlic, parsley, and red pepper flakes. The bottarga was once the fishermen food but nowadays it is served in restaurants as delicious hors' d'ouvre.

Bottle The traditional wine bottle holds 700, 720, or 750 mL of wine, depending on the variety; within the EU wine bottles are being standardized at 700 mL.

A two-bottle size is a magnum; four-bottle is a Jeroboam or double magnum, six is a Methuselah, twelve a Salmanzar, and twenty is a Nebuchadnezzar.

Bottle house An old English term for a manufacturer of glass containers (bottles and jars) as distinct from tableware.

Botulinum cook The degree of heat required to ensure destruction of (virtually) all spores of Clostridium botulinum, the causative organism of botulism, which are the most resistant of bacterial spores.

Botulinum toxin A toxin produced by the bacterium Clostridium botulinum, which can cause fatal food poisoning. It is the most toxic substance known to man.

Botulism A rare and serious form of food poisoning from foods containing the toxin produced by the bacterium Clostridium botulinum . The toxin can affect the cardiac and respiratory centres of the brain and may result in death by heart or lung failure. The bacterium thrives in improperly preserved foods, such as tinned raw meats. The toxin is invariably destroyed in cooking.

Boucanning A Caribbean process by which meat was preserved by sun-drying and smoking while resting on a wooden grid known as a boucan.

Bouchees Puff pastry shells, used for holding fillings and stuffings. Large bouchees are called voul au vents in France, and patty shells in the United States.

Boudin blanc 1. Also called white boudin, it is a wonderful Cajun sausage stuffed with pork and rice. It's one of those food products that originated in frugality; the rice was meant to stretch the meat. Now, it's a unique and delicious treat all its own.

2. This term in French means, "white pudding." It is a delicate sausage made with pork, chicken, fat, eggs, cream, breadcrumbs, and seasonings.

Bouillabaisse The name probably derives from the French phrase bouillepeis, meaning "bubble of fish." Although called a soup, this is really a main dish or a stew, a full meal in itself. Bouillabaisse has many regional variations based on the different local fish. The favourite place for bouillabaisse in Marseilles, France is the cabanon, a modest shed erected along the seashore by local people who used it for fishing, and gatherings with family and close friends.

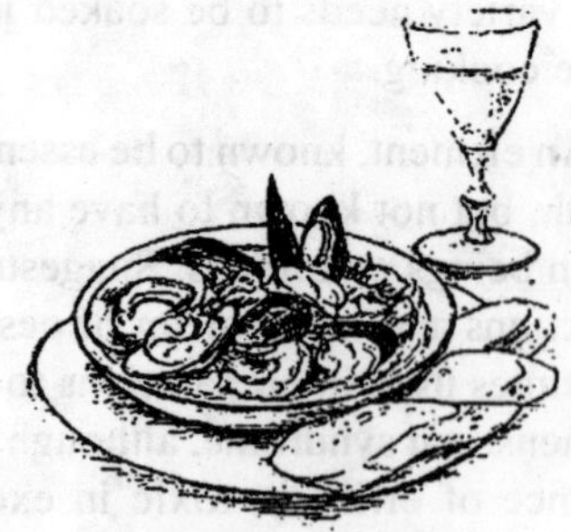

Fig. Bouillabaisse

Bouillabaisse is a soup that came from the Provence region of France in and around Marseilles, the seafood capital of Provence, France. The soup was based on local fish, usually those unsold at the daily market, with other local shellfish added. It was a "fisherman's" dish, and never contained any expensive ingredients such as lobster.

Bouillon It is the French word for broth. It is a clear soup made from cooking meat, vegetables, poultry, or fish in water. The liquid that is strained after cooking is the bouillon, which can form the base for soups and sauces. The Duke of Godefry, who was born in 1061 and died in the year of 1100, in his castle at Bouillon, Belgium, invented this clear, delicious soup, which is now called bouillon. He became the first European King of Jerusalem.

Bouquet garni It is generally a triad of herbs. The literal translation from the French is "nosegay trimmings." It is a small bunch of herbs, which traditionally consist of a bay leaf, sprig of thyme, and a sprig of parsley. When fresh herbs are used, the three herb sprigs can be tied together with kitchen twine and tossed into the sauce "as is". When the cooking is done, the bouquet is removed and discarded. If the herbs are dried, they can be crushed and added directly to the pot in roughly equal proportions. In Britain it is sometimes called an herbal faggot.

Bourbon American whiskey made by distilling fermented maize mash. Sour mash bourbon is made from mash that has yeast left in it from a previous fermentation.

Bournvita Trade name for a preparation of malt, milk, sugar, cocoa, eggs, and flavouring, to make a beverage when mixed with milk.

Bovine somatotropin (BST) The natural growth hormone of cattle; biosynthetic BST is used in some dairy herds to increase milk production.

Bovine spongiform encephalopathy (BSE) Bovine spongiform encephalopathy, or BSE, is also known as "mad cow disease." It is a rare, chronic degenerative disease affecting the brain and central nervous system of cattle. Cattle with BSE lose their coordination, develop abnormal posture and experience changes in behaviour. Clinical symptoms take 4 5 years to develop, followed by death in a period of several weeks to months unless the affected animal is destroyed sooner.

Bovril Trade name for a preparation of meat extract, hydrolysed beef, beef powder and yeast extract, used as a beverage, a flavouring agent, and for spreading on bread. A 10-g portion is a good source of vitamin B2 and a source of niacin.

Boysenberry Similar to loganberry.

Bozbash Russian; mutton soup.

Bracken Young unopened leaves (fronds) of bracken (Pteridium spp.), eaten as a vegetable and regarded as a delicacy in the Far East. Known as fiddleheads in Canada. They contain an antagonist of vitamin B1; cattle and horses eating large amounts suffer from blind staggers due to acute vitamin B 1 deficiency; also contain a number of known or suspected carcinogens.

Bradycardia An unusually slow heartbeat, less than 60 beats/min. Such a low rate may be normal in trained athletes.

Bradyphagia Eating very slowly.

Brain Traditionally the brains of sheep and calves are stewed and eaten; probably not advisable because of the risk of transmitting the agents responsible for various degenerative brain diseases, including scrapie and bovine spongiform encephalopathy (BSE).

Brain-gut axis The continuous bi-directional flow of information and feedback that takes place between the gastrointestinal tract, and the brain and spinal cord (which together comprise the central nervous system).

Braise Braising is basically a slow-cooking method for tough cuts of meat or poultry and even stringy vegetables. They are cooked slowly in a small amount of liquid in a covered pan. Stews and pot roasts are among the dishes prepared this way. Braising may be done in a covered container in the oven, on the range, or in a covered steam kettle or fry pan. In all the moist-heats methods of cooking, the moisture or liquid not only conducts heat to a product, but it interacts with the food being cooked and can influence the final taste and texture of a product.

Bran The outer layers of cereal grain, which are largely removed when the grain is milled (i.e. in the preparation of white flour or white rice). The germ is discarded at the same time, and there is a considerable loss of iron and other minerals, and particularly of the B vitamins, as well as of dietary fibre. A 30-g portion of wheat bran is a rich source of niacin, iron, and zinc; a good source of vitamin B1; a source of vitamin B2; provides 12 g of dietary fibre; supplies 70 kcal (295 kJ). See also flour, extraction rate; wheatfeed.

Brandy A spirit distilled from wine, and containing 37-44% (most usually 40%) alcohol by volume. The name is derived from the German brandtwein, meaning burnt wine, corrupted to brandy wine. Most wine-producing countries also make brandy.

The age of brandy is generally designated as 3-star (3-5 years old before bottling); VSOP (very special old pale, aged 4-10 or more years, the name indicating that it has not been heavily coloured with caramel); Napoleon (premium blend aged 6-20 years); XO, Extraordinary Old (Extra or Grand Reserve, possibly 50 years old). Cognac and Armagnac are brandies made in defined regions of France.

Fruit brandies are either distilled from fruit wines (e.g. plum and apple brandies) or are prepared by soaking fruit in brandy (e.g. cherry and apricot brandies). See also eau de vie; marc.

Brandy butter Hard sauce made from butter, caster sugar, and brandy, traditionally served with Christmas pudding and mince pies.

Brandy sauce English; sauce made from egg yolk, cream, sugar, and brandy, traditionally served with Christmas pudding.

Brandy snaps Crisp toffee-like biscuits made from flour, butter, syrup, and powdered ginger, baked, then rolled into cylinders while still warm and pliable.

Brassica Genus of vegetables that includes broccoli, Brussels sprouts, cabbage, cauliflower, kale, kohl rabi, mustard, and swedes.

Bratwurst German; pork sausage with many regional specialist varieties; may be served boiled, grilled, or fried.

Brawn Made from pig meat, particularly the head, boiled with peppercorns and herbs, minced and pressed into a mould. Mock brawn (head cheese) differs in that other meat by-products are used. A 150-g portion is a rich source of protein; a good source of niacin and iron; contains 18 g of fat; supplies 230 kcal.

Brazil nut A large nut with a very hard shell, cultivated in Brazil and Paraguay. They tend to be expensive because commercial supplies are derived entirely from wild trees. They're tough nuts to crack so buy shelled brazils if you can. The creamy, white kernel is very nutritious with a high fat content. Brazil nuts can be eaten raw or used in cooking. Whole, they're used in confectionery and are good for decorating fruitcakes or larger cakes because of their nice shape and size. Roughly ground, they make good toppings for desserts and add crunch to rice or vegetable dishes. Ground brazil nuts can be stirred into cakes and cheesecake bases.

Bread Bread is the name given to the oldest, commonest, and cheapest form of human food. Bread is made of the flour or meal of one or more kinds of cereals, which can be obtained from some grasses, seeds, and rootstocks other than cereals. Grain cultivation most likely began around 10,000 B.C, and bread was baked on hot stones into loaves of flatbread. Evidence of ovens was found dating back as far as 25,000 B.C. in the Ukraine. Historians think that the first combination of bread ingredients and yeast happened by accident. Probably when an alcoholic drink or fermented honey was accidentally added to flatbread dough. This more likely happened in a brewery in ancient Egypt where archaeologists have found ruins and drawings of bakeries and breweries. The Egyptians had supplies of mead, beer, and primitive wines. By the third century B.C., Romans had created ovens made from dried and hardened mud, and by 200 B.C. there were more than 200 bakeries in Rome. Roman Emperor Trajan (98-117 A.D.) founded the first bakers' school in Rome. Once a man became a baker, he was not allowed to change work. They taught their sons the trade, passing baking secrets down from generation to generation. There are many stories of wars being won or lost and favours being granted by the barter of freshly baked bread. French soldiers demanded white bread to give them courage, and Greek women were said to have tucked a piece of bread into their husbands' clothing as he went off to war. Bakers in local communities celebrated political victories or "saved a country" by introducing a specific shape or type of bread.

Bread sauce Thick white sauce made from bread and milk in which an onion has been boiled; a traditional accompaniment to poultry.

Bread, starch-reduced Bread is normally 9-10% protein and about 50% starch; if the starch is reduced, either by washing some of it out of the dough or by adding extra protein, the bread is referred to as starchreduced, and is often claimed to be of value in slimming and diabetic diets. Legally, the name 'starch-reduced bread' may be applied only to bread containing less than 50% carbohydrate, and any claims for its value as a slimming aid are strictly controlled.

Breadfruit Although it is a fruit, it's light yellow flesh has the starchy consistency of unripe potatoes, which makes it seem more like a vegetable weighing between two to five pounds. As the breadfruit ripens it softens to about the consistency of a mango but without the sweetness. The reason for the name "breadfruit" is that when eaten before it is ripe, breadfruit not only feels like fresh bread, but also tastes like it. Not only are breadfruit trees in the Pacific prized for their fruits but their wood is also highly valuable. In Hawaii, the wood of breadfruit trees was made into fine quality canoes, drums, and surfboards. In Guam and Samoa, the bark was used for making tapa cloth. A starchy staple of the Caribbean and Pacific islands, breadfruit is fried, baked, boiled, and sometimes mixed with coconut milk to make a pudding. It is used like a potato—in stews, whipped, and diced, and in a salad resembling potato salad. Probably native to the Malay Archipelago, breadfruit either drifted on the sea or was carried by early peoples to the Pacific Islands well before written history. The plant has been cultivated there for thousands of years. Breadfruits were traditionally baked with hot stones in pits dug into the ground. The wood of the trees—which grew as high as 60 feet—was also used for canoes, and the bark was made into cloth on Guam and the islands of Samoa. In Hawaii the wood was prized for making drums and surfboards. In the 1700's the British began to establish breadfruit crops in the West Indies, as a staple with which to feed the African slaves who worked the huge sugar plantations. During his voyage to Tahiti in 1769, Captain James Cook was introduced to breadfruit when he brought it back to England. King George III was convinced of the necessity of transporting breadfruit from the Pacific to the Caribbean and in 1787 Captain Bligh and his ship HMS Bounty was sent to Tahiti with the mission of delivering the breadfruit trees to the Caribbean. Records indicate that 347 breadfruit trees arrived on the HMS Providence on the fifth of February 1793, and were distributed throughout the island.

Breakfast cereal Legally defined as any food obtained by the swelling, roasting, grinding, rolling, or flaking of any cereal. Products are described under their individual names.

Breast The breast refers to the front of the chest or, more specifically, to the mammary gland. The mammary gland is a milk producing gland. It is composed largely of fat. Within the mammary gland is a complex network of branching ducts. These ducts exit from sac-like structures called lobules, which can produce milk in females. The ducts exit the breast at the nipple.

Breastfeeding The series of nutritional, behavioural and physiological processes that result in the child's ingestion, either directly at the breast or through artificial extraction, of milk produced by the mother herself.

Breast-milk substitute Any food being marketed or otherwise represented as a partial or total replacement for breast-milk, whether or not suitable for that purpose.

Breathing Of red wine, opening the bottle some time before serving to allow oxidation and development of the full mature flavour.

Bredsoy Trade name for an unheated (i.e. enzyme active) full-fat soya flour.

Bretonne sauce used with eggs and fish, made with onions or leeks and white wine.

Brewers' grains Cereal residue from brewing, containing about 25% protein; used as animal feed.

Brewing The process by which beers, ales, and lagers are made. In the West the basic ingredient of beer is barley, while in Africa millet or maize may be used, and rice beer is made in Japan . In beer-making the barley or other grain is germinated, and the young seedlings are then dried to produce malt. The malt is ground, and placed in a mash tub with water and cereal, where enzymes in the malt convert the starch into fermentable sugars. The resulting liquid, called wort, is transferred to a brewing kettle, where flavourings, particularly hops, are added, and the mixture is boiled. The mixture is then filtered, and fermentation is stimulated by the introduction of yeast. Traditionally, the liquid at this stage is filtered again and placed in wooden barrels, where fermentation continues. Ales and stouts are usually fermented at 15-20°C, while lagers are fermented at 6-8°C for longer periods. In keg beers and lagers, fermentation is stopped after only a short period by placing the liquid in sealed metal barrels and introducing carbon dioxide.

Brie Soft white cheese originally from the Brie region of France, made from cows' milk and moulded into a flat disc; it has a white rind, is ripened for 3-4 weeks, and deteriorates rapidly. A 30-g portion is a rich source of vitamin B 12, a source of protein and vitamin A, contains 8 g of fat of which 70% is saturated, 200 mg sodium, and 160 mg calcium; supplies 100 kcal (400 kJ).

Brie cheese One of the most popular of imported cheeses, brie has been called the "king of all cheeses." This cheese is made from whole, skim, or partially skim cow's milk (the quality varies with the kind of milk used). It is described as creamy, smooth, and very delicate. The natural white rind of the brie cheese is edible; so don't discard it when serving brie as an appetizer. Brie cheese originated in France centuries ago. It is named after La Brie, the province in northern France where it was first made.

Brillat-savarin A French gourmet (1755-1826) whose name is given to a consommı, baba, and several other dishes.

Brine Salt solutions of varying concentrations used in pickling. 'Fresh' brine may have added nitrite; 'live' brine contains micro-organisms that convert nitrate to nitrite (pickling salts).

Brining The process of soaking vegetables in brine before pickling in vinegar, in order to remove some of the water, and retain a crisp texture. Dry brining is when the vegetables are covered with dry salt, rather than immersed in a salt solution.

Brioche A slightly sweet French yeast bread, rich with butter and eggs. The traditional shape has a fluted bottom and a topknot and is made in a special mould. Good as a sweet bread or served with cheese or pβtı. Use it in place of plain bread when making bread and butter pudding. It's also delicious pan-fried in butter and served with a fruit coulis and crome fracche.

Brioli Corsican; chestnut meal, prepared in the same way as polenta.

Brisket A cut of beef taken from just below the shoulder along the length of the chest/breast. It's a fairly firm cut, so it's inexpensive, and benefits from long, slow cooking. Sold on the bone, or boned and rolled, it's often cooked in one piece. Delicious pot-roasted, poached or braised and used in casseroles or stews.

Brislings Young sprats, Clupea sprattus. A 100-g portion is an extremely rich source of vitamin D and a rich source of vitamin A.

Brix A table of specific gravity based on the Balling tables, calculated in grams of cane sugar in 100 g of solution at 20 °C; degree Brix = % sugar. It is used to refer to the concentration of sugar syrups used in canned fruits.

Broad beans Broad beans are also called fava beans, particularly in the US.

Fresh broad beans only have a short natural season during the summer and are often sold frozen or canned. They're sweet and delicious with a smooth creamy texture. Fresh beans are more popular than the dried variety, which tend to be quite floury. Young thin beans are eaten pods and all, but larger, older broad beans need to have the tough pods removed.

After boiling or steaming them (for about five minutes), peel away the thin, pale sheath covering the bean. Dried broad beans don't hold their shape very well, so they're often used to make spreads or puries. They're also good for flavouring meat stews or lamb dishes. Egyptian ful medames is a dish of cooked broad beans (a dried variety called 'ful') flavoured with garlic and lemon.

Broaster, broasted, and broasting Broaster and broasted are registered trademarks of the Broaster Co. in Beloit, Wisc. that has been broasting chickens since 1954. It is a registered process that builds pressure in the pot, which seals in the natural juices while sealing out almost 100% of the cooking oil. It is not only the process of frying chickens under pressure, but includes a special marinating process. The Broasters and the seasonings are sold only to restaurants and the food trade, so Broasted chicken is available to you only when you dine out.

Broasting A cooking method in which the food is deep fried under pressure, which is quicker than without pressure, and the food absorbs less fat.

Broccoli It is a member of the Cruciferae family and is a relative of cabbage, brussels sprouts, and cauliflower. It has tight clusters of tiny buds that sit on stout, edible stems. It's available year-round. The word broccoli comes from the Italian word "brocco" meaning "arm branch." Broccoli has been around for more than 2000 years. During the 16th century, the plant was grown in France and Italy. Little was known about broccoli in the United States until the 1920s, when the first commercially grown broccoli was grown in Brooklyn, New York. In 1923, broccoli was first planted in California.

Broccoli rabe Also known as rapini, broccoli raab, broccoletti di rape, and broccoletto. It is related to the turnip and cabbage families and has very little resemblance to broccoli. It has a thin, leafy, dark green stock with few buds, and has a pungent-bitter flavor. It gives a lift to bland foods and a nice accent to spicy foods. If served alone, blanch in salt water before further cooking to remove some of the bitterness. When choosing broccoli rabe, it should be firm with small stems and few buds. It is best to keep it wrapped and in the vegetable crisper for no more than five days. Broccoli rabe is available all year, but it most plentiful from spring to late fall. It is a great source of vitamins A, C and K, and a good source of potassium and folic acid.

Broccoli, chinese Brassica oleracea var. alboglabra; similar to calabrese and purple sprouting broccoli.

Broccoli, sprouting Member of the cabbage family, Brassica oleracea Italica group with purple and white clusters of flower buds (which turn green when boiled) with smaller heads than calabrese. (Italian broccoli means 'little shoots'.) A 100-g portion, boiled, is a rich source of vitamin C; a source of vitamin A (500 μg carotene); provides 3 g of dietary fibre; supplies 25 kcal.

Broccolini A new hybrid vegetable that is sure to make a statement at your dinner table. Technically a cross between broccoli and Chinese kale, this vegetable looks more like a broccoli-asparagus mix. Broccolini comes in bunches of 17-20 stalks and has a shelf life of 2 weeks in the refrigerator from date of purchase. Broccolini is a great source of Vitamin C, Vitamin A and potassium, and has no fat. It can be cooked and eaten the same as broccoli: blanched, steamed, sautied, poached, roasted, fried or grilled. It is 100% edible, so there's no need to remove any of the stems, making a wonderful presentation on the plate with its long slender stems.

Brochette Brochette is the French name for a skewer, and in cookery refers to cubes of meat or fish and vegetables threaded onto a skewer and then grilled or barbecued. In Turkey it is a 'shish', hence shish kebab. Invest in some metal skewers as the bamboo ones tend to burn (unless you soak them in cold water for at least half an hour before you're ready to cook).

Broil, broiling In this method of cooking, the heat source is above the food. In home cooking, an oven is often used for broiling by setting it so that only the top element comes on. Broiling is a high-heat method of cooking in which food is placed on a rack below, and the speed with which it cooks depends on how far away it is from the element. As with grilling, food has to be watched carefully, so it does not overcook.

Broiling Cooking by direct heat over a flame, as in a barbecue; American term for grilling. Pan broiling is cooking through hot dry metal over direct heat.

Bromatology The science of foods, from the Greek broma, food.

Bromelains Enzymes in the pineapple and related plants of the family Bromelidaceae, which hydrolyse proteins. They are available as by-products from commercial pineapple production, usually from the stems, and are used to tenderize meat, to treat sausage casings, and to .chill-proof beer. Similar enzymes are found in figs (ficin) and pawpaw (papain).

Brominated oils Oils from a variety of sources, including peach and apricot kernels, olive and soya oils which have been reacted with bromine. They are used to help to stabilize emulsions of flavouring substances in soft drinks. Also known as weighting oils.

Bromine An element, chemically related to iodine, chlorine, and fluorine, not known to have any function in the body, and not a dietary essential.

Bronchopulmonary dysplasia (BPD) A chronic lung disorder that is most common among children who were born prematurely, with low birthweights, and who received prolonged mechanical ventilation; nutritional consequences can include feeding difficulties, slow growth and increased energy needs

Brooklime A wild plant (Veronica beccabunga) that grows in very wet marshy conditions. The large, round, fleshy leaves can be added to salads.

Brose A Scottish dish made by pouring boiling water onto oatmeal or barley meal; fish, meat, and vegetables may be added.

Broth Broth is a flavorful liquid resulting from the long simmering of meat, vegetables, poultry or fish. The French call if "bouillon."

Brown adipose tissue Metabolically highly active adipose tissue, which is involved in heat production to maintain body temperature, as opposed to white adipose tissue, which is storage fat and has a relatively low rate of metabolic activity.

Brown betty American; pudding made from apple and breadcrumbs; similar to apple charlotte.

Brown butter Is made by cooking butter over low heat until it turns light brown. If allowed to darken further, is called Black Butter.

Brown sugar Brown sugar has a molasses film on the sugar crystals, which imparts the brown colour and characteristics flavour of this sugar. It contains approximately 2% moisture and requires storage protection against moisture loss.

Brownie A dense, chewy cake, usually made with chocolate in a large tin and cut into squares.

Brownie, brownies A chocolate bar cookie. The name comes from the deep-brown colour of the cookie. The origins of the chocolate brownies is uncertain but it is felt that it was probably created by accident, the result of a forgetful cook neglecting to add baking powder to chocolate cake batter. Sears, Roebuck catalog in 1897 published the first known recipe for the brownies, and it quickly became very popular (so popular that a brownie mix was even sold in the catalog).

Browning reactions Chemical reactions in foods which result in the formation of a brown colour.

Brugnon Hybrid fruit, a cross between plum and peach. Resembles nectarine, and name sometimes used in France for nectarines.

Brule Literally 'burnt'; food grilled or otherwise heated sufficiently to give it a good brown colour.

Brunch A combination of the words for breakfast and lunch, and which is neither breakfast nor lunch, which combines some of the features of both and is served mid-morning. Brunch first appeared in England at the end of the 19th century. In August 1896, the word appeared in the magazine called Punch. The magazine reported on a company breakfast by Mr. Guy Beringer of the defunct Hunter's Weekly about a combined breakfast and lunch that was served after guests returned home from a morning of hunting. The article went on to say "To be fashionable nowadays, we much brunch." It wasn't until the 1930s in the United States that the idea of brunch became popular in restaurants and hotels. Customers became know as "pilers."

Brunoise It is a French word used to describe a mixture of vegetables, usually onion, celery, and carrot, which has been very finely diced, then cooked slowly in butter. This classic mixture is used as a base to flavor soups, stews and sauces.

Brunswick stew This famous stew was originally a game stew and not a domestic meat stew as it is today. According to one story, it began as a squirrel stew created by "Uncle" Jimmy Matthews and named after Brunswick County, Virginia (which was named for Braunschweig in Germany). In 1828, Dr. Creed Haskins, a member of the Virginia state legislature, wanted something special for a political rally he was sponsoring. He persuaded Matthews to part with his recipe. The stew remained, for many years, one of the main attractions at political rallies conducted by both the Whigs and the Democrats. Gradually more vegetables were added and chicken replaced squirrel as the major ingredient. Virginians insist that the dish was invented in Brunswick County, VA. A county of the same name in North Carolina and some citizens of Brunswick, GA., also lay claim to have originated the stew.

Bruschetta Italian bread (usually ciabatta), that's sliced and grilled or toasted, then rubbed with a clove of garlic and drizzled with extra virgin olive oil, before being finished off with a variety of toppings (ripe plum tomatoes and fresh basil is a classic combination). Bruschetta can be served with drinks before a meal, or as a light starter.

Brussels sprouts They are the buds of a cultivated variety of the common cabbage plant. In appearance, brussel sprouts resemble miniature cabbages, but have a much stronger flavor than their larger cousins.

Brut Very dry (unsweet) reference to Champagne or sparkling wine.

BS 5750 British Standard of excellence in quality management; originally an engineering standard but applicable to food companies, hospitals, etc.; incorporates the EU equivalent ISO 9002.

BSE Bovine spongiform encephalopathy; a degenerative disease of the brain, transmitted between animals by feeding slaughter-house waste from infected animals. Commonly known as 'mad cow disease'. The infective agent is believed to be a prion. It is not known whether it can be transmitted to human beings, but similar infectious agents cause scrapie in sheep and Kreutzfeld-Jacob disease (and possibly other dementias) in human beings.

BT (Bacillus thuringiensis) One of the most common microorganisms used in biologically based pesticides is the Bacillus thuringiensis or Bt bacterium. Several of the proteins produced by the Bt, principally in the coating the bacteria forms around itself, are lethal to individual species of insects. By using Bt in pesticide formulations, target insects can be controlled using an environmentally benign, biologically based agent. Bt based insecticides have been widely used by home gardeners for many years as well as on farms.

Bubble and Squeak An English dish of equal parts mashed potatoes and chopped cooked cabbage mixed together and fried until well browned. Originally, the dish included chopped boiled beef. The name is said to come from the sounds the potato-cabbage mixture makes as it cooks (some say it's from the sounds one's stomach makes after eating bubble and squeak).

Bubble Tea Bubble Tea is the catch-all name for endless unusual names of this drink such as: tapioca pearl drink, tapioca ball drink, pearl shake, pearl tea, black pearl tea, big pearl, boba tea, boba ice tea, boba nai cha, milk tea, bubble drink, zhen zhu nai cha, momi, momi milk tea, QQ, BBT, PT, and possibly many other names. This drink is far from the plain-looking tea that you are generally familiar with and it. It is non-alcoholic and non-carbonated. The tea is sweet, thought it has less sugar than a typical soft drink. There are a huge variety of flavors to try; depending on the teahouse or stand you visit. The drink is usually a mix of tea, milk, sugar, and giant black tapioca balls. The "bubble" refers to the foam created by shaking the freshly brewed tea with ice (the drink must always be shaken and not stirred). The unique ingredient of Bubble Tea is the tapioca pearl. About the size of pearls or small marbles, they have a consistency like gummy candy (soft and chewy). Being heavier than the drink they tend to always stay near the bottom of the glass. These drinks are usually served in large see-through plastic containers with an extra-wide straw to sip these jumbo pearls.

Buckle Also called crumble. Is a type of cake made in a single layer with berries added to the batter. It is usually made with blueberries. The topping is similar to a streusel, which gives it a buckled or crumpled appearance.

Buckling A hot-smoked herring (the kipper is cold-smoked).

Buck's fizz Sparkling wine mixed with orange juice; known in the USA as a mimosa.

Buckwheat A type of grain used extensively in Eastern European cooking. Buckwheat flour is traditionally used to make blinis - small pancakes eaten with caviar. In Italy it's sometimes used to make gnocchi; buckwheat pasta is the basis of the famous pizzocheri, a northern Italian dish traditionally made with potatoes, cabbage and cheese. Buckwheat can be purchased from larger supermarkets or health-food shops.

Buffalo chicken wings They are deep-fried chicken wing serve with a hot sauce, celery stalks, and blue cheese dressing. Because the residents of Buffalo are so enamored with these chicken wings, the city of Buffalo, New York has declared July 19th as the "Official Chicken Wing Day." The city's proclamation noted that, because of Mrs. Bellissimo's kitchen, "thousands of chicken wings are consumed by buffalonians in restaurants and taverns throughout the city each week." This famous chicken wings were created a the Frank & Teressa's Anchor Bar in Buffalo, New York on October 30 1962, by owner Teressa Bellissimo. According to the story by the restaurant, her son, Dom Bellissimo, asked Teressa Bellissimo to fix something for his group of hungry friends. To make a long story short, as she was about to put them in the stockpot for soup, she looked at them and said, "It's a shame to put such beautiful wings in a stock pot." So she battered and then deep-fried the chicken wings. The rest is history!

Buffalo currant Two varieties of N. American currant: Ribes odoratum, which has a distinctive smell, and R. aureum, the golden or Missouri currant.

Buffer Substances that prevent a change in the pH when acid or alkali is added. Salts of weak acids and bases are buffers and are commonly used to control the acidity of foods. Amino acids and proteins also act as buffers. The pH of blood (acid-base balance) is maintained by physiological buffers including phosphates, bicarbonate, and proteins.

Bulgogi Bulgogi is marinated strips of beef cooked over charcoal on a grill. It is the best known and most popular of all Korean foods. Beef is most often identified with bulgogi, but even pork, chicken, lamb, squid, and octopus can be cooked bulgogi style. Foreigners consider it the national dish of Korea. It is often prepared at the table on small grills and accompanied by kimchi, a spicy pickled cabbage. In Korean, the word bul means "fire" and gogi means "meat." The word is commonly translated as Korean barbecue, thought it literally means "fire meat."

Bulgur The oldest processed food known. Prepared precooked wheat, originally from the Middle East. Wheat is soaked, cooked, and dried, then lightly milled to remove the outer bran and cracked. It is eaten in soups and cooked with meat (when it is known as kibbe). Also called ala, burghul, cracked wheat, and American rice.

Bulimia Nervosa An eating disorder characterized by rapid consumption of a large amount of food in a short period of time, with a sense of lack of control during the episode and self evaluation unduly influenced by body weight and shape. There are two forms of the condition, purging and non purging. The first type regularly engages in purging through self induced vomiting or the excessive use of laxatives or diuretics. Alternatively, the non purging type controls weight through strict dieting, fasting or excessive exercise.

Buljol Caribbean; salad of salt cod, chilli, tomato, and avocado.

Bulking agents Non-nutritive substances (commonly non-starch polysaccharides) added to foods to increase the bulk and hence sense of satiety, especially in foods designed for weight reduction.

Bullace Fruit of the wild damson, Prunus insititia; similar to sloe (P. spinosa), and very acidic.

Bully beef The name given by troops during the First World War to corned beef (canned salted beef).

Bulrush A wild plant common in ponds and marshes (correctly the false bulrush or common reedmace, Typha latifola). The young sprouts and shoots can be eaten in salads, the pollen is used as a flavouring, and the roots and unripe flower heads may be boiled as a vegetable.

Bun Sweetened bread roll; correctly made with yeast dough, although sometimes applied to small cakes made with baking powder, or to cream buns, which are made with choux pastry. Also applied to the rolls used for hamburgers (burger buns).

Buni Coffee beans left in the field to dry; generally hard and of poor quality.

Burgoo Burgoo is a savory stew made from a varying array of ingredients that is popular in Kentucky. It is often cooked in enormous iron kettles outdoors over an open flame. Cooking can take as long as 30 hours and flavor improves as it ages. It has been said that burgoo is more of a concept than a recipe. This is because there are as many different ways to prepare burgoo as there are people who prepare it. The meats could include any or all of the following meats: mutton (sheep/lamb), beef, pork, chicken, veal or opossum. You will also find some combination of these vegetables: potatoes, corn, lima beans, tomatoes, or okra. Of course there are also many spices to choose from as well. As you might imagine there are many people who keep their recipes a closely guarded secret.

Burgundy Red and white wines produced in the Burgundy region of France (Bourgogne).

Burnet Salad burnet, a wild plant (Poterium sanguisorba) growing in grassland on chalky soil. The leaves have the flavour of cucumber, and can be used to flavour fruit wines, vinegar, and butter, and are used in salads. Also called pimpernel.

Burning foot syndrome Nutritional melalgia (neuralgic pain); severe aching, throbbing, and burning pain in the feet, associated with nerve damage, observed in severely under-nourished prisoners of war in the Far East. It results from long periods on a diet poor in protein and B vitamins, and may (doubtfully) be due specifically to a deficiency of pantothenic acid.

Burnt cream It is sometimes known as Trinity Cream since it is generally believed to have originated at Trinity College, Cambridge, in the 18th century. It is the English relation (and predecessor) of the French Crθme Brulee.

Burrito A large (10") flour tortilla filled with any number of ingredients, which can include beans, beef, or pork. The tortillas are rolled and then sealed by tucking the ends under. They can be eaten like this or topped with salsa, lettuce, tomato, cheese, and guacamole.

Bushel A traditional dry measure of capacity, equivalent to 80 lb of distilled water at 17 °C with a barometer reading of 30 inches, i.e. 8 imperial gallons (36.4 L); used as a measure of corn, potatoes, etc. The American (Winchester) bushel is 3% larger.

The weight of a bushel varies with the product: wheat 27 kg, maize and rye 25 kg, barley 22 kg, paddy rice 20 kg, oats 14.5 kg.

Butifarra Spanish (Catalan and Mallorquin); spiced pork sausage containing pine nuts, almonds, cumin seed, and cinnamon. Butifarrones are smaller.

Butt A cask for beer or wine, containing 108 imperial gallons.

Butter Made from separated cream by churning (sweet cream butter); legally not less than 80% fat (and not more than 16% water) of which around 60% is saturated, a small proportion (3%) polyunsaturated, the rest being mono-unsaturated. Lactic butter, which is preferred in some countries, is made by first ripening the cream with a bacterial culture to produce lactic acid and increase the flavour (due to diacetyl). This is normally unsalted or up to 0.5% salt added. Sweet cream butter may be salted up to 2%. Butter supplies 72 kcal (300 kJ) per g; a 40-g portion (as spread on 4 slices of bread) is a rich source of vitamin A and contains 32 g of fat, of which two-thirds is saturated; supplies 300 kcal.

Butter, whey Butter made from the small amount of fat left in whey; it has a slightly different fatty acid composition from ordinary butter.

Buttermilk The residue left after churning butter, 0.1-2% fat, with the other constituents of milk proportionally increased. It is slightly acidic, with a distinctive flavour due to the presence of diacetyl and other substances. Usually made by adding lactic bacteria to skim milk; 90-92% water, 4% lactose with acidic flavour from lactic acid, it is similar to skim milk in composition. Dried buttermilk is used in bakery products and ice cream.

Butylated hydroxyanisole (BHA) A phenolic chemical compound used to preserve foods by preventing rancidity. It may also be used as a defoaming agent for yeast. BHA is found in foods high in fats and oils; also in meats, cereals, baked goods, beer, and snack foods.

Butylated hydroxytoluene (BHT) A phenolic chemical compound used to keep food from changing flavor, odor and/or colour. It is added to foods high in fats and oils and cereals.

Butyric acid A short-chain saturated fatty acid containing four carbon atoms. It occurs as the triglyceride in 5-6% of butter fat, and in small amounts in other fats and oils.

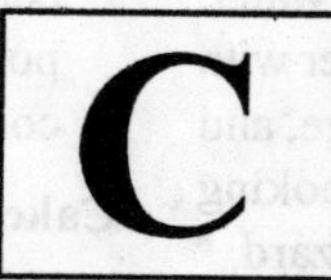

Cabbage There are over 70 varieties of cabbage. Broccoli, Brussels sprouts, cauliflower, kohlrabi, collards, kale, turnips, and many more are all a member of the cabbage family. These plants are all known botanically as members of the species Brassica oleracea, and they native to the Mediterranean region of Europe

Cabbie-claw Scottish (Shetland); fresh codling, salted and hung in the open air for 1-2 days, then simmered with horseradish. The name derives from the Shetland dialect name for young cod, kabbilow (from the German Kabbeljau).

Cabernet franc A grape variety widely used for wine making, although not one of the classic varieties. Also known as bouchet.

Cabernet sauvignon One of the 9 'classic' grape varieties used for wine making, used for some of the great red wines of Bordeaux, and widely grown throughout the world.

Cabinet pudding Moulded pudding made from bread and butter or sponge cake, with custard; sometimes glace cherries and egg are added.

Cacciatora, alla Italian; in the hunter's style, generally game or poultry with onions, herbs, and tomatoes in a wine sauce.

Cachelos Spanish (Galician) dish of potatoes, cabbage, ham, and chorizo (spiced sausage).

Cachexia The condition of extreme emaciation and wasting seen in patients with advanced diseases such as cancer and AIDS. Due to both an inadequate intake of food and the effects of the disease in increasing metabolic rate (hypermetabolism) and the breakdown of tissue protein.

Cachou Small scented tablets for sweetening the breath.

Caciocavallo cheese This cheese is said to date back to the 14th century, and believed by some to have originally been made from mare's milk. Today, Caciocavallo cheese is made from cow's milk, though its cryptic name literally means "horse cheese" - the Sicilian word "cacio" sharing the same root as casein while "cavallo" means horse. (There's a theory that the cheese owes its name to the manner in which two bulbs were attached by a string and suspended from a beam "a cavallo" as though astride a horse.) It takes at least eight months to age Caciocavallo cheese properly, achieving a sharper flavor in about two years. Caciocavallo is a good complement to stronger wines, and widely used for grating over pasta. It is a favourite of Sicilian chefs for use with pasta. It's usually shaped as a large wheel. "Caciovacchino" was a similar product made in times past.

Cadmium A mineral of no known function in the body, and therefore not a dietary essential. It accumulates in the body throughout life, reaching a total body content of 20-30 mg (200-300 µmol). It is toxic, and cadmium poisoning is a recognized industrial disease. In Japan cadmium poisoning has been implicated in itai-itai disease, a severe and sometimes fatal loss of calcium from the bones, as the disease occurred in an area where rice was grown on land irrigated with contaminated waste water. Accidental contamination of drinking water with cadmium salts also leads to kidney damage, and enough cadmium can leach out from cooking vessels with cadmium glaze to pose a hazard.

Caecum The first part of the large intestine, separated from the small intestine by the ileo-colic sphincter. It is small in carnivorous animals and very large in herbivores, since it is involved in the digestion of cellulose. In omnivorous animals, including man, it is of intermediate size. See also gastro-intestinal tract.

Caesar Salad The salad consists of greens (classically romaine lettuce) with a garlic vinaigrette dressing. The Caesar salad was once voted by the International Society of Epicures in Paris as the "greatest recipe to originate from the Americas in fifty years."

Caffeic acid A type of phenol found in various fruits, vegetables and citrus fruits which has antioxidant like activities that may reduce the risk of degenerative diseases, heart disease and eye disease.

Caffeine Caffeine is a naturally occurring substance found in the leaves, seeds or fruits of over 63 plant species worldwide and is part of a group of compounds known as methylxanthines. The most commonly known sources of caffeine are coffee and cocoa beans, cola nuts and tea leaves. Caffeine is a pharmacologically active substance and, depending on the dose, can be a mild central nervous system stimulant. Caffeine does not accumulate in the body over the course of time and is normally excreted within several hours of consumption.

Cajun cuisine Cajun food is essentially the poor cousin to Creole. Today it tends to be spicier and more robust than Creole, utilizing regionally available resources and less of the foods gained through trade. Some popular Cajun dishes include pork based sausages such as andouille and boudin; various jambalayas and gumbos; coush-coush (a creamed corn dish) and etouffee. The true art of Louisiana seasonings is in the unique blend of herbs and spices that serve to enhance the flavor of vegetables, seafood, meats, poúltry and wild game, along with a "Cajun" cook that knows how to blend these spices.

Cake Baked from flour with added fat (butter or margarine), sugar, and eggs. Plain cakes are made by rubbing the fat and sugar into the flour, with no egg; sponge cakes by whipping with or without fat; rich cakes contain dried fruit.

A 100-g portion of typical rich fruit cake is a source of calcium and iron; contains 10 g of fat of which one-third is saturated and onequarter polyunsaturated; supplies 340 kcal. A 100-g portion of sponge made without added fat ('fatless sponge') is a good source of protein; a source of vitamin B2, niacin, and iron; contains 6 g of fat; supplies 300 kcal.

Cake flour Cake flour is very finely ground soft wheat used to make tender, fine-textured cakes. It is bleached with chlorine gas, which, besides whitening the flour, also makes it slightly acidic. This acidity makes cakes set faster and have a finer texture.

Calabasa West Indian or green pumpkin, with yellow flesh.

Calabrese An annual plant (Brassica olearacea italica), a variety of broccoli which yields a crop in the same year as it is sown. Also called American, Italian, or green sprouting broccoli. A 75-g portion is a rich source of vitamin A (as carotene), folate, and vitamin C; provides 3 g of dietary fibre; supplies 25 kcal.

Calamari Calamari are squid. This cephalopod has a long body with swimming fins at the rear, two tentacles, and eight arms. Calamari takes their name from the Latin word "calamus," which refers to the inky liquid excreted by the squid and used in pastas and sauces.

Calas Calas are fried balls of rice and dough that are eaten covered with powdered sugar, not unlike rice-filled beignets. It is said that long ago, on cold mornings in New Orleans, women would walk the streets of the French Quarter selling these warm fried cakes for breakfast. "Calas! Calas, Tout Chaud!" as the Creole women used to shout when they sold them in the French Quarter of New Orleans.

Calcidiol The 25-hydroxy-derivative of vitamin D, also known as 25-hydroxycholecalciferol, the main storage and circulating form of the vitamin in the body.

Calciferol Used at one time as a name for ercalciol (ergocalciferol or vitamin D 2), made by the ultra-violet irradiation of ergosterol. Also used as a general term to include both vitamers of vitamin D (vitamins D 2 and D 3).

Calcium A mineral found mainly in the hard part of bones, where it is stored. Calcium is added to bones by cells called osteoblasts and is removed from bones by cells called osteoclasts. Calcium is essential for healthy bones. It is also important for muscle contraction, heart action, nervous system maintenance, and normal blood clotting. Food sources of calcium include dairy foods, some leafy green vegetables such as broccoli and collards, canned salmon, clams, oysters, calcium-fortified foods, and tofu. According to the National Academy of Sciences, adequate intake of calcium is 1,200 milligrams a day (four glasses of milk) for men and women 51 and older, 1,000 milligrams a day for adults 19 through 50, and 1,300 milligrams a day for children 9 through 18. The upper limit for calcium intake is 2.5 grams daily.

Calcium acid phosphate Also known as monocalcium phosphate and acid calcium phosphate or ACP, $Ca(H_2 PO_4)$ 2. Used as the acid ingredient of baking powder and self-raising flour, since it reacts with bicarbonate to liberate carbon dioxide. Calcium phosphates are permitted food additives.

Calculi Stones formed in tissues such as the gall bladder (biliary calculus or gallstone), kidney (renal calculus), or ureters. Renal calculi may consist of uric acid and its salts (especially in gout) or of oxalic acid salts. Oxalate calculi may be of metabolic or dietary origin and people at metabolic risk of forming oxalate renal calculi are advised to avoid dietary sources of oxalic acid and its precursors. Rarely, renal calculi may consist of the amino acid cystine.

Caldereta Spanish; stewed fish or meat, named from the caldera or cauldron in which it is cooked.

Calfos Trade name for a prepared 'bone meal (i.e. calcium phosphate) used as a source of calcium and phosphate in foods.

Calf's foot jelly Stock made by boiling calves' feet in water; it sets to a stiff jelly on cooling; largely water, so of little nutritional value.

California roll A California roll is a slender mat-rolled sushi roll containing crab, avocado, and cucumber. Today, in California and Hawaii, sushi reigns supreme, and the most popular sushi today are the California Rolls. Most people in Japan have never heard of the California Roll.

Calipash The gelatinous green fat attached to the upper shell (carapace) of the turtle; the yellow fat attached to the lower shell is calipee.

Caliper An instrument with two hinged jaws used for measuring the thickness or diameter of an object; often used to measure skinfold thickness

Calisay Spanish (Catalan); liqueur made from chinchona (cinchona) bark, aged in oak casks.

Call to stool Feeling the need to have a bowel movement.

Callaloo Caribbean name for leaves of both taro and Chinese spinach (Amaranthus gangeticus), and for the soup made from them.

Calorie A unit of food energy. In nutrition terms, the word calorie is used instead of the more precise scientific term kilocalorie which represents the amount of energy required to raise the temperature of a liter of water one degree centigrade at sea level. The common usage of the word calorie of food energy is understood to refer to a kilocalorie and actually represents, therefore, 1000 true calories of energy. A calorie is also known as cal, gram calorie, or small calorie.

Calories, empty A term used to describe foods that provide energy but little, if any, of the nutrients.

Calorimeter An instrument for measuring the amount of oxidizable energy in a substance, by burning it in oxygen and measuring the heat produced. The energy yield of a foodstuff in the body is equal to that obtained in a bomb calorimeter only when the metabolic end-products are the same as those obtained by combustion. Thus, proteins liberate 5.65 kcal (23.64 kJ)/g in a calorimeter, when the nitrogen is oxidized to the dioxide, but only 4.4 kcal (18.4 1kJ)/g in the body, when the nitrogen is excreted as urea (which has a heat of combustion equal to the 'missing' 1.25 kcal). See also energy conversion factors.

Calorimetry The measurement of energy expenditure by the body. Direct calorimetry is the direct measurement of heat output from the body, as an index of energy expenditure, and hence energy requirements. The subject is placed inside a small, thermally insulated room, and the heat produced is measured. Few such difficult studies have been performed, and only a limited range of activities can be studied under these confined conditions.

Indirect calorimetry is a means of estimating energy expenditure indirectly, rather than by direct measurement of heat production. There are two methods in use: 1. Measurement of the rate of oxygen consumption, using a spirometer, permits calculation of energy expenditure. Most studies of the energy cost of activities have been performed by this method.

2. Estimation of the total production of carbon dioxide over a period of 7-10 days, after consumption of dual isotopically labelled water.

Calphos Trade name for a prepared bone-meal used as a source of calcium and phosphate in foods.

Calvados Calvados is an apple brandy made in Normandy, northern France. It's produced from distilled cider and matured in oak barrels. In Normandy it's traditionally served as a digestif during (yes, during) the meal. It's good in cocktails and makes an excellent mulled cider mixed with apple juice, cider, cinnamon, cloves and brown sugar. It can be used in cooking, particularly in Norman specialities such as chicken with cream and calvados, crкpes flambı or apple-based dishes.

Calzone A pizza that's folded in half and baked so that the filling is enclosed completely - similar to a Cornish pasty or turnover. Calzones are usually made as a single serving. It's popular street food in Italy, particularly in Naples where pizza is said to have originated. People fold them in quarters and eat them with their hands while they're on the go.

Cambridge sauce English; substitute for mayonnaise, made with oil, vinegar, and pounded yolk of hard-boiled eggs, flavoured with capers, anchovies, and herbs. See also salad dressing.

Camembert A major soft, French cheese made from cows' milk, originating from Auge, Normandy, France. Covered with a white mould (Penicillium candidum or P. camembertii) which participates in the ripening process; deteriorates after a few days.

Commonly in the UK it contains 50% water and 25% fat (= '50% fat in dry matter'); a 30-g portion is a rich source of vitamin B 12, a source of protein, vitamins A, B 2, and niacin, contains 8 g of fat, 100 mg of calcium and 200 mg of sodium; supplies 90 kcal (370 kJ). Also made with '30% fat in dry matter' (= 13% of total), '40', '45' and '60% fat in dry matter' (= 18% of total).

Camembert cheese Soft and ripened (tastes much like Brie cheese), but more pointed in flavor and richer in texture. It is made from 100% cow's milk. The most widely marketed of all French cheeses. It is used for dessert and snacks.

Camomile Either of two herbs, Anthemis nobilis or Matricaria recutica. The essential oil is used to flavour liqueurs; camomile tea is a tisane prepared by infusion of the dried flower heads, and the whole herb can be used to make a herb beer.

Campden process The preservation of food by the addition of sodium bisulphite (E-222), which liberates sulphur dioxide. Also known as cold preservation, since it replaces heat sterilization.

Campden tablets Tablets of sodium bisulphite (E-222), used for sterilization of bottles and other containers and in the preservation of foods (the Campden process).

Campylobacter A genus of pathogenic organisms which are the most commonly reported cause of gastro-enteritis in the UK, although it is not known what proportion of cases are foodborne. Campylobacteriosis has been associated with the consumption of undercooked meats, milk that has been inadequately pasteurized or contaminated by birds, and contaminated water. Helicobacter pyloris was formerly classified as a campylobacter.

Canada's food guide to healthy eating The Food Guide is a tool to help individuals make wise food choices. Using a rainbow pictorial, it identifies the recommended number of daily serving from four foods groups for healthy eating.

Canadian bacon It is a lean, boneless pork loin roast that is smoked. Called back bacon in Canada, Canadian bacon is pre-cooked and can be fried, baked, or added to casseroles or salads.

Canapes The term 'canapt' means sofa or settee in French - so traditionally canapts were little platforms of pastry or buttered, fried or toasted bread for tasty things to sit on. It now encompasses all kinds of bite-sized appetisers that can be eaten with the fingers, leaving the other hand free to hold a drink.

Canbra oil Oil extracted from selected strains of rapeseed containing not more than 2% erucic acid.

Cancer A wide variety of diseases characterized by uncontrolled growth of tissue. Dietary factors may be involved in the initiation of some forms of cancer, and a high-fat diet has been especially implicated. There is some evidence that antioxidant nutrients such as carotene, vitamins C and E, and the mineral selenium may be protective. See also carcinogen.

Patients with advanced cancer are frequently malnourished, the condition of cachexia.

Canderel Trade name for tablets of the sweetener aspartame.

Candied peel Preserved fruit peel, commonly of citrus fruits, used in confectionery and cake making. It is prepared by softening the peel, then boiling with sugar syrup.

Candlenut Candlenut is the name of a tropical nut used in Malaysian cuisine. It derives its peculiar name from the fact that the oil of the nut is also used to make candles. Candlenuts are available only roasted, whole, or in pieces, because raw they are highly toxic. The function of the candlenut in satays or curries is to flavor and thicken.

Candy 1. Crystallized sugar made by repeated boiling and slow evaporation.

2. USA; a general term for sugar confectionery.

Candy bar At the 1893 Columbian Exposition, a World's Fair held in Chicago, chocolate-making machinery made in Dresden, Germany, was displayed. Milton S. Hershey, who had made his fortune in caramels, saw the potential for chocolate and installed chocolate machinery in his factory in Lancaster, and produced his first chocolate bars in 1894. Other Americans began mixing in other ingredients to make up new candy bars throughout the end of the 1890's and the early 1900's. It was World War I that really brought attention to the candy bar. The U.S. Army Quartermaster Corps commissioned various American chocolate manufacturers to provide 20 to 40 pound blocks of chocolate to be shipped to quartermaster bases. The blocks were chopped up into smaller pieces and distributed to doughboys in Europe. Eventually the task of making smaller pieces was turned back to the manufacturers. As a result, from that time on and through the 1920s, candy bar manufacturers became established throughout the United States, and as many as 40,000 different candy bars appeared on the scene. The Twenties became the decade that among other things was the high point of the candy bar industry. The original candy bar industry had its start on the eastern seaboard in such cities as Philadelphia, Boston, and New York. The industry soon spread to the Midwest, because shipping and raw materials such as sugar, corn syrup, and milk were easily available. Chicago became the seat of the candy bar industry and is even today an important base.

Candy cane The symbol of the shepherds' crook is an ancient one, representing the humble shepherds who were the first to worship the newborn Christ. Its counterpart is our candy cane (so old as a symbol that we have nearly forgotten its humble origin). In 1670, the choirmaster at the Cologne Cathedral handed out sugar sticks among his young singers to keep them quiet during the long Living Creche ceremony. In honour of the occasion, he had the candies bent into shepherds' crooks. In 1847, a German-Swedish immigrant named August Imgard of Wooster, Ohio, decorated a small blue spruce with paper ornaments and candy canes. It wasn't until the turn of the century that the red and white stripes and peppermint flavors became the norm. The body of the cane is white, representing the life that is pure. The broad red stripe is symbolic of the Lord's sacrifice for man. In the 1920s, Bob McCormack began making candy canes as special Christmas treats for his children, friends and local shopkeepers in Albany, Georgia. It was a laborious process pulling, twisting, cutting and bending the candy by hand. It could only be done on a local scale. In the 1950s, Bob's brother-in-law, Gregory Keller, a Catholic priest, invented a machine to automate candy cane production. Packaging innovations by the younger McCormack made it possible to transport the delicate canes on a scale that transformed Bobs Candies, Inc. into the largest producer of candy canes in the world. Although modern technology has made candy canes accessible and plentiful, they've not lost their purity and simplicity as a traditional holiday food and symbol of the humble roots of Christianity.

Cane sugar Sucrose extracted from the sugar cane Saccharum officinarum; identical with sucrose prepared from any other source, such as sugar beet.

Canning The process of preserving food by sterilization and cooking in a sealed metal can, which destroys bacteria and protects from recontamination. If foods are sterilized and cooked in glass jars which are then closed with hermetically sealed lids, the process is known as bottling. Canned foods are sometimes known as tinned foods, because the cans are sometimes made using tin-plated steel. More commonly now they are made of lacquered steel or aluminium. In aseptic canning, foods are pre-sterilized at a very high temperature (150-175 °C) for a few seconds, and then sealed into cans under sterile (aseptic) conditions. The flavour, colour, and retention of vitamins are superior with this short-time, high-temperature process than with conventional canning.

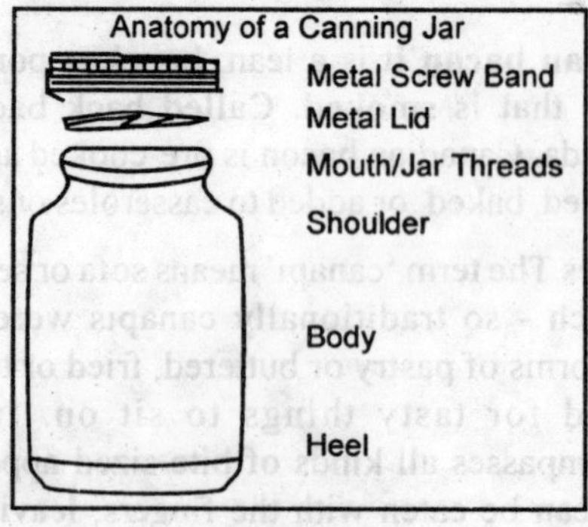

Fig. Canning

Cannoli/cannola They are sometimes called "Turkish hats." The cannoli is perhaps the best-known Sicilian pastry and is part of Sicily's ancient tradition of pastry and dessert making. It is made by stuffing cylinders of fried dough (wafer shells) with a mixture of ricotta or custard, candied fruit, chocolate, and other ingredients. Originally, the pastry was flavored with wine, and in Sicily this is still done. They are traditionally prepared for festivities at Carnival time (though nowadays they are to be found all year round).

Canola oil Canola's history goes back to the rapeseed plant, but canola and rapeseed are not the same. Because canola and rapeseed have different chemical compositions, the names cannot be used interchangeably. Canola is an oilseed crop, which is grown primarily in regions of Western Canada, with some acreage being planted in Ontario and the Pacific Northwest, north central, and southeast United States.

Cantaloupe A variety of muskmelon. . It is found in many shapes and sizes. Because of trade usage, cantaloupe has become the name commonly applied to muskmelons grown in the U.S.

Canthaxanthin A red carotenoid pigment which is not a precursor of vitamin A. It is used as a food colour (E-161g), and can be added to the diet of broiler chickens to colour the skin and shanks, and to the diet of farmed trout to produce the same bright colour as is seen in wild trout. These colours are normally derived from carotenoids in natural foodstuffs. Canthaxanthin is also used to maintain the colour of flamingos kept in captivity.

Cape gooseberries Also known as physalis, this is a small, smooth round fruit wrapped in its own papery case that resembles a Chinese lantern. The fruit itself is a pretty orange-gold colour and can be unwrapped and eaten as is, or dipped in melted chocolate and served after dinner with coffee. They have a delicate sweet-sour taste - sort of a cross between a gooseberry and a cherry tomato. They make excellent jams, jellies and puries, and can be used in exotic fruit salads, pavlovas or roulades, or simmered in water with a little sugar and used in fruit pies or crumbles.

Capellini In Italian, capellini means, "thin hair." This is one of the very thin varieties of flat spaghetti. Also called angel hair pasta.

Caper Unopened flower buds of the subtropical shrub Capparis spinosa or C. inermis with a peppery flavour; commonly used in pickles and sauces. Unripe seeds of the nasturtium (Tropaeolum majus) can be pickled and used as a substitute.

Capercaillie A large game bird (Tetrao urogallus), also known as wood grouse or cock of the wood.

Capers The pickled flower buds of the caper bush, which grows wild all over the Mediterranean. Fresh capers are picked and immediately preserved in brine or wine vinegar, or are packed in salt (these should be rinsed before use to remove any excess salt). Their tangy, bitter flavour adds piquancy to many sauces and condiments, such as tartare sauce, and they're a good match for fish. They can be used as a garnish for meat and vegetable dishes and in tapenade. Caperberries are well developed capers, slightly larger and a little sweeter. They're often sold with the stalk left on and can be used in the same way as capers.

Capon A 6 to 8 pound castrated male chicken (an unsexed rooster). More richly flavored than regular chicken and with a denser texture. It was under a Roman prohibition that the capon was created. The law prohibited eating any fowl except a hen, and this bird was not to be fattened. A surgeon, looking for a way around this law, transformed a rooster into a capon by the now old and well-known surgical trick. Neither hen nor rooster, the capon was a huge success. It was perfectly safe to eat him because he was "within the law."

Caponata Sicilian; fried aubergine, in a tomato sauce containing capers, olives, celery, and anchovy, garnished with slices of tuna, crawfish, etc.

Caponate A Sicilian vegetable dish made of various ingredients, but usually includes cooked eggplant, celery, capers, anchovies, chile peppers, olives, tomatoes, vinegar, and onions. Sailors' taverns in Sicily were called "caupone," where the dish was usually made and served with sea biscuits. The dish seems to have gotten its name from this word suggesting the kind of robust food served at a tavern or inn.

Cappuccino Coffee made by topping espresso with the creamy foam from steamed milk. A small amount of the steamed milk is also added to the cup. The foam's surface is sometimes dusted with sweetened cocoa powder, nutmeg or cinnamon.

Caprese In the style of Capri. such a sauce is usually made from lightly cooked tomatoes, basil, olive oil, and mozzarella, to use on pastas, meats, fish, or salads.

Caprylic acid One of the medium-chain fatty acids, containing eight carbon atoms, found in the triglycerides of goat and cow butter, coconut oil, and human fat.

Capsicum This is the generic name for the pepper family, which includes the large, sweet, mild peppers (green, yellow, orange and red are the most common), which are also called bell peppers or sweet peppers, as well as any of the hundreds of hot chilli peppers. Peppers have many culinary uses.

They can be used raw in salads, marinated and tossed into pasta, cooked and sieved and transformed into pepper sauce, stuffed with meats or other vegetables and rice or used in classic dishes such as ratatouille or the classic Spanish dish, pisto - peppers fried in a large pan with onion, garlic, tomatoes, herbs and a couple of eggs cracked in the centre.

Carambola Or star fruit, long (8-12 cm) ribbed fruit of Averrhoa carambola and A. bilimbi; a 50-g portion is a rich source of vitamin C.

Caramel Brown material formed by heating carbohydrates in the presence of acid or alkali (sulfite or ammonia); also known as burnt sugar. It can be manufactured from various sugars, starches, and starch hydrolysates and is used as a flavour and colour (E-150a-d) in a wide variety of foods: soft drinks, alcoholic beverages, baked goods, sauces, canned meats, and stews.

Caramel cream A dessert made either by gently heating eggs in milk and allowing to cool (egg custard) or by using cornflour and milk, topped with a caramel sauce. Also known as crθme caramel and (in Spain) as flαn.

Caramelise The process of either heating sugar to a point when it melts and resets as a hard glaze, as on the top of a crθme brϋlte, or cooking small or cut fruit or vegetables in water and sugar until they become brown and glazed. You can invest in a cook's blow torch to caramelise the tops of desserts, but a very hot preheated grill is usually adequate to do the job.

Caraway seed They are the fruit of the "carum carvi" a biennial plant, which grows in northern and central Europe and Asia, and have been cultivated in England and America for its seeds. They are available whole; if desired, grind or pound before using. Caraway seeds can become bitter during long cooking. When preparing soups and stews, add the crushed or whole seeds only 15 minutes before you take the pot off the stove.

Carbohydrate Carbohydrates are organic compounds that consist of carbon, hydrogen and oxygen. They vary from simple sugars containing from three to seven carbon atoms to very complex polymers. Only the hexoses (sugars with six carbon atoms) and pentoses (sugars with five carbon atoms) and their polymers play important roles in nutrition. Carbohydrates in food provide 4 calories per gram.

Plants manufacture and store carbohydrates as their chief source of energy. The glucose synthesized in the leaves of plants is used as the basis for more complex forms of carbohydrates. Classification of carbohydrates relates to their structural core of simple sugars, saccharides. Principal monosaccharides that occur in food are glucose and fructose. Three common disaccharides are sucrose, maltose and lactose. Polysaccharides of interest in nutrition include starch, dextrin, glycogen and cellulose.

Carbohydrate loading Practice of some endurance athletes (e.g. marathon runners) in training for a major event; it consists of exercising to exhaustion, so depleting muscle glycogen, then eating a large carbohydrate-rich meal so as to replenish glycogen reserves with a higher than normal proportion of straight-chain glycogen.

Carbohydrates Carbohydrates are a group of organic compounds that contain carbon in combination with the same proportion of hydrogen and oxygen (as in water). All starches and sugars are carbohydrates. The body receives a large amount of heat and energy from carbohydrate foods. The body changes all carbohydrates into simple sugar and the surplus is stored in the body as fat (and in the liver as glycogen). A large excess of sugar is normally elimated by the kidneys. The usual "sweet tooth" of people is the result of body hunger for carbohydrates. Children require more carbohydrates than adults because they must satisfy the needs of growing bodies.

Carbonara Carbonara in Italian means "charcoal" or "coal," and "alla carbonara" means "in the manner of the coal miners." In Italy, the names of dishes generally tell us where or with whom they originated: dishes called Bolognese come from Bologna, alla Romana from Rome, Neapolitan from Naples; anything marinara is prepared in the manner of sailors, puttanesca is favoured by hookers, and carbonara comes to us from the charcoal makers or wood cutters. A classic Roman dish is Spaghetti alla Carbonara. Most of the ingredients for Spaghetti alla Carbonara could easily be carried by charcoal makers traveling to the forests of the Abruzzi to get wood, and the rest could be bought or "found" along the way. The town now called Aquilonia, was originally named Carbonara during the Samnite and Roman period. Carbonara most likely derived its name from the principal activity of coal mining in the nearby woods. Carbonara was destroyed by the barbarians and rebuilt on its ruins by the Longobard in the 6th century. 1. There are several ideas that one hears from time to time. It is thought that a coal miner's wife first cooked pasta this way that probably cooked over a coal or charcoal cooking fire, and it was popular among coal miners' families before it spread to the general public.

2. Another story suggests that the abundant black pepper in Pasta alla Carbonara symbolized the charcoal that inevitably fell from the artisan onto the plate. The other, that the pepper simply camouflaged the flecks of charcoal on the plate.

3. Carbonara Americana was invented as a way to use bacon and eggs bought on the black market from American service personnel during the Second World War. After World War II when the GIs tasted the original Spaghetti alla Carbonara, they "Americanized" it in the mess halls by tossing in peas, mushrooms, and using American bacon that the Army shipped over.

Carboxypeptidase An enzyme secreted in the pancreatic juice which is involved in the digestion of proteins.

Carcinogen In pathology, a carcinogen is any substance or agent that promotes cancer. Carcinogens are also often, but not necessarily, mutagens or teratogens.Carcinogens may cause cancer by altering cellular metabolism or damaging DNA directly in cells, which interferes with normal biological processes. Aflatoxin B1, which is produced by the fungus Aspergillus flavus growing on stored grains, nuts and peanut butter, is an example of a potent, naturally-occurring microbial carcinogen.

Carcinogenesis The complex, multistep process of cancer causation.Cardiovascular disease (CVD)Any one of numerous abnormal conditions characterised by dysfunction of the heart and blood vessels (see also coronary heart disease and stroke). Other types of CVD mentioned in this blood are congestive heart failure and sudden cardiac death.

Carcinogens, natural and synthetic The basic mechanism involved in the entire process of carcinogenisis—from exposure to the organism to expression of tumors—are qualitatively similar, if not identical, for the synthetic and naturally occurring carcinogens. Consequently, both naturally occurring and synthetic chemicals can be evaluated by the same epidemiologic or experimental methods and procedures.

Cardamom An aromatic spice indigenous to south India and Sri Lanka, cardamom seeds come from a plant belonging to the ginger family. They're contained in small pods about the size of a cranberry.

Cardamom pods are usually green in colour, but they're sometimes bleached white, although the flavour remains the same. You may also come across brown or black 'cardamom', which are slightly larger and have a different flavour and aroma. They add a smoky note to cooked foods and are more frequently used with meat than with vegetable dishes. Cardamom has a wonderful aroma and an enticing warm, spicy-sweet flavour. It's widely used in Indian cooking and in Scandinavian baking. Cardamom can be bought in the pod, as seeds or ground but, as the ground seeds soon lose their flavour, it's preferable to use the pods, either removing the seeds and grinding them or grinding the whole pod - quickly done with a pestle and mortar. If you're using cardamom to flavour dishes such as stews and curries, lightly crush the whole pod and add it to the mixture the shell can be removed after cooking. Cardamom also has an affinity with chocolate. A little cardamom goes a long way, though, so use it sparingly.

Cardoon A large stalky vegetable related to the artichoke, the cardoon is popular in France, Italy and Spain but less known or used in the UK. Cardoons can be found in markets from midwinter to early spring. Look for stalks that are firm and have a silvery grey-green colour. To prepare, remove the tough outer ribs, cut the inner ribs into 8cm (3in) slices and soak in acidulated water to prevent browning. Cardoons can be boiled, braised or baked. Pre-cooking for about 30 minutes in boiling water is suggested in many recipes. Though high in sodium, cardoons are a good source of potassium, calcium and iron.

They were very popular with the Victorians and have a similar taste to globe artichokes. Raw cardoon is eaten with bagna cauda in Piedmont and boiled cardoon is delicious with cheese sauce.

Carignan A grape variety widely used for wine making, although not one of the classic varieties. Probably the commonest grape of France, a prolific cropper producing uninspiring wines.

Cariogenic Causing tooth decay (caries) by stimulating the growth of acid-forming bacteria on the teeth. The term is applied to sucrose and other fermentable carbohydrates.

Carnitine A derivative of the amino acid lysine, required for the transport of fatty acids into mitochondria for oxidation. There is no evidence that it is a dietary essential for human beings, since it can readily be formed from lysine in the body, although there is some evidence that increased intake may enhance the work capacity of muscles. It is a dietary essential for some insects, and was at one time called vitamin B T.

Carob The fruits of this evergreen tree, native to the Middle East, grow in large pods that look similar to broad beans until they ripen from green to brown. They contain a very sweet pulp and hard, brown seeds.

In the Middle East, the sweet pods are chewed raw, and are used as animal feed. Carob beans are also ground and used as a healthier alternative to chocolate and coffee as they contain no caffeine or oxalic acid, and only half the fat of cocoa. The flavour is sweet and treacly, so is excellent in baking.

Carob powder can be substituted for cocoa powder in any recipe. Carob is also available in bars, drops and confectionery. Carob products are available in health food shops and larger supermarkets.

Carotene The red and orange pigments of many plants, obvious in carrots, red palm oil, and yellow maize, but masked by chlorophyll in leaves. Three main types of carotene in foods are important as precursors of vitamin A: [alpha]-, [beta]- and [gamma]-carotene, which are also used as food colours (E-160a). Plant foods contain a considerable number of other carotenes, most of which are not precursors of vitamin A. Carotene is mostly converted into vitamin A (retinol) in the wall of the intestine, but some is absorbed unchanged. 6 [mu]g of [beta]-carotene, and 12 [mu]g of other provitamin A carotenoids, are nutritionally equivalent to 1 [mu]g of preformed vitamin A. About 30% of the vitamin A in Western diets, and considerably more in diets in less-developed countries, comes from carotene.

Carotenoids 1. A group of red, orange and yellow pigments found in plant food and in the tissues of organisms that consume plants. Carotenoids have antioxidant activity. Some, but not all, can act as precursors of vitamin A; the principal of these is fs0 carotene, the most common of the carotenoids.

2. Carotenoids are organic pigments that are naturally occurring in plants and some other photosynthetic organisms like algae, some types of fungus and some bacteria. There are over 600 known carotenoids; they are split into two classes, xanthophylls and carotenes.

Carpaccio A classic Italian dish, served as a starter, of very thin shavings of raw beef fillet, served cold with olive oil and lemon juice or with a mayonnaise or mustard sauce. The dish is often topped with capers and sometimes onions. Although true carpaccio is made with beef, 'carpaccios' of other thinly sliced raw meats, fish or even fruits are becoming more frequently sighted on restaurant menus.

Carpal tunnel syndrome Painful disorder of wrist and hand due to compression of the median nerve in the carpal tunnel. Claimed to be relieved by high intakes of vitamin B6, some 50-100 times the reference intake, but there is little evidence. See also tenosynovitis; vitamin B6 toxicity.

Carrageen Edible seaweeds, Chondrus crispus, also known as Iberian moss or Irish sea moss, and Gigartina stellata; stewed in milk to make a jelly or blancmange. A source of carrageenan.

Carrageenan A compound extracted from Irish moss (a type of seaweed) that is used in puddings, milk shakes and ice cream to stabilize and keep colour and flavor even.

Carrot Carrots are a member of the parsley family and are the roots of the plant. Other root crops are celeriac, parsnip, beets, potatoes, and turnips. Carrots are always in season and can be found with their curly green tops, pre-trimmed for easy use, cut into sticks for use as snacks, or in packages of miniature varieties perfect for school lunches.

Cartilage, The hard connective tissue of the body, composed mainly of collagen, together with chondromucoid (a protein combined with chondroitin sulphate) and chondroalbuminoid (a protein similar to elastin). New bone growth consists of cartilage on which calcium salts are deposited as it develops.

Cartose Trade name for a steam hydrolysate of maize starch, used as a carbohydrate modifier in milk preparations for infant feeding. It consists of a mixture of dextrin, maltose, and glucose.

Case-control Case-control studies are one type of epidemiological study design.Case-control studies are a less-expensive and often-used type of epidemiological study that can be carried out by small teams or individual researchers in single facilities, in a way which more structured trials often cannot. They have pointed the way to a number of important discoveries and advances, but their very success has led some to place excessive faith in them to the point where their credibility has been significantly undermined. This is largely the result of misconceptions regarding the nature of such studies. These misconceptions are particularly widespread in the medical community.

Case-control study A study that compares two groups of people: those with the disease or condition under study (cases) and a very similar group ofpeople who do not have the disease or condition (controls). Researchers study the medical and lifestyle histories of the people in each group to learn what factors may be associated with the disease or condition. For example, one group may have been exposed to a particular substance that the other was not. Also called a retrospective study.

Casein About 75% of the proteins of milk are classified as caseins; a group of 12-15 different proteins. Often used as a protein supplement, since the casein fraction from milk is more than 90% protein.

Caseinogen An obsolete name for the form in which casein is present in solution in milk; when it was precipitated it was then called casein.

Cashew The cashew nut has a very unusual growth habit. It grows on a small tree, dangling beneath a fleshy stalk known as the cashew apple, or cashew pear. The 'pear' can be used for juices, syrups and liqueurs but the cashew nut is much more widely used. Cashews are thought to have originated in Brazil and were taken to India by Portuguese traders. The nut has a shell which contains an irritant oil that can burn human skin - hence cashews are never sold in their shells. The smooth creamy-white kidney-shaped kernel is rich in vitamin A and has a high fat content. In Europe cashews are usually eaten dried, roasted and salted as a snack or in salads. Unsalted cashews are generally used for cooking and they're particularly popular in south Indian cuisine, used whole or ground and often added just before serving. They're also used in Chinese cookery, in main dishes such as noodle salads and stir-fries. They're particularly good with chicken or prawn dishes and can be used in meat or vegetable stews or curries. Roughly chopped, they can be thrown in to rice dishes to add texture.

Cashew nut Fruit of the tropical tree Anacardium occidentale, generally eaten roasted and salted. The nut hangs from the true fruit, a large fleshy but sour apple-like fruit, which is very rich in vitamin C. A 30-g portion of roasted salted nuts (30 nuts) is a source of protein, niacin, iron, and zinc; contains 15 g of fat, of which 20% is saturated and 60% mono-unsaturated; provides 180 kcal.

Cassareep Caribbean; boiled-down juice squeezed from grated cassava root, flavoured with cinnamon, cloves, and brown sugar; used as a base for sauces. It can also be fermented with molasses.

Cassata There are two theories on where cassata derives it name from; 1. A term in Arabic, "quas at," meaning the round bowl in which this sweet was originally made.

2. Other sources say that the word derives from the Latin word caseus (cheese) which would clearly refer to the ricotta cheese, one of the main ingredients needed for making cassata. Cassata is a spectacular Sicilian dessert of ricotta, candied fruit, pistachios, sugar, chocolate, liqueur soaked sponge cake and green pistachio icing.

Cassatella A miniature versions of cassata, perfectly domed and frosted white with a cherry on top, is said to recall St Agata, the patron saint of Catania, who was martyred by being rolled in hot coals and having her breasts cut off. Catanians, with their intense emotional inner life and love of melodramatic gesture, are proud of their little cakes. The rationale is that if you eat the body of Christ in communion, why not the breasts of a saint.

Cassava The tuber of the tropical plant Manihot utilissima. It is the dietary staple in many tropical countries, although it is an extremely poor source of protein; the plant grows well even in poor soil, and is extremely hardy, withstanding considerable drought. It is one of the most prolific crops, yielding, e.g. in Nigeria, 13 million kcal/acre, compared with yam, 9 million, and sorghum or maize, 1 million. A 150-g portion is a rich source of vitamin C; a source of iron and vitamin B1; supplies 150 kcal.

Cassava root contains cyanide, and before it can be eaten it must be grated and left in the open to allow the cyanide to evaporate. The leaves can be eaten as a vegetable, and the tuber is the source of tapioca. See also cassareep.

Casserole The word casserole is derived from the Old French word casse and the Latin word cattia meaning a "frying pan or saucepan." As often happens in history, the name of the cooking utensil was used for the dish name. 1. A casserole is an ovenproof or flameproof dish or pan that has a tight lid. It is used to cook meat and vegetables slowly.

2. A casserole is also a stew or ragout consisting of meat and vegetables, which are put in a casserole dish at the same time and cooked by stewing.

Cassia The inner bark of a tree grown in the Far East (Cinnamomium cassia), used as a flavouring, similar to cinnamon.

Cassina A tea-like beverage made from cured leaves of a holly bush, Ilex cassine, containing 1-1.6% caffeine and 8% tannin.

Cassis Extract of blackcurrants (French: cassis); about 15% alcohol by volume, sweetened with sugar. Mixed with about 10 parts of white wine to make kir, or with sparkling wine to make kir royale.

Cassolette 1. Cassolette means a small dish for food sufficient for one person (a one-portion dish), which is usually made from earthenware.

2. It can also mean a very small case made from fried bread, pastry, egg, and breadcrumbs that are filled with a savory mixture (these are served as snacks or appetizers).

Cassoulet A cassoulet (which was first made in Languedoc in the southwest of France) is a casserole, which consists of different kinds of meat (usually five different kinds), one of which should be pork and another a bird (such as goose, duck, or chicken). The dish also includes white haricot beans, sausage, and garlic. It is covered while cooking and cooked very slowly.

Castor oil Oil from the seeds of the castor oil plant, Ricinus spp. The oil itself is not irritating, but in the small intestine it is hydrolysed by lipase to release ricinoleic acid, which is irritant to the intestinal mucosa and therefore acts as a purgative. The seeds also contain the toxic lettin, ricin.

Catabolic The aspect of metabolism which converts nutrients or complex substances in living cells into simpler compounds with the release of energy, such as cortisol catabolizing muscle protein into glucose for quick energy.

Catabolism Those pathways of metabolism concerned with the breakdown and oxidation of fuels and hence provision of metabolic energy. People who are undernourished or suffering from cachexia are sometimes said to be in a catabolic state, in that they are catabolizing their body tissues, without replacing them.

Catadromous fish Fish that live in fresh water and go to sea to spawn, such as eels.

Catalase An enzyme that splits hydrogen peroxide to yield oxygen and water; an important part of the body's antioxidant defences.

Catalyst An agent that participates in a chemical reaction, speeding the rate, but itself remains unchanged. Catalysts are used, for example, in the hydrogenation of vegetable oils. Enzymes and coenzymes are biological catalysts.

Cataract 1. For other uses, see . A cataract is an opacity that develops in the, crystalline lens of the eye or in its envelope. Early on in the development of senile cataract the power of the crystaline lens may be increased, causing myopia, and the accumulation of brown pigment within the lens may reduce the perception of blue colours. Cataracts typically progress slowly to cause vision loss and are potentially blinding if left untreated. Moreover, with time the cataract cortex liquefies to form a milky white fluid in a Morgagnian Cataract, and can cause severe inflammation if lens capsule ruptures & leaks. Untreated, the cataract can cause phacomorphic glaucoma. Very advanced cataracts with weak zonules are liable for dislocation anteriorly or posteriorly. Such spontaneous posterior dislocations (akin to earliest surgical procedure of couching) in ancient times were regarded as a blessing from heavens, because it restored some perception of light in the bilaterally affected patients. 2. A clouding or loss of transparency of the eye lens. There are many causes of cataracts including aging, diabetes, cortisone medication, trauma, or other diseases. Cataracts will affect most people if they live long enough. Symptoms include double or blurred vision and sensitivity to light and glare. Cataracts can be diagnosed when the doctor examines the eyes with a viewing instrument. The ideal treatment for cataracts is surgical implantation of a new lens. Sunglasses can help to prevent cataracts.

Catechins A type of flavonoid found in tea which provides the health benefits of neutralizing free radicals and possibly reducing the risk of cancer.

Categorical Eligibility Refers to an individual's eligibility for one program based upon his or her eligibility and participation in another program. Households participating in cash assistance programs of the Temporary Assistance for Needy Families Program (TANF) or receiving SSI or General Assistance are categorically eligible to participate in the Food Stamp Program, but still must have net income at or below the federal poverty level and complete the Food Stamp Program application process in order to receive food stamp benefits. States may also treat as categorically eligible for food stamps families receiving certain TANF-funded services even if the households do not receive TANF cash assistance. Categorical eligibility in the child nutrition programs varies by program. In general, homeless, runaway, and migrant youth and children from households participating in the Food Stamp Program, the Food Distribution Program in Indian Reservations (FDPIR), or TANF are categorically eligible to receive free meals.

Catfish A mostly freshwater fish with long, cat-like whiskers (like feelers) around the mouth. Most catfish are farmed. The U.S. leads all other nations in the consumption of catfish. It is particularly popular in the southern and central states. Catfish have skin that is similar to that of an eel, which is thick, slippery, and strong. All catfish should be skinned before cooking. The most common and easiest method to skin a catfish is to nail the head of the dead fish to a board, hold on to its tail, and pull the skin off with pliers. There are 2,000 species of catfish, whose name (probably due to the "whiskers") first appeared in print in 1612. North America has 28 species of catfish, over a dozen of which are eaten. The most popular edible catfish are the "channel catfish", the "white catfish", and "blue catfish". Of all the catfish grown in the United States, eighty percent comes from Mississippi, where more than 102,000 acres are devoted to catfish farms.

Catmint The wild catmint (Nepeta cataria) is distinct from the cultivated catmint (Nepeta spp.) of gardens; both have a minty smell which is liked by cats. The leaves are used to prepare herb teas and may be added to stews; young shoots can be eaten raw in salads.

Caul fat The lacy, fatty membrane encasing the internal organs of an animal. Pork caul is often used for wrapping faggots or pβtεs. It comes in thin sheets and you can buy it from traditional butchers.

Caul Membrane enclosing the foetus; that from sheep or pig used to cover meat while roasting.

Cauliflower The edible flower of Brassica olearacea bortytis, normally creamy-white in colour, although some cultivars have green or purple flowers. Horticulturally, varieties that mature in summer and autumn are called cauliflower, and those that mature in winter broccoli, but commonly both are called cauliflower. A 90-g portion is a rich source of vitamin C; a good source of folate; a source of vitamin B6; provides 1.8 g of dietary fibre and supplies 8 kcal (33 kJ).

Caviar True caviar is the salted and matured eggs or roe of the female sturgeon. Most caviar comes from the Caspian Sea and is processed in Russia and Iran. Beluga is the most expensive variety, followed by Oscietra and Sevruga, all of which are produced from different species of sturgeon. You can buy caviar in tins or jars. The eggs are usually a pearly greyish-black in colour and vary in size. They should be firm but soft and moist and never dry. Keep it well chilled in the fridge and take it out just before you're ready to serve. Because it's so costly caviar is usually served in small portions - on thin slices of toast with butter or a squeeze of lemon, or on blinis with a spoonful of soured cream. It's also traditional to serve it with a glass of chilled neat vodka.

Sturgeon populations in the Caspian are under extreme pressure, with breeding stocks of some species critically low. Consequently, environmentally minded chefs and consumers have been exploring other types of fish roe as an alternative. 'Avruga' is a caviar substitute made from herring roe; lumpfish roe and salmon roe are other alternatives.

Caviar/Caviare Caviar is from the Persian word "khav-yar" meaning "cake of strength," because it was thought that caviar had restorative powers and the power to give one long life. Caviar is from the salted roe (eggs) of several species of sturgeon (it was originally prepared in China from carp eggs). The carp is really a goldfish and is the only fish besides the sturgeon that has gray coloured eggs. Up until 1966, any fish roe that could be coloured black was called caviar. Then the Food and Drug Administration defined the product, limiting it to sturgeon eggs. It takes up to twenty years for the female sturgeon fish to mature before it produces eggs (called berries). Serving caviar begins with buying. The most important think to look for is that each berry is whole, uncrushed, and well coated with its own glistening fat. The best caviar is generally eaten as is, au natural, on a piece of freshly made thin toast, with or without butter (though the caviar itself should be fat enough not to require butter). It can also be sprinkled lightly with some finely chopped hard-cooked egg, and onions or chives.

Cavolo nero An Italian cabbage with dark green leaves that have a good, strong flavour. It can be used in all cabbage recipes but it's particularly good in soups - such as the classic Tuscan soup, ribolitta, which is traditionally left to sit for a day before serving to allow the soup to thicken and the flavours to develop. Cavolo nero is delicious cooked simply, just fried in olive oil with garlic and chillies.

Cayenne pepper A red, fiery hot spice ground from the pod and seeds of dried chillies. A pinch of cayenne over devilled kidneys or stirred through gravy for game birds adds a gutsy kick and heightens the flavour of the dish. It's also good used sparingly in vegetable or lentil soups, in curries or sprinkled over stir-fried prawns or over crispy whitebait. If you like a little heat then add some to shepherd's pie, chilli con carne or to cheese fondue.

Cayenne pepper The cayenne is one of the most widely used peppers in the world. The cayenne is about 3 to 5 times hotter than the jalapeno, and when ripe, has it's own distinct, slightly fruity flavor. Heat range is 6-7.

Celacol Trade name for methyl, hydroxyethyl, and other cellulose derivatives. celeriac A variety of celery with a thick root which is eaten grated in salads or cooked as a vegetable, Apium graveolens var. rapaceum, also known as turnip-rooted or knob celery. A 40-g portion provides 1.2 g of dietary fibre and supplies 5 kcal.

Celeriac Also known as celery knob, celery root, celeri-rave, and turnip-rooted celery. Though known by many names, celeriac or celery root is easily identified where specialty vegetables or root crops (such as turnips and parsnips) are found. A member of the celery family, celery root is a brown-to-beige-coloured, rough, gnarled looking vegetable. It hints of celery with an earthy pungency (its aroma is a sure indicator of its membership in the celery family). It is in season from late fall through early spring. Look for as smooth a surface as you can find to aid in peeling. A one-pound weight is preferred. It should be firm with no indication of a soft or spongy centre.

Celery Celery is ordinarily marketed as the whole stalk, which contains the outer branches and leaves. Sometimes the outer branches are removed and the hearts are sold in bunches. The ancient Chinese credited celery with medicinal qualities and used it as a blood purifier. The Romans like to use it to decorate coffins at funerals. The Romans also felt that wearing crowns of celery helped to ward of headaches after a lot of drinking and partying.

Celery salt Celery salt is a mixture of fine white salt and ground celery seeds.

Celery seed Celery seeds are the fruit of a plant related to the parsley family and are not to be confused with the plant we recognize and serve as a vegetable. They are now grown extensively in France, Holland, India, and the United States. Celery seeds are tiny and brown in colour. They taste strongly of the vegetable and are aromatic and slightly bitter. They are sometimes used where celery itself would not be appropriate.

Celiac disease A disease characterized by sensitivity to gluten, with chronic inflammation of intestinal mucosa; symptoms include diarrhea, malabsorption, and steatorrhea

Cell The basic unit of any living organism. It is a small, watery, compartment filled with chemicals and a complete copy of the organism's genome.

Cellofas Trade name for derivatives of cellulose: Cellofas A is methylethylcellulose, Cellofas B is sodium carboxymethylcellulose.

Cellophane or glass noodles Also known as bean thread noodles, these are made from mung bean flour. They are usually softened by soaking in hot water for 10 -15 minutes before cooking with other ingredients.

Cellophane Trade name for the first of the transparent, non-porous films, made from wood pulp (cellulose) (1925). Still widely used for wrapping foods and other commodities.

Cellulase An enzyme that hydroiyses cellulose to its constituent monosaccharide (glucose) and disaccharide (cellobiose) units. It is present in the digestive juices of some wood-boring insects and in various micro-organisms, but not in mammals.

Cellulose A polysaccharide of glucose units which is not hydrolysed by mammalian digestive enzymes. It is the main component of plant cell walls, but does not occur in animal tissues. It is digested by the bacterial enzyme cellulase, and hence only ruminants and animals that have a large intestine have an adequate population of intestinal bacteria to permit them to digest cellulose to any significant extent. There is little digestion of cellulose in the human large intestine; nevertheless, it serves a valuable purpose in providing bulk to the intestinal contents, and is one of the major components of dietary fibre or non-starch polysaccharides.

Cellulose derivatives A number of chemically modified forms of cellulose are used in food processing for their special properties, including:

1. Carboxymethylcellulose (E-466), which is prepared from the pure cellulose of cotton or wood. It absorbs up to fifty times its own weight of water to form a stable colloidal mass. It is used, together with stabilizers, as a whipping agent, in ice-cream, confectionery, jellies, etc., and as an inert filler in 'slimming aids'.

2. Methylcellulose (E-461), which differs from carboxymethylcellulose (and other gums) since its viscosity increases rather than decreases with increasing temperature. Hence it is soluble in cold water and forms a gel on heating. It is used

as a thickener and emulsifier, and in foods formulated to be low in gluten.

3. Other cellulose derivatives used as emulsifiers and stabilizers are hydroxypropylcellulose (E-463), hydroxypropyl-methylcellulose (E-464), and ethyl-methylcellulose (E-465).

Celtuce Stem lettuce, Lactuca sativa; enlarged stem eaten raw or cooked, with a flavour between celery and lettuce; the leaves are not palatable.

Centre for Disease Control and Prevention (CDC) The CDC, composed of 11 Centres, Institutes and Offices, aims to promote health and quality of life by preventing and controlling disease, injury and disability.

Central amplification Changes that occur in the central nervous system (brain and spinal cord) that affect cell transmitters and receptors, thereby increasing the excitability of neurons and resulting in heightened perception of signals from the gastrointestinal tract.

Centrifuge A machine that exerts a force many thousand times that of gravity, by spinning. Commonly used to clarify liquids by settling the heavier solids in a few minutes, a process that might take several days under gravity. Liquids of different density can also be separated by centrifugation, e.g. cream from milk.

Ceplapro A protein-rich baby food (18-20% protein) in a granular form, made from degerminated maize flour, wheat, defatted soya flour, and skim milk powder, with added vitamins and minerals.

Cereal Any grain or edible seed of the grass family which may be used as food; e.g. wheat, rice, oats, barley, rye, maize, and millet. Collectively known as corn in the UK, although in the USA corn is specifically maize. Cereals provide the largest single foodstuff in almost all diets; in some less-developed countries up to 90% of the total diet may be cereal, and in the UK bread and flour provide 25-30% of the total energy and protein of the average diet. See also flour, extraction rate.

Cerebral palsy A motor nerve disorder caused by injury to the central nervous system; symptoms depend on the area of the brain involved and the severity of the damage; major types include spastic, athetoid and ataxic quadriplegia or diplegia

Cerebrosides Complex lipids, containing the carbohydrate galactose, which is important in nerve membranes and the myelin sheath of nerves.

Ceruloplasmin A copper-containing protein in blood plasma, the main circulating form of copper in the body.

Ceviche A South American dish of raw white fish, marinated and effectively 'cooked' in lemon or lime juice - the acid in the juices breaks down the fish and after a few hours it will eventually become opaque like ordinary cooked fish. It's typically served with sweet limes, raw onion rings, tomatoes and boiled sweet corn.

Chafing dish The chafing dish is a metal pan, with a water basin, which is heated by an alcohol lamp and used for cooking at the table.

Chai tea Chai is the word used for tea in many parts of the world. It is a fragrant milk tea that is growing more popular in the U.S. The tea originated in India, where those in the cooler regions add spices to their tea (not only for flavoring but to induce heat in the body). It is a centuries-old beverage, which has played an important role in many cultures. It's generally made up of rich black tea, milk, a combination of various spices, and a sweetener. The spices used vary from region to region. The most common are cardamom, cinnamon, ginger, cloves, and pepper. It can be served following a meal or anytime. Though some Americans serve Chai tea chilled or even iced, Bengal custom is to serve Chai tea hot.

Chakalaka A very hot and spicy South African cooked vegetable relish/sauce/salad (in some ways it is like a Mexican salsa) that usually includes tomatoes, garlic, chile peppers, grated carrots, and grated cabbage with beans or diced cauliflower. Preparing chakalaka is very much an individual thing, and depends on what you have available. A traditional dish with the black community that is now popular in the urban areas as well as a side dish at barbeques.

Chalazae Ropey strands of egg white which anchor the yolk in place in the centre of the thick white. They are neither imperfections nor beginning embryos. The more prominent the chalazae, the fresher the egg. Chalazae do not interfere with the cooking or beating of the white and need not be removed, although some cooks like to strain them from stirred custard.

Challenge test Reintroduction of a food previously eliminated from the diet on suspicion that it caused an adverse reaction.

Chambre Red wines brought to room temperature (15-18°C, 59-65°F) before serving.

Champagne Champagne is a sparkling wine. Only wines produced in Champagne, France can legally be called champagne. Otherwise it is called sparkling wine. It is considered the most glamorous of all wines (the name has become synonymous with expensive living).

Champignon French word for an edible mushroom. In Greece, around 400 B.C. Hippocrates makes mention of the delicacy of mushrooms that were consumed by the wealthy. The mushroom was thought to possess divine and magical powers. The first written reference to eating mushrooms is the death of a mother and her three children from mushroom poisoning in about 450 B.C. In ancient Rome, the easiest way to get rid of an enemy was to invite him to a disguised mushroom meal using the deadly mushroom from the Borgia family.

Chanterelle mushrooms These trumpet-shaped mushrooms flourish in the wilderness areas of the Pacific Northwest and a few places on the east coast. The European and Asian varieties are usually about the size of a thumb. But on the west coast, Chanterelles can be larger than a foot wide and heavier than two pounds. They smell a bit like apricots, have a mild, nutty flavor, and a chewy texture.

Chantilly cream Sweetened, vanilla-flavoured, whipped cream used for desserts and puddings. It's sometimes flavoured with liqueur. Chantilly is a medieval French market town just north of Paris, famous for its whipped cream, and there's no shortage of patisseries serving pastries piped full of Chantilly cream!

Chapatti Indian; unleavened whole-grain wheat or millet bread, baked on an ungreased griddle. Phulka are small chapattis; roti are chapattis prepared with maize flour. Two chapattis (60 g) are a source of vitamin B 1 and copper; provide 4.2 g of dietary fibre; if made with added fat contain 8 g of fat; supply 210 kcal; if made without added fat contain 0.6 g of fat; supply 130 kcal.

Chapon A small piece from end of French loaf, a slice, or a cube of bread that has been rubbed over with a clove of garlic, first dipped in salt. Placed in bottom of salad bowl before arranging salad. A chapon is often used in vegetable salads and gives an agreeable additional flavor.

Chaptalization Addition of sugar to grape must during fermentation to increase the alcohol content of the final wine.

Charcoal Finely divided carbon, obtained by heating bones (bone charcoal) or wood in a closed retort to carbonize the organic matter. Used to purify solutions because it will absorb colouring matter and other impurities; wood charcoal is commonly used as a fuel for barbecues.

Charcuterie Charcuterie is a generic term for the products traditionally sold by charcutiers (pork butchers), and includes all products based on pork meat or offal, including cured and cooked meats, fresh and smoked sausages, pβtts, black puddings and salamis. It also refers to the shop itself that sells these kinds of products. Order charcuterie in a restaurant and you'll be served a platter of cuts of meats and sausages prepared in various ways.

Chardonnay One of the nine 'classic' grape varieties used for wine making, widely grown throughout the world. Chardonnay wines are among the white wines best adapted to maturing in oak barrels.

Charlotte 1. Small, waxy potato with a pale yellow skin and buttery yellow flesh. Excellent in salads, eaten hot or cold, and in Spanish omelettes. Also good for boiling, pan-frying and using in gratins.

2. A pudding made in a mould lined with sponge fingers or bread slices. Apple charlotte is probably the best-known example. Charlottes can be baked or unbaked.

Charlotte Malakoff It has a lining of ladyfingers and a centre filling of a souffle mixture of cream, butter, sugar, a liqueur, chopped almonds, and whipped cream. It is decorated with strawberries.

Charlotte russe A cake is which the mold is lined with sponge fingers and custard replaces the apples. It is served cold with cream.

Charqui South American (especially Brazilian); dried meat, normally prepared from beef, but may also be made from sheep, llama, and alpaca in Peru. Strips of meat cut lengthways and pressed after salting, then air-dried. The final form is flat, thin, flaky sheets, so differing from the long strips of biltong. Also called jerky.

Chasseur sauce Chasseur is French for hunter. It is a hunter-style brown sauce consisting of mushrooms, shallots, and white wine (sometimes tomatoes and parsley). It is most often served with game and other meats.

Chat/chaat/chatt The word literally means, "to lick" in Hindu. Chaat belongs to the traditional Hindu cuisine. In India, chaat refers to both a spice blend and a cold, spicy salad-like appetizer or snack that uses the spice blend. It can be made with chopped vegetables or fruits, or both. Indian Chaat is usually vegetarian. Chat is considered a "street-corner food" in India. Today there isn't a town in India where one would not find some form of Chaat. It is tasty, pungent and really spicy, traditionally eaten from roadside stalls in banana leaves or even newspaper. Different regions of India have their different chats. A supplier of chaat is called a "chaatwallah."

Chateaubriand It is a recipe, not a cut of meat. The choice (centre section or eye) of the beef tenderloin is generally broiled or grilled and served with a sauce. There is generally sufficient meat for two people and traditionally the fillet is cut at the table.

Chaurice This is a Creole pork sausage that is a local favourite in Louisiana. The term is similar to the Spanish "chorizo." It is an old local favourite dating back to the 19th Century, but isn't as easy to find as it once was. It would seem to have come to Louisiana with the Spanish, where it was adapted to local custom and ingredients.

Chayote The chayote is a pear-shaped member of the gourd family. Also called vegetable pear, mirliton (southern United States), choko (Australia and New Zealand) Several varieties of chayote exist, but the commonly available one has thick apple-green skin and generally weighs 1/2 to 1 pound. Its crisp flesh is mild in flavor, falling somewhere between cucumber and summer squash. It is prominent in the cuisine of Mexico, and today is a mainstay in the cuisines of all of South and Central America, as well as the West Indies, Africa, India, Indonesia, Australia, and New Zealand. In the United States, it's grown in the Southwest, in Louisiana and in Florida. Though the chayote can be prepared many ways, it is always cooked, never eaten raw (even if used in salad). Its thick skin is edible, but many cooks prefer to remove it (it can be chewy unless used in a long cooking preparation). The large seed is also edible (many of the vegetable's proponents insisting that the seed is the best part).

Cheddar cheese Cheddar, the most widely imitated cheese in the world. Mature English Farmhouse Cheddar is aged over nine months. Cheddar cheese stands by itself at the end of the meal, as a companion to well-aged Burgundy. It is also marvelous shredded over salads, melted over omelets, served with fruit pies and cobblers, or nibbled with crusty rye bread and a hearty beer.

Cheddar Hard cheese dating from sixteenth century prepared by a particular method (cheddaring); originally from the Cheddar area of Somerset, England; matured for several months or even years. Red Cheddar is coloured with annatto; fat-reduced versions are now made. A 30-g portion is a rich source of vitamin B12, a source of protein, niacin, and vitamin A; contains 10 g of fat, 200 mg of calcium, 200 mg of sodium; supplies 120 kcal.

Cheddaring In the manufacture of cheese, after coagulation of the milk, heating of the curd, and draining, the curds are piled along the floor of the vat, where they consolidate to a rubbery sheet of curd. This is the cheddaring process; for cheeses with a more crumbly texture the curd is not allowed to settle so densely.

Cheese Cheese is a food made from the curds of milk pressed together to form a solid. Through the centuries, cheese has been made from the milk of any milk-producing animal, from the ass to the zebra. Today it is most commonly made from milk of cows, goats, or sheep, with a small fraction from water buffaloes. The differences in cheeses come from the way the curds are drained, cut, flavored, pressed, the bacteria involved, the type and length of curing in caves, cellars, or under refrigeration, and a host of other subtle to severe variations. Generally cheese is grouped into four categories:

Soft cheese These include the fresh, unripened cheeses such as cottage, cream, farmer, or pot cheese that need only a starter, perhaps buttermilk, and a few hours before they're ready to eat. More complex soft cheeses include quickly ripened brie and camembert, as well as those made with added cream, known as double-cremes and triple-cremes; all have thin, white edible rinds with creamy to runny interiors and are ready to eat within a few days or weeks.

Semi-soft cheese With this group are cheeses ripened three ways: bacteria- or yeast-ripened mildly flavored cheeses such as Italian fontina and Danish havarti. Also included are blue-veined cheeses such as gorgonzola, Roquefort, and English Stilton that are ripened by the presence of "penicillium" molds.

Firm cheese Originally termed "farmhouse cheese" but now mostly made in factories, these cheeses are formed into wheels or blocks, usually with a wax coating to seal out molds and external bacteria. This category includes cheddar, edam, gouda, Swiss cheese, jarlsberg, etc. These are generally aged a few weeks to more than a year.

Hard cheese These are the carefully aged cheeses with grainy textures that are primarily intended for grating. These include Asia go, parmesan, and Romano. The aging process takes form one year to over seven years. It is likely that nomadic tribes of Central Asia found animal skin bags a useful way to carry milk on animal backs when on the move. Fermentation of the milk sugars would cause the milk to curdle and the swaying motion would break up the curd to provide a refreshing whey drink. The curds would then be removed, drained and lightly salted to provide a tasty and nourishing high protein food, i.e. a welcome supplement to meat protein. The earliest type was a form of sour milk, which came into being when it was discovered that domesticated animals could be milked. According to legend, cheese was discovered 4,000 years ago when an Arabian merchant journeyed across the desert carrying a supply of milk in a pouch made of a sheep's stomach. The rennet in the lining of the pouch, combined with the heat of the sun, caused the milk to separate into curd and whey. That night he drank the whey and ate the cheese, and thus, so the story goes, cheese was born. The ancient Sumerians knew cheese four thousand years before the birth of Christ. The ancient Greeks credited Aristaeus, a son of Apollo and Cyrene, with its discovery; it is mentioned in the Old Testament. In the Roman era cheese really came into its own. Cheese making was done with skill and knowledge and reached a high standard. By this time the ripening process had been developed and it was known that various treatments and conditions under storage resulted in different flavors and characteristics. Cheese making, thus, gradually evolved from two main streams. The first was the liquid fermented milks such as yogurt, koumiss and kefir. The second through allowing the milk to acidify to form curds and whey. Whey could then be drained either through perforated earthenware bowls or through woven reed baskets or similar material.

The art of cheese making traveled from Asia to Europe and flourished. When the Pilgrims voyaged to America (in 1620), they made sure the Mayflower was stocked with cheese. In 1801, an enterprising cheese maker delivered a mammoth 1,235-pound wheel of cheese to Thomas Jefferson. Intrigued citizens dubbed it the "big cheese," coining the phrase, which has since come to describe someone of importance. Cheese making quickly grew in the New World, but remained a local farm industry until 1851. In that year, the Jesse Williams in Oneida County, New York built the first United States cheese factory. As the U.S. population increased, so did the appetite for cheese. The industry moved westward, centreing on the rich farmlands of Wisconsin, where the American cheese industry really took off. Most Wisconsin farmers believed their survival was tied to cheese. They opened their first cheese factory, Limburger, in 1868.

Cheese curds Cheese curds, a uniquely Wisconsin delicacy, are formed as a by-product of the cheese making process. They are little "nubs" of cheese, which if very fresh, squeak when you bite down on them. Unlike aged cheese, curds lose their desirable qualities if refrigerated or if not eaten within a few days. The squeak disappears and they turn dry and salty. Every restaurant or bar in Wisconsin seems to serve them, as they are listed on most appetizer sections of restaurant menus in the state.

Cheesecake Now days there are hundreds of different cheesecake recipes. The ingredients are what make one cheesecake different from another. The most essential ingredient in any cheesecake is cheese (the most commonly used are cream cheese, Neufchatel, cottage cheese, and ricotta.)

Chef de Partie Also known as a "station chef" or "line cook", is in charge of a particular area of production. In large kitchens, each station chef might have several cooks and/or assistants. In most kitchens however, the station chef is the only worker in that department. Line cooks are often divided into a hierarchy of their own, starting with "First Cook", then "Second Cook", and so on as needed. The Chef de Partie is in charge of any of the following kitchen positions:

Chemical-nutritional composition tables Tables that provide information concerning tha contents of foods in terms od proteins, fats, carboydrates, vitamins and minerals significant to human nutrition.

Chenin blanc A widely produced white wine. It is often used as a blending wine in generic blends and jug wine.

Chenopods Seeds of two species of Chenopodium eaten in the Peruvian Andes: C. quinoa (quinoa) and C. pallidicaule (canihua). Other species of Chenopodium have been considered for poultry feed, including Russian thistle, summer cypress, and garden orache.

Cherimoya The heart-shaped cherimoya is sometimes referred to as a custard apple, which describes its appearance and texture. The taste, however, is uniquely its own. Cherimoya combines the flavors of pineapple, mango, banana, and papaya into a slightly fermented flavor of the tropics. They are available November through April with the largest supply in February and March. Ripe cherimoyas are dull brownish-green in colour and give to pressure when gently squeezed. Eat within a day or two. If fruit is pale green and firm, store at room temperature until slightly soft and then refrigerate, carefully wrapped individually in paper towels, for up to 4 days. Peel fruit with a sharp knife and cut into cubes, discarding the dark black seeds. Add to fruit salads or puree and incorporate into a mousse, custard, or pie filling.

Cherries jubilee It is a dessert that consists of cherries flamed tableside with sugar and Kirsch (cherry brandy) spooned over vanilla ice cream. Cherries Jubilee was created by Chef Auguste Escoffier (1847-1935) in honour of Queen Victoria's Jubilee celebration. There seems to be some conflict as if it was her 1887 Golden Jubilee or her 1897 Diamond Jubilee. Then, as now, the British public delighted in every detail of the Royal Family's life and everyone know that cherries were the queen's favourite fruit. The whole nation celebrated at her Golden Jubilee in 1887. The original dish did not call for ice cream at all. Sweet cherries poached in simple syrup that was slightly thickened, were poured into fireproof dishes, and then warmed brandy was added and set on flame at the moment of serving.

Cherry There are now 250 different kinds, which vary in colour, size, and taste. There are two main groups of cherries, -sweet and sour.

Sweet cherry It is the larger of the two types and they are firm, heart-shaped sweet cherries. The most popular varieties range from the dark red to the black Bing, to the golden red-blushed Royal Ann. Some varieties are Bing cherry, Rainier cherry, Lambert cherry, and Van cherry.

Cherry pepper Also called cherry bombs. They are very thick fleshed and about the size and shape of a small red ripe tomato. They also pack a considerable punch. Heat range is 4-6.

Chervil Chervil is a mild-flavored herb and a member of the parsley family. It has dark green curly leaves that have parsley-like flavor with overtones of anise. Chervil is generally used fresh rather than dried, although it is available in dried form. Though most chervil is cultivated for its leaves alone, the root is edible and was, in fact, enjoyed by early Greeks and Romans. It is one of the main classic ingredients in Fines Herbes (along with chives, parsley and tarragon), a finely chopped herb mixture that should be added to cooked foods shortly before serving because their delicate flavor can be diminished when boiled.

Cheshire cheese Oldest English cheese dating from Roman Britain; crumbly, may be pale yellow, blue-veined, or coloured orange with annatto; matured 2-6 weeks; approx. 30% water, 24% protein, 30% fat. Cheshire cat is an old English measure of cheese.

Chess Pie Chess pies are a Southern specialty that has a simple filling of eggs, sugar, butter, and a small amount of flour. Some recipes include cornmeal and others are made with vinegar. Flavorings, such as vanilla, lemon juice, or chocolate are also added to vary the basic recipe.

Chest sweetbread The thymus of an animal, as distinct from the gut sweetbread (sometimes called simply sweetbread), which is the pancreas.

Chestnut 1. Spanish or sweet chestnut from trees of Castanea spp. Unlike other common nuts it contains very little fat, being largely starch and water. Seven nuts (75 g) provide 5.3 g of dietary fibre and are a good source of copper; a source of vitamins B 1 and B6; contain 2 g of fat of which 18% is saturated; supply 135 kcal (570 kJ).

2. Water chestnut, seeds of Trapa natans, also called caltrops or sinharanut; eaten raw or roasted.

3. Chinese water chestnut, also called matai or waternut; tuber of the sedge, Eleocharis tuberosa or dulcis; white flesh in a black, horned shell.

Chestnut flour Chestnut flour is used primarily in Italian and Hungarian cake and pastry making. The chestnut flour used in Italian cakes and pancakes is made from pulverized raw chestnuts, whereas in Hungary it is made from dried chestnuts.

Chestnut Known as castagne in Italy. There are many varieties of chestnuts and the trees are common throughout Europe, Asia, and the

United States. Chestnuts can be roasted, boiled, pureed, preserved, and candied. Choose unblemished shells that show no sign of drying.

Chevre cheese Chevre is the French word for goat and for the fresh goat's milk cheese. Goat cheeses are not usually aged, so they are fresh and creamy looking with a fairly mild, salty flavor. They are French in origin. This cheese can be molded into any shape. They come plain or coated with herbs and pepper. Used for relishes, appetizers, sauces, and compliments any cheese board.

Chevre The French word for 'goat' has come to be used to refer to all French cheeses made from pasteurised goats' milk. Chθvres can vary in maturity and strength of flavour, and they range in texture from moist and creamy to dry and semi-firm. They come in a variety of shapes including cylinders, discs, cones and pyramids, and are often coated in edible ash or leaves, herbs or pepper.

Chewing gum When Antonio Lopez de Santa Anna, the Mexican leader of the Alamo attack, was in exile on Staten Island, N.Y, in 1869, he brought with him a large lump of chicle, the elastic sap of the sapodilla tree, which Mayan Indians had been chewing for centuries. He hoped that Thomas Adams, an inventor, could refine the chicle for a rubber substitute. Adams experimented with the stuff, but it remained lifeless. By chance, he saw a little girl buying paraffin a "pretty poor gum" at a drug store. Adams asked the druggist if he would be willing to try a new kind of gum. He said yes. Adams rushed home, soaked and kneaded the chicle into small grayish balls. The druggist sold all of them the next day. With $55, Adams went into business making Adams New York Gum #1 and set the world to chewing and snapping!

Chianti A classic dry red wine of Tuscany. Often called "pizza wine" as it is often served in wicker-wrapped bottles.

Chicago Deep-Dish Pizza Chicago deep-dish pizza is different from the regular thin crust pizza as it has a thicker crust with more ingredients topping it. It is almost like a casserole on bread crust.

Chicken Domestic fowl, Gallus domesticus. A 150-g portion is a rich source of protein and niacin; a good source of copper and selenium; a source of iron and vitamins B1, B2, and B6. There are differences between the white (breast) and dark (leg) meat, the former being lower in fat but also lower in iron and vitamin B2. Of a 150-g portion of boiled chicken, the white meat supplies 0.9 mg of iron, 0.09 mg of vitamin B1, 0.18 mg of vitamin B2, 7.5 g of fat of which one-third is saturated; the dark meat supplies 3.8 mg of iron, 0.1 mg of vitamin B1, 0.4 mg of vitamin B2, 15 g of fat of which one-third is saturated.

Chicken A' La King This is a rich chicken dish that uses lots of cream with pimentos and sherry. It is served either on hot buttered toast, pastry shells, or in a nest of noodles.

Chicken Booyah A super "stick to your ribs" soup-stew made with chicken. While chicken soup is universal and variations of this dish can be found in many cultures world wide, northeastern Wisconsin is the only place in the world where Chicken Booyah is found. It is a favourite at the many festivals, church picnics, bazaars, and any other large gathering in the northeast part of Wisconsin. Restaurants have their own special recipe. Booyah is lovingly called "Belgian Penicillin." It is believed that the word "Booyah" comes from the word "bouillon."

Chicken Cacciatora Cacciatore means "hunter's style." See cacciatore. This dish developed in central Italy and has many variations. It is considered a country-style dish in which chicken pieces are simmered together with tomatoes and mushrooms. The dish originated in the Renaissance period (1450-1600) when the only people who could afford to enjoy poultry and the sport of hunting were the well to do, This dish developed in central Italy and has many variations.

Chicken Divan A chicken casserole dish with broccoli and mornay or hollandaise sauce.

Chicken Kiev Also called Tsiplenokovo Po-Kievski. A boned and flattened chicken breast that is then rolled around a chilled piece of herbed butter. It is then breaded and fried. This poultry dish is also called "Chicken Supreme."

Chicken Marengo Originally made with crayfish and chicken. Today, the crayfish is usually left out. Chicken Marengo today is chicken cut into pieces, browned in oil, and then cooked slowly with peeled tomatoes, crushed garlic, parsley, white wine and cognac, seasoned with crushed pepper and served with fried eggs on the side (with or without crayfish, also on the side) and toast or croutons, doubling as Dunand's army bread.

Chicken Rochambeau This Louisiana Creole dish is half a chicken (breast, leg, thigh), which is boned and not skinned. It's grilled, then served as a layered dish -first a slice of baked ham, then the brown Rochambeau sauce (chicken stock and brown sugar), then the chicken is covered with a Bıarnaise sauce. Antoine's restaurant in New Orleans, Louisiana is famous for this chicken dish.

Chicken-Fried Steak It is also known as Country-Fried Steak and affectionately called "CFS" by Texans. There is no chicken in Chicken-Fried Steak. It is tenderized round steak (a cheap and tough piece of beef) made like fried chicken with a milk gravy made from the drippings left in the pan. Although not official, the dish is considered the state dish of Texas. According to a Texas Restaurant Associate, it is estimated that 800,000 orders of Chicken-Fried Steak are served in Texas every day, not counting any prepared at home. Every city, town, and village in Texas takes prides in their CFS. Some, admittedly, are better than others. Texans have a unique way of rating restaurants that serve CFS. The restaurants are rated by the number of pickup trucks that is parked out in front. Never stop at a one pickup place, as the steak will have been frozen and factory breaded. A two and three pickup restaurant is not much better. A four and five pickup place is a must stop restaurants, as the CFS will be fresh and tender with good sopping gravy.

Chickpea A small legume that was first grown in the Levant and ancient Egypt, and is now used in cuisines all around the world. In Indian cookery, finely milled chickpea flour, called gram flour or besan flour, is used to make some kinds of batter.

Chickpeas are a major ingredient in many Middle Eastern dishes, such as hummus (the Arabic word for chickpea), a paste made from chickpeas and tahini (sesame paste) mixed with garlic and lemon, and falafel. In Spain and some parts of the US, chickpeas are known as 'garbanzos'. Chickpeas are usually sold in dried form, whether split or not, or canned, but may also be eaten fresh. If using dried chickpeas, soak them overnight before use.

Chicle The partially evaporated milky latex of the evergreen sapodilla tree (Achra sapota); it contains gutta (which has elastic properties) and resin, together with carbohydrates, waxes, and tannins. The same tree also produces the sapodilla plum.

Chicory A vegetable and/or salad leaf comprising a white bulb of tightly packed elongated cones of overlapping white leaves with pale yellow leaf tips. Although we call it chicory here, it's more commonly known as witloof (meaning white leaf) in Belgium and is called Belgian endive in the US. It's essentially a salad vegetable with a mildly bitter taste, but it can be cooked too. It's particularly good wrapped in ham, covered with a bıchamel sauce and oven baked.

Chiffon cake It is the first really new development in cake making in many years. It uses vegetable oil in place of conventional shortening.

Chiffonade 1. This is a French word, which comes from the word "chiffon" which means, "rag". In culinary terms, a chiffonade describes a way of cutting herbs and lettuces into thin strips or shreds, which look a bit like rags.

2. Chiffonade is also a dish consisting of a mixture of green vegetables (such as spinach,

lettuce, and sorrel) which are shredded or cut finely into ribbons (sometimes melted butter is added). It is used to form a bed for a dish such as egg mayonnaise or as a garnish for soups.

Child and Adult Care Food Program (CACFP) This USDA program provides subsidized meals to children and adults cared for by participating child care centres, family child care homes, and adult day care centres.

Child nutrition act The Child Nutrition Act and the National School Lunch Act are the two pieces of authorizing legislation for the child nutrition and WIC programs. These laws were most recently reauthorized through 2009 by the Child Nutrition and WIC Reauthorization Act of 2004, P.L. 108-265.

Child nutrition programs The five USDA domestic food assistance programs that primarily serve the nutritional needs of children. These programs include: the National School Lunch Program, School Breakfast Program, Summer Food Service Program, Child and Adult Care Food Program, and the Special Milk Program.

Chile, chilie, chili pepper Chile peppers are all members of the capsicum family. There are more than 200 varieties available today. They vary in length from 1/2-inch to 12 inches long with the shortest and smallest peppers being the hottest. Always take caution when handling them (wear rubber gloves when seeding a fresh one). Colours range from yellow to green to red to black. The best antidote for a "chile burn" in the mouth is sugar or hard candy. The heat of chiles comes from a compound called capsaicin. It is located in the "ribs" of the chile. Seeds do contain some heat, but not at the same intensity as the ribs. Chiles are called peppers, but are not related to black pepper. Botanically, they are berries and horticulturally, they are fruits. When fresh, we use them as vegetables. When dried, we use them as spices. Scoville unit is the thermometer of the chile business. Established by Wilbur Scoville, these are the units of heat of a chile's burn. A habanero is considered 100 times hotter than a jalapeno! Units rank from 0 to 300,000.

Chiles Relleno A Mexican and Southwest dish of stuffed chile peppers.

Chilli Chilli peppers are much smaller than sweet peppers (see capsicum) and can be green, yellow, orange, red or black. Don't be fooled by their small size - they pack a fiery punch! There are more than 200 known varieties and they differ greatly in size, colour and level of hotness. The seeds and flesh of the chilli can both be eaten; removing the seeds reduces the heat of the chilli. It's very important to avoid contact with the eyes or any sensitive skin - even washing your hands after preparing chillies may not be enough to remove all the capsaicin, the volatile oil in the fruit that gives it its hot taste. There's an official heat scale for chillies known as the Scoville scale, developed by Wilbur Scoville in 1912. To give you an idea of the range of heat in various chillies, a sweet pepper scores 0 on the scale, Jalapeño and chipotle chillies score anything between 2,500 to 10,000 and habanero and Scotch bonnet score 80,000 to 300,000 plus! Types of chilli you should be able to find quite easily include bird's-eye, which is frequently used in Asian cooking - it's hot but usually bearable for most tastes; habanero, small and blow-your-head-off hot with a smoked, dried version called chipotle; and Scotch bonnet which is yellow, green or red and lethally hot. You can buy chillies fresh, dried (whole chilli flakes or chillies ground into powder), preserved in oil or made into condiments such as Tabasco. Fresh chillies sold in packets in supermarkets usually have a heat scale on them which is helpful. Mild chillies can be stuffed in the same way you would a sweet pepper. Poblano chillies are used in the Mexican speciality 'chiles rellenos' - stuffed with cheese and fried.

Chillies are an essential part of Mexican and Tex-Mex dishes, North African cooking (harissa is a thick, fiery paste made from chillies and spices) and many Asian dishes. They're the basis of a good salsa and can be combined with herbs and other spices to form a dry rub for meat or fish.

Chillproofing A treatment to prevent the development of haziness or cloudiness due to precipitation of proteins when beer is chilled. Treatments include the addition of tannins to precipitate proteins, materials such as bentonite to adsorb them and proteolytic enzymes to hydrolyse them.

Chimichanga A burrito prepared with your choice of meat, vegetables, and spices that are rolled up to form a large spring roll, either deep fried or grilled deep-fried, and served on a bed of lettuce with cheese and mild sauce. The chimichanga or "chimi" is the quintessential Tucson, Arizona food item, which has achieved a cult status in that city. The residents of Tucson take their "chimis" very seriously and would prefer to pay more money so as not to be served a smaller one with fewer ingredients. They love the large, gigantic ones. Every restaurant and Mom and Pop eatery has his or her own version of this favourite dish. Culinary historians argue about exactly where in Tucson chimichangas were invented. Several restaurants claim the bragging rights of being the first to serve one. The strongest claim comes from Tucson's El Charro Cake, the oldest Mexican restaurant in Tucson. Family legend says that, Monica Flin, who started the restaurant in 1922, cussed in the kitchen when a burrito flipped into the deep fryer. As young nieces and nephews were in the kitchen with her, she hanged the swear word to chimichanga, the Spanish equivalent of "thingamagig."

Chine A joint of meat containing the whole or part of the backbone of the animal. See also chining.

Chinese eggs Known as pidan, houeidan, and dsaoudan, depending on variations in the method of preparation. Prepared by covering fresh duck eggs with a mixture of caustic soda, burnt straw ash, and slaked lime, then storing for several months (they are sometimes referred to as 'hundred year old eggs'). The white and yolk coagulate and become discoloured, with partial decomposition of the protein and phospholipids.

Chinese gooseberry It is now called kiwi fruit and it is a native of China. It was introduced into New .Zealand in 1906 and has been commercially cultivated there ever since. Since Chinese gooseberry is a rather un-enchanting name, they decided to rename the fruit "kiwi." This name not only identifies New Zealand but also describes the tiny New Zealand Kiwi bird.

Chinese parsley Chinese parsley is also called coriander, cilantro, and dhania (fresh coriander in India). Cilantro is the fresh green leaves and stems of the herb coriander. It can be used to flavor Chinese and Indian recipes and can also be used in Mexican and southwestern cooking.

Chinese restaurant syndrome Flushing, palpitations, numbness associated at one time with the consumption of monosodium glutamate, and then with histamine, but the cause of these symptoms after eating various foods is not known.

Chining To sever the rib bones from the backbone by sawing through the ribs close to the spine.

Chinois A fine metal conical strainer with a long handle, used for straining soups and sauces to give them a professional sheen and finish, as well as sorting out any lumps! It has a finer mesh than a standard sieve.

Chipotle A mild, dried chilli with a deep smoky flavour, commonly used in Mexican cooking and in the cooking of the American south-west. It's frequently used in commercially produced chilli sauces.

Chipotle chile A chipotle pepper is simply a smoked jalapeno pepper. These chilies are usually a dull tan to coffee colour and measure approximately 2 to 4 inches in length and about an inch wide. It is sold either dried or canned with adobo sauce. Most of the natural heat of the jalapeno is retained in the process. Chipotle peppers are very hot, and they can easily over power dishes and recipes. Chipotles are available dried whole, powdered, pickled, and canned in Adobo sauce.

Chips Chipped potatoes; pieces of potato deep fried in fat or oil. Known in French as pommes frites or just frites; in the USApotato crisps are known as chips, and chips are called French fries or just fries. A 200-g portion is a rich source of vitamins C and B1; a source of protein, niacin, and iron; fat content depends on the size of the chip and the process: commonly about 25 g, but can be 40 g in fine-cut chips and as little as 8 g in frozen, oven-baked chips. Degree of saturation of the fat depends on the frying oil: 10% in blended oils, and up to 60% in dripping. A 200-g portion with an average of 25 g of fat supplies 500 kcal (2100 kJ); with 40 g of fat, supplies 700 kcal (2900 kJ); low-fat, oven-baked supplies 300 kcal.

Chirga Indian; skinned chicken rubbed with cayenne, paprika, and lime juice, coated with a sauce of ginger, onion, and pimiento in yoghurt, then roasted, basting with ghee. It has a red colour.

Chitin The organic matrix of the hard parts of the exoskeleton of insects and crustaceans, and present in small amounts in mushrooms. It is an insoluble and indigestible non-starch polysaccharide, similar to cellulose, but composed of N-acetylglucosamine units rather than glucose. Partial deacetylation results in the formation of chitosans, which are used as protein-flocculating agents.

Chitterlings/chitlins Chitterlings are the middle section or small intestines of animals (hot intestines or guts). Chitterlings are the more formal name, but most people call them chitlins. Some people turn up their noses at the mention of chitlins, as they are a food that you either love or hate. Others leave the house while they are cooking, driven away by their earthly odor. The volume sold for New Year's dinners, with Christmas and Thanksgiving not far behind, attests to chitlins' popularity in the United States. In colonial slave days of the sold South of the United States, December was the time when the hogs were slaughtered. The hams and all the better cuts went to the plantation owners, while the leftovers or garbage (chitterlings) were given to the slaves. Because of the West African traditional of cooking all edible part of plants and animals, these foods helped the slaves survive in the United States. Animal innards have long been treasured foods around the world Scotland has their national dish of haggis (sheep's stomach stuffed with animal's minced heart, liver, and lungs); Throughout Europe, tripe 9cow or ox stomach) is popular, and French chefs in upscale restaurants serve dishes based on cow's brains and kidneys.

Chive Chives are a member of the onion family. They are used to delicately flavor soups, salads, dips, cheeses, eggs, sauces, and dressings. They make an eye-catching garnish when sprinkled on top of a favourite recipe. Their lavender flowers are an attractive and tasty addition to salads. Chives are almost always used fresh or added to hot foods at the last minute so they retain their flavor. Chives have been respected for their culinary versatility for more than 3000 years. In Ancient China, raw chives were prescribed to control internal bleeding. But when chives made their way to Europe, herbalists had a different opinion. They warned that eating the herb raw would induce evil vapors in the brain. Despite the admonishments, chives became everyday sights in European households; bunches of them were hung in houses to ward off evil spirits. Gypsies used chives for their fortune-telling rituals and also hung them from the ceiling to drive away diseases and evil spirits.

Chloride The major anion (negatively charged substance) in the blood and extracellular fluid (the body fluid that lies outside cells). Blood and other body fluids have almost the same concentration of chloride ion as sea water. The balance of chloride ion (Cl^-) is closely regulated by the body.

Chlorophyll The green pigment of plant materials which is responsible for the trapping of light energy for photosynthesis, the formation of carbohydrates from carbon dioxide and water. Both [alpha]- and [beta]-chlorophylls occur in leaves, together with the carioteniods xanthophyll and carotene. Chlorophyll has no nutritional value, although it does contain magnesium as part of its molecule, and although it is used in breath-fresheners and toothpaste, there is no evidence that it has any useful action.

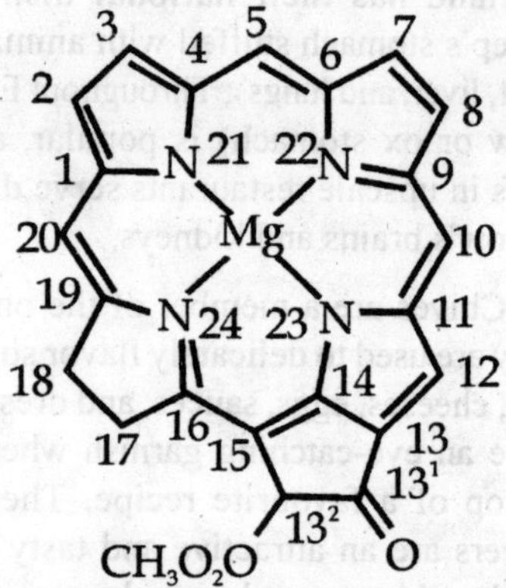

Fig. Structure of Chlorophyll

Chocolate A delicate tree, cacao, it is only grown in rain forests in the tropics, usually on large plantations, where it must be protected from wind and intense sunlight. The cacao bean is harvested twice a year.

Bittersweet chocolate Still dark, but a little sweeter than unsweetened. Bittersweet has become the sophisticated choice of chefs.

Milk chocolate or sweet chocolate Candy bar chocolate. Chocolate to which whole and/or skim milk powder has been added. Rarely used in cooking because the protein in the added milk solids interferes with the texture of the baked products.

Semisweet chocolate Slightly sweetened during processing and most often used in frostings, sauces, fillings, and mousses. They are interchangeable in most recipes. The favourite of most home bakers.

German chocolate Dark, but sweeter than semisweet. German chocolate is the predecessor to bittersweet. It has no connection to Germany; a man named German developed it.

Unsweetened chocolate It is also called baking chocolate or plain chocolate. This is the most common type used in baking and is the only true baking chocolate.

White chocolate According to the FDA, "white chocolate" cannot legally be called chocolate because it contains no cocoa powder, a component of chocolate. True chocolate contains pulverized roasted cocoa bean, consisting of cocoa butter and cocoa solids. White chocolate contains no cocoa solids and thus technically is white confectionery coating. Beware—some white confectionery coatings don't even contain cocoa butter. Even in "real" white chocolate the chocolate flavor is subtle at best, being to real chocolate what white soul is to soul.

Chocolate chip cookie Today the chocolate chip cookie remains a favourite choice among cookie connoisseurs. The term "toll house" has become a part of the American language.

Chocolate chips In 1939, Nestle created the convenient, ready-to-use chocolate pieces, introducing chocolate chips. In the 1940s, Mrs. Wakefield sold all legal rights to the use of the Toll House trademark to Nestle. In 1983, the Nestle Company lost its exclusive rights to the trademark in federal court. Toll house is now a descriptive term for a cookie. See chocolate chip cookie.

Chocolate, drinking Partially solubilized cocoa powder for preparation of a chocolate-flavoured milk drink, containing about 75% sucrose.

Cholagogue A substance that stimulates the secretion of bile from the gall bladder into the duodenum.

Cholent Cholent is traditional Jewish cuisine served on the Sabbath. Whether the hamin of Sephardic communities, the cholent of Ashkenazic ones, or a fusion of the two, it is still favoured by many for Shabbat, particularly on a cold winter day. It was born of Orthodox Jewish observance of the Sabbath, when fires could not be kindled. Instead, families would either leave a real low oven going at home or take their pots to the village baker and let the food cook overnight. Some contend that every slow-cooking dish made with beans derives from this Jewish technique. There is no doubt that, in Hungary, it evolved into shalet, one of the national dishes, while the Pilgrims, after spending time with Sephardic Jews in Holland, adopted it prior to sailing to the New World. The substitutions they later had to make for some ingredients resulted in Boston baked beans. The origin of cholent is likely in the pre-Inquisition Sephardic kitchen. From there, it probably traveled to Alsace, where it is believed to have been called chault-lent, Old French for hot and slow. When it was then brought to Germany and Eastern Europe, it took on the basic composition, which characterizes it today.

Cholesterol A fat-like substance that is made by the body and is found naturally in animal foods such as meat, fish, poultry, eggs, and dairy products. Foods high in cholesterol include liver and organ meats, egg yolks, and dairy fats. Cholesterol is carried in the blood. When cholesterol levels are too high, some of the cholesterol is deposited on the walls of the blood vessels. Over time, the deposits can build up causing the blood vessels to narrow and blood flow to decrease. The cholesterol in food, like saturated fat, tends to raise blood cholesterol, which increases the risk for heart disease. Total blood cholesterol levels above 240 mg/dl are considered high. Levels between 200-239 mg/dl are considered borderline high. Levels under 200 mg/dl are considered desirable.

Choline A derivative of the amino acid serine, formed in the body; an important component of cell membranes. Phosphatidylcholine is also known as lecithine, and preparations of mixed phospholipids rich in phosphatidylcholine are generally called lecithin, although they also contain other phospholipids; lecithin from peanuts and soya beans is widely used as an emulsifying agent (E-322). Choline released from membrane phospholipids is important for the formation of the neurotransmitter acetylcholine, and choline is also important in the metabolism of methyl groups.

Chondroitin A polysaccharide, classified as a mucopolysaccharide, a polymer of galactosamine and glucuronic acid. Chondroitin sulphate is a component of cartilage and the organic matrix of bone.

Chop To cut food into irregular pieces. The size is specified if it is critical to the outcome of the recipe.

Chop Suey Chop Suey is the English pronunciation of the Cantonese words tsap seui (tsa-sui in Mandarin), which means, "mixed pieces." It is a Chinese-American dish consisting of bits of meat or chicken, bean sprouts, onions, mushrooms, etc., cooked in its own juices and served with rice. Most Chinese are not fond of Chop Suey as it is mainly popular with non Chinese-Americans. According to the Chinese-Americans, its presence on a restaurant's menu is often times a harbinger of bad food to come. It is only served in Chinese restaurants that cater to American customers. An American dish that Chinese immigrants in the 1860s, who were untrained as cooks, created out of meat and vegetables fried together in their own juices and served over rice. In the 1860s, a pattern of discrimination emerged that prevented the Chinese from working their own gold mining claims, causing them to take work as laborers and cooks for the Transcontinental Railway. It was this Chinese influence that gave us the totally American Chop Suey, as these dishes were created to feed the workers with what food was on hand. Constrained by the lack of Asian vegetables, and trying to produce a Chinese dish palatable to Westerners, the cook stir-fried whatever vegetables were handy, thus Chop Suey is a mixture of odds and ends of large pieces of vegetables and meat. After World War II, Chop Suey became as American as apple pie to the non-Chinese population.

Chopsticks Eating utensils, about eight inches long, rectangular at the top and tapered at the eating ends. Today, chopsticks are used in Japan, Korea, and Vietnam, as well as China, making them the world's second-most popular method of conveying food to mouth, the most popular being the fingers. Chopsticks are never made of metal because metal may react with the acids found in food and taint its taste. Usually made out of wood, some of the more fancy ones are intricately carved out of bone or ivory. Bamboo is used also. It is not known when chopsticks first began to be used, although it is fairly certain that they were invented in China, where they have been traced back at least as far as the 3rd century BC. Knives, with all their associations with war and death, were not brought to the dinner table, as they were in the West.

Chinese chopsticks In China, chopsticks are usually made of bamboo or other wood. Chinese chopsticks were once referred to as chu, meaning, "help in eating." Today, they are called k'uai-tzu, meaning "something fast." This phrase is said to have originated among boatmen, who renamed the utensils, originally called chu, which means, "help," because the word sounded so much like their word for a slow or becalmed ship. This struck them as particularly inappropriate for such an efficient eating tool. The word with which we are all familiar came into being during the 19th century, when traders into Pidgin English translated Chinese words. The word chop means fast, as in the phrase "chop chop!"

Japanese chopsticks The Japanese word for chopsticks, hashi, means "bridge." Unlike Chinese chopsticks, which are squared-off and blunt at the end, the Japanese utensils are rounded and tapered to a point. It has been suggested that this is in order to facilitate the removal of bones from fish, which makes up a great part of the Japanese diet.

Chopsuey Chinese dishes based on bean sprouts and shredded vegetables, cooked with shredded quick-fried meat, capped with a thin omelette. Not authentically Chinese, but an invention of Chinese restaurateurs in Western countries. Unlike true Chinese food, the flavours of a chopsuey are all mixed together; one translation is 'savoury mess'.

Chorizo A spicy Spanish sausage with new-found popularity. Pronounced 'chor-eetho', it's made all over Spain, as well as in Portugal, where it's spelled 'chouriηo'. There are lots of regional varieties but all are made with pork and flavoured with pimenton (smoked paprika).

There are two main types - an air-dried sausage that can be sliced and eaten like salami and smaller fresh sausages that must be cooked before eating. Chorizo is made in lots of countries, but buy Spanish or Portuguese ones for the real thing.

It's available smoked or unsmoked, mild or spicy and is sometimes flavoured with garlic or wine. Fresh chorizo sausages are delicious fried or grilled and are perfect for barbecuing, or try them skinned and crumbled into stews. Sliced and grilled they're a popular tapas dish.

Serve the air-dried chorizo cut up in salads, or as a starter with other sliced meats, olives and cheeses, or stirred into rice or pasta dishes. Store both types in the fridge wrapped in foil or waxed paper.

Chorley cake Chorley cakes are a British pastry made with dried fruit similar to the cakes and buns common in Banbury, Eccles, Coventry, and Clifton. A typical recipe consists of a pie crust (like pastry cut into small rounds) filled with a mixture of dried currants, peel, brown sugar, butter, and spices such as nutmeg. The pastry is folded, and then rolled out until the fruit begins to show through. They are baked, then eaten fresh with butter, or kept for several days.

Choux pastry A very light, double-cooked pastry usually used for sweets and buns. It's made with plain flour, salt, butter, eggs, milk and a little sugar (if it's being used for a sweet dish). It's used to make profiteroles, eclairs and choux puffs and is the basis of the dramatic dessert gβteau St Honorι - a shortcrust pastry base topped with a ring of choux pastry, then a layer of choux balls filled with whipped cream and glazed with caramel - definite wow factor! It can be used for savoury pastries too, such as gougθre, a large ring of choux flavoured with gruyθre or emmental cheese. Choux pastry has a reputation for being difficult to master, but in fact it's really no bother once you know the technique. A preheated hot oven is essential to raise and set choux and if you take it out of the oven before it's cooked thoroughly (firm to the touch) it will collapse. Filling shouldn't be added until the last possible moment before serving because it will make the choux sag.

Chow An American slang term for food. The named is credited to American servicemen for have to stand in line and wait for their food. The word is thought to be from the Chinese word "ch'ao" meaning "to fry or cook" during 1850s when Chinese laborers worked on the Pacific railroads.

Chow line A line of people waiting for food, as in a cafeteria.

Chow mein A Chinese-American dish consisting of stewed vegetables and meat with fried noodles. It comes from the Mandarin Chinese words ch'ao mien meaning "fried noodles." It is thought that this Chinese dish was brought to America by the Chinese laborers and cooks for the Transcontinental Railway in the 1850s.

Chow-chow Chinese; preserve of ginger, orange peel and fruit in syrup, or a mixed vegetable pickle containing mustard and spices.

Chowder A thick, chunky seafood soup from North America, of which clam chowder is the best known. The word chowder comes from the French 'chaudiθre' - a heavy, three-legged iron cauldron in which fishermen made stews fresh from their day's catch. Chowder is believed to have originated in French Canada and made its way down the coast to New England. As with many classic dishes, opinions on the ingredients and how it should be cooked vary from region to region. New England chowder tends to be made with milk but further down the coast it's made with tomatoes and water and there are all kinds of different additions - potatoes, bacon, clams, cockles, sweet corn. Whatever the variations, chowder is essentially a rich, gutsy soup, often served as a main course.

Chromium A metallic element that is a dietary essential. It forms an organic complex with nicotinic acid, known as the glucose tolerance factor, which facilitates the interaction of insulin with receptors on cell surfaces. Deficiency results in impaired glucose tolerance.

There is little evidence on which to base estimates of requirements; deficiency has been observed at intakes below 6 µg (0.12 µol)day, and the safe and adequate level of intake is estimated at about 25 µg (0.5 gmol)/day. High intakes of inorganic chromium salts (in excess of 1-2 g/day) are associated with kidney and liver damage.

Chromoproteins Proteins conjugated with a metal-containing group, such as the haem group of haemoglobin, which contains iron.

Chromosome One of the threadlike structures that carry the genetic information of living organisms and are found in the nuclei of their cells. Chromosomes consist of a central axis of DNA with associated RNA and proteins.

Chronic disease A disease that persists for a long time. A chronic disease is one lasting 3 months or more, by the definition of the U.S. National Centre for Health Statistics. Chronic diseases generally cannot be prevented by vaccines or cured by medication, nor do they just disappear. Eighty-eight percent of Americans over 65 years of age have at least one chronic health condition (as of 1998). Health damaging behaviours - particularly tobacco use, lack of physical activity, and poor eating habits - are major contributors to the leading chronic diseases.

Chronic malnutrition Deprivational process of long duration, characteristically expressed in insuficient height.

Chronic This important term in medicine comes from the Greek chronos, time and means lasting a long time.

Chuck and blade This is a cut of beef from the shoulder. Because it's a part that has worked hard during the animal's life, this is one of the tougher cuts. Although it's less expensive and has lots of flavour, it needs long, gentle cooking. Ideal for casseroles and stews.

Chump A cut of either lamb or pork taken from the lower back. Sold as chops, or with the bone removed as steaks, it's ideal for grilling and barbecues but also delicious if baked slowly in the oven.

Chuno Traditional dried potato prepared in the highlands of Peru and Bolivia. The tubers are crushed, pressed, frozen during the night, then dried in the sunshine during the day, a process of freeze-drying.

Chutney From the Hindi word 'chatni' meaning strong spices, chutney is a preserved or fresh relish made from fruit or vegetables with vinegar, sugar, herbs and spices. British-style chutneys tend to be preserved by being cooked and are usually quite sweet, whereas Indian-style chutneys are fresh (uncooked) and are usually hotter and quite sour. It can range in texture from chunky to smooth, and in degrees of spiciness from mild to hot. Chutney is a delicious accompaniment to curries. The sweeter chutneys also make interesting spreads for bread and are the perfect accompaniment to cheese with their tangy flavour helping to cut through the creaminess of the cheese.

Chylomicron Chylomicrons are large lipoprotein particles (having a diameter of 75 to 1,200nm) that are created by the absorptive cells of the small intestine. Chylomicrons transport exogenous lipids to adipose, cardiac and skeletal tissue where they are broken down by lipoprotein lipase. The chylomicrons are released by exocytosis from enterocytes into lacteals, lymphatic vessels originating in the villi of the small intestine, and are then secreted into the bloodstream at the thoracic duct's connection with the left subclavian vein.

Chymosin In the abomasums of calves and the stomach of human infants which clots milk by precipitation of the casein. There is no evidence that it plays any part in digestion in the adult. Also known as rennin; however, to avoid confusion with the kidney enzyme renin the name rennin should be replaced by chymosin. Biosynthetic chymosin is used in cheese making (vegetable rennet).

Ciabatta Ciabatta means 'slipper' in Italian and describes the appearance of this oval, flattish yeast bread with an open texture and a crisp, floury crust. It's flavoured with olive oil and is often used as the base for bruschetta. Slice it at an angle and serve with olive oil, salt and freshly ground black pepper for dipping or make sandwiches filled with Italian meats, cheese and tomatoes. It's best eaten on the day of purchase but it does keep for a couple of days in a bread bin or can be frozen for a couple of months.

Cider Cider is fermented apple juice that is made by pressing the juice from fruit. Although apples are the most common fruit from which cider is made, pears and sweet cherries are often pressed for cider as well. It can be drunk straight or diluted with water.

Ciguatera Poisoning from eating fish feeding in the region of coral reefs in the Caribbean and the Indian and Pacific Oceans. The species of fish are normally edible, and appear to derive the toxins, ciguatoxins, from their diet. Reported in seafarers' tales in the sixteenth century.

Cilantro Cilantro is the Spanish word for coriander leaves. It is also sometimes called Chinese or Mexican parsley. Technically, coriander refers to the entire plant. It is a member of the carrot family. Chopped fresh leaves are widely used in Mexican and Tex-Mex cooking, where they are combined with chiles and added to salsas, guacamoles, and seasoned rice dishes. Most people either love it or hate it. Taste experts aren't sure why, but for some people the smell of fresh coriander is fetid and the taste soapy. In other words, while most people love coriander, for some people, coriander just doesn't taste good. When purchasing, look for leaves that are tender, aromatic, and very green. If it has no aroma, it will have no flavor. Avoid wilted bunches with yellowing leaves.

Cincinnati Chili The main differences between Cincinnati and Texas chili is that the Cincinnati Chili calls for some sweet spices and the way you start cooking the meat. The sauce has a thinner consistency that is more like a topping and is mixed with an unusual and secret blend of spices that includes cinnamon, chocolate, or cocoa, allspice, and Worcestershire sauce. Cincinnati Chili is truly the unofficial food of the city of Cincinnati, Ohio, and is the most chili-crazed city in the United States. Cincinnati prides itself on being a true chili capital with over 180 chili parlors.

If you choose "the works," you are eating what they call "Five-Way Chili." Make sure to pile on the toppings that is what sets it apart from any other chili dish. To test a restaurant for authenticity, ask for a Four-Way. If tney ask you whether you want the bean or onion option, you have a fake Cincinnati Chili as Four-Way comes with onions.

Cinnamon This warm, sweet spice comes from the bark of a tree native to Sri Lanka. The bark is removed, dried and rolled up to make a tube.

Cinnamon is sold dry as sticks and as a powder. You can try to grind your own cinnamon from the bark but it's difficult to get it fine enough. It's best to buy ground cinnamon in small quantities because the freshness and flavour quickly disappear. The warm, sweet flavour of cinnamon is an essential ingredient in many sweet dishes, but it's also used in savoury dishes. It's gorgeous in baked goods, used to flavour buns, cakes, sweet pastries and puddings. Baked apples or apple pies wouldn't be the same without the flavour of cinnamon.

Mexicans used cinnamon to flavour chocolate in cooking and in drinks. Cinnamon bark is used to flavour meat, poultry and vegetable stews and it can be added to spicy marinades or to spice up rice dishes. Break a stick in half and add to a poaching syrup for fruits such as pears, plums and bananas or use it to infuse wine or punch.

Cinsaut A grape variety widely used for wine making, although not one of the classic varieties. The common bulk wine producing grape of southern France. In South Africa it has been crossed with the pinot noir to produce the pinotage grape.

Cioppino It is a fish stew that is considered San Francisco's signature dish. It is a descendant of the various regional fish soups and stews of Italian cooking. The best way to make Cioppino, is as you like it. It can by prepared with as many as a dozen kinds of fish and shellfish. It all depends on what the day's catch is like and what your own personal choice is. The origin of the word is something of a mystery and many historians believe that it is Italian-American for "chip in." It is also believed that the name comes form a Genoese fish stew called cioppin. This fish stew first became popular on the docks of San Francisco's Fisherman's Wharf in the 1930s. It is thought to be the result of Italian fishermen adding something from their day's catch to the communal stew kettle on the wharf. After World War II, Cioppino migrated to the East Coast.

Cirrhosis 1. Cirrhosis is a consequence of chronic liver disease characterized by replacement of liver tissue by fibrotic scar tissue as well as regenerative nodules, leading to progressive loss of liver function. Cirrhosis is most commonly caused by alcoholism and hepatitis C, and was the 12th leading cause of death in the United States in 2000. Ascites is the most common complication of cirrhosis and is associated with a poor quality of life, increased risk of infections, and a poor long term outcome. In advanced stages of cirrhosis, the condition is irreversible and the only option would be a liver transplant.

2. An abnormal liver condition characterized by irreversible scarring of the liver. Alcohol and viral hepatitis B and C are among the many causes of cirrhosis. Cirrhosis can cause yellowing of the skin (jaundice), itching, and

fatigue. Diagnosis of cirrhosis can be suggested by physical examination and blood tests, and can be confirmed by liver biopsy in some patients. Complications of cirrhosis include mental confusion, coma, fluid accumulation (ascites), internal bleeding, and kidney failure. Treatment of cirrhosis is designed to limit any further damage to the liver as well as complications. Liver transplantation is becoming an important option for patients with advanced cirrhosis.

Cis A chemical prefix sometimes found on food labels to designate the precise chemical form of polyunsaturated fatty acids (as in the phrase 'cis-cis methylene interrupted'). This is used because some compounds can exist in two forms with the same chemical structure but with different shapes and so have different biological activities. The opposite conformation to cis- is the trans-form.

Cis fatty acid The form of most naturally occurring unsaturated fatty acids, where the hydrogen bonds are on adjacent sides of double bonds, resulting in a bend in the hydrocarbon chain at that point.

Cissa An unnatural desire for foods; alternative words, cittosis, allotriophagy, and pica.

Citral An important constituent of many essential oils, especially lemon. Used as the starting material for the synthesis of ionone (the synthetic perfume with an odour of violets), which is an intermediate in the chemical synthesis of retinol.

Citrange An American citrus fruit resulting from a cross between the ordinary orange and the trifoliate orange, Poncirus trifoliata. citric acid An organic acid (chemically a tricarboxylic acid) which is widely distributed in plant and animal tissues; it is an important metabolic intermediate, and yields 2.47 kcal (10.9 kJ)/g. It is used as a flavouring and acidifying agent (E-330), and its salts (citrates) are used as acidity regulators (E-331, 332, 333). Commercially it is either prepared by the fermentation of sugars by the mould Aspergillus niger or extracted from citrus fruits (lemon juice contains 5-8% citric acid).

Citranin A flavonone glycoside from the peel of immature Ponderosa lemons; see flavonoids.

Citrin A mixture of two flavonones found in citrus pith, hesperidin and eriodictin. A constituent of what is sometimes called vitamin P.

Citron 1. Citron is a semi-tropical citrus fruit like a lemon, but larger and less acidic. It grows as an irregular, open-headed shrub or small tree with large, light green leaves. The flowers are purple on the outside and are followed by large, oblong or ellipsoid fruits. The peel is very thick and is rough and yellow on the outside and white inside. They were originally grown in Europe out of interest for its fragrant fruits, but later, the white pulp was used raw, being served as a salad or with fish. A method of candying the peel was developed and candied peel is now the main Citron product. This plant is never eaten raw but is harvested for usage of its peel. The plant is soaked in a brine solution to extract the oil, which is used in liqueurs. The peel is then candied. This product is used in many baking dishes and desserts.

Citronella It is also known as lemongrass. It is a stiff tropical grass that resembles a large fibrous green onion. It is an essential herb in southeast Asian cooking. It adds a lemony flavor to dishes.

Citrovorum factor The name given to a growth factor for the microorganism Leuconostoc citrovorum, now known to be one of the main forms of the vitamin folic acid (chemically formyltetrahydropteroylglutamic acid).

Citroxanthin A yellow carotenoid pigment in orange peel which has vitamin A activity. Also known as mutachrome.

Citrullinaemia A genetic disease affecting the formation of urea, and hence the elimination of end-products of protein metabolism. The defect may be mild, or so severe that affected infants become comatose and may die after a moderately high intake of protein. Treatment is usually by restriction of protein intake and feeding supplements of the. amino acid arginine. Sodium benzoate may be given to increase the excretion of nitrogenous waste as hippuric acid. See also benzoic acid.

Citrulline An amino acid formed as a metabolic intermediate, but not involved in proteins, and of no nutritional importanc.

Citrus fruits Citrus fruits are native to the southern and southeastern mainland of Asia and the bordering Malayan islands. Their flowers smell sweet and they have five petals that are white and some kinds have purple staining the outer surfaces. The fruits are spherical or egg-shaped and have 8-14 juicy sections containing large, white or greenish seed leaves (cotyledons). These trees are cultivated in orchards or groves and in gardens where the climate and soil are suitable and as greenhouse plants. Florida and California produce an abundant supply of Citrus fruits. Citrus trees require a minimum winter temperature of 45-50 degrees. Citrus fruits are native to Southern China and Southeast Asia where they have been cultivated for approximately 4,000 years. In fact, the oldest Oriental literature includes stories about these fruits. The citron was carried to the Middle East sometime between 400 and 600 BC. Arab traders in Asia carried lemons, limes, and oranges to eastern Africa and the Middle East between AD 100 and 700. During the Arab occupation of Spain, citrus fruits arrived in southern Europe. From Europe they were carried to the New World by Christopher Columbus and Portuguese and Spanish explorers and were well known in Florida and Brazil by the 16th century. Superior varieties from Southeast Asia also arrived in Europe with the Portuguese traders in the 16th century

Citrus Genus of trees with fleshy, juicy fruits; there is considerable confusion over the names because of hybridization and mutations. Sweet orange Citrus sinensis; various cultivars including Valencia, Washington navel, Jaffa, Shamouti. Sour, bitter, or Seville orange, C. aurantium, is too bitter to eat and is used for marmalade. Lemon, C. limon. Lime, C. aurantifolia. Citron, C. medica, has thick, white inner skin and is used mainly to make candied peel. Pomelo (shaddock), C. grandis, is the parent of the grapefruit. Grapefruit, C. paradisi, is a hybrid of pomelo and sweet orange. Tangerine, satsuma, mandarin, calamondin, naartje (S. Africa), are small citrus fruits with loose skins. Clementine, a hybrid of tangerine and bitter orange, is sometimes regarded as a variety of tangerine. Mineola is a hybrid of grapefruit and tangerine. Ortanique is a hybrid of orange and tangerine, unique to Jamaica. Citrange is a hybrid of citron and orange. Tangors are hybrids of tangerine and sweet orange (e.g. Variety Temple). Ugli fruit is a hybrid of grapefruit and tangerine. Tangelo is a hybrid of tangerine and pomelo. All are a rich source of vitamin C and contain up to 10% sugars (glucose and fructose).

Cittosis An unnatural desire for foods; alternative words are, cissa, allotriophagy, and pica.

Clabbered milk Unpasteurized milk that has soured naturally, becoming thick and curdy. Clabber cheese is curd or cottage cheese.

Clafoutis French; batter pudding with black cherries or other fruit. claims, misleading descriptions There are no restrictions on the sales of foods so long as they are not harmful and do not transgress the regulations. What is controlled by law is any claim (on the label, leaflets, or in advertisements). It is illegal to claim that a food is capable of preventing, treating, or curing a disease unless it has a specific Product Licence under the Medicines Act. Misleading claims are illegal even if, strictly speaking, they are true.

Clams All clams are mollusks that live in the sediments of bays, estuaries, or the ocean floor. Clams are sold in the shell or shucked. There are three major types of clams.

Soft-shell clams Known as steamers, manninoses, or squirts. They have brittle shells that break easily.

Hard-shell clams Known as quahog, littleneck, cherrystone, and hard clam.

Surf clams These make up the bulk of the commercial catch. They are used for preparing chowders, clam sauces, and fried clam strips.

Clapshot Scottish (Orkney); mashed potato and turnip, seasoned with chives and bacon fat.

Claret Name given in the UK to red wines from the Bordeaux region of France.

Clarete Portuguese, Spanish; light red wines.

Clarification The process of clearing a liquid of suspended particles. It may be carried out by filtration, centrifugation, the addition of enzymes to hydrolyse and solubilize particulate matter (proteolytic or pectolytic enzymes), or the addition of flocculating agents.

Clarified butter This is butter that has had the water, milk solids and salt removed. Butter browns and burns at lower temperatures than many other fats do, but by clarifying it you leave pure butter fat which is more stable and can be cooked at a higher temperature.

Clarified butter also stores better than ordinary butter, for about two months in the fridge. You can make it at home by gently heating butter (cut into smallish pieces) up to boiling point, then allowing it to separate, straining off the pure melted butter. Transfer it to a suitable storage jar, leave to cool then cover and refrigerate. Ghee is a form of clarified butter used in Indian cookery.

Clarify To clear a liquid of all solid particles using a special cooking process. 1. To clarify butter means to melt it and pour off the clear top layer from the milky residue at the bottom of the pan. The resulting clear liquid can be used at a higher cooking temperature and will not go rancid as quickly as unclarified butter.

2. To clarify stock, egg whites and/or eggshells are commonly added and simmered for about 15 minutes. The egg whites attract and trap particles from the liquid. After cooling, strain the mixture through a cloth-lined sieve to remove residue.

3. To clarify rendered fat, add hot water and boil for about 15 minutes. The mixture should then be strained through several layers of cheesecloth and chilled. The resulting layer of fat should be completely clear of residue.

Clay A dried mineral clay under the names of sikor, mithi, pakhuri, and khatta, is sometimes used by Asians as a treatment for indigestion and as a vitamin supplement, but can be toxic since it contains varying amounts of arsenic and lead.

Cleft palate A "hole" in the palate (roof of the mouth) caused by a failure of the palate to close during gestation; surgical repair of the cleft is generally done after one to two years of age

Clementine A citrus fruit, Citrus nobilis var. deliciosa; regarded by some as a variety of tangerine and by others as a cross between the tangerine and a wild North African orange.

Clinical science The approach aimed at understanding the diagnosis and treatment of diseases and disorders through studies involving people, usually carried out in clinical settings.

Clinical significance A conclusion that an intervention has an effect that is of practical meaning to patients and health care providers.

Clinical trials Clinical trials undertake experimental study of human subjects. Trials may attempt to determine whether the finds of basic research are applicable to humans, or to confirm the results of epidemiological research. Studies may be small, with a limited number of participants, or they may be large intervention trials that seek to discover the outcome of treatments on entire populations. The "gold standard" clinical trials are double-blind, placebo-controlled studies which employ random assignment of subjects to experimental and control groups unknown to the subject or the researcher.

Clostridium A genus of bacteria, of which C. botulinum is responsible for botulism, a rare but often fatal form of food poisoning. It is found widely distributed in soil; during growth on favourable food materials, the organism synthesizes an extremely potent neurotoxin which is released into the food when the cell dies. The spores are the most heat-resistant food-poisoning organism encountered and their thermal death time is used as a minimum standard for processing foods with pH values higher than 4.5.

Clotted cream Thick, rich and indulgent with the consistency of soft butter, clotted cream is made by heating normal cream to evaporate some of the liquids. It has at least 55 per cent butter fat giving it a pale yellow colour, often topped with a deeper yellow crust. It's traditionally made in Devon and Cornwall and served with scones or desserts or made into ice cream. If you buy an ice cream in Devon or Cornwall it's usual for your ice cream to be topped off with a spoonful of clotted cream.

Cloudberry An orange-yellow fruit resembling the raspberry in shape; Rubus chamaemorus, known as avron in Scotland, and baked-apple berry in Canada. It is an extremely rich natural source of benzoic acid and will not ferment; it remains fresh for many months without preservation.

Cloves Cloves are the dried flower buds of an evergreen tree native to eastern Indonesia. It's a versatile spice that can be used in drinks and in sweet and savoury dishes. The pungent, sweet flavour of the clove lends itself perfectly to meats such as beef or venison, as well as fruits such as apples, oranges and plums and to pickled vegetables. Spike an onion with cloves and place it into a meat stew or casserole, add a few cloves to chilli con carne, spice up boiled rice or pop a clove into a bouquet garni. When baking a ham, spike the boiled ham with cloves so that the flavour permeates the meat during baking. Apples and cloves are a perfect combination and cloves are also an essential ingredient of mulled wine or warm punches.

Club Sandwich It is a sandwich with cooked chicken breast and bacon, along with juicy ripe tomatoes and crisp lettuce layered between two or three slices of toasted bread with mayonnaise.

Coacervation The heat-reversible aggregation of the amylopectin form of starch, which is believed to be one of the mechanisms involved in the staling of bread.

Coagulation The process in which colloidal particles come together irreversibly to form larger masses. Coagulation can be brought about by adding ions to change the ionic strength of the solution and thus destabilize the colloid. Ions with a high charge are particularly effective (e.g. alum, containing Al3+, is used in styptics to coagulate blood). Alum and iron(III) sulphate are also used for coagulation in sewage treatment. Heating is another way of coagulating certain colloids (e.g. boiling an egg coagulates the albumin).

Cobb Salad Typically a Cobb Salad consists of chopped chicken or turkey, bacon, hard cooked eggs, tomatoes, avocado, cheddar cheese, and lettuce. It is served with crumbled blue cheese and vinaigrette dressing. The original recipe for Cobb salad included avocado, celery, tomato, chives, watercress, hard-boiled eggs, chicken, bacon, and Roquefort cheese.

Cobbler Cobblers are an American deep-dish fruit dessert or pie with a thick crust (usually a biscuit crust) and a fruit filling (such as peaches, apples, berries). Some versions are enclosed in the crust, while others have a drop-biscuit or crumb topping.

These desserts have been and are still called by various names such as cobbler, tart, pie, torte, pandowdy, grunt, slump, buckles, crisp, croustade, upside-down cakes, bird's nest pudding or crow's nest pudding. They are all simple variations of cobblers, and they are all based on seasonal fruits and berries. Whatever fresh ingredients are readily at hand. They are all homemade and simple to make and rely more on taste than fancy pastry preparation. Early settlers were very good at improvising. When they first arrived, they bought their favourite recipes with the. Not finding their favourite ingredients, they used whatever was available. That's how all these traditional American dishes came about with such unusual names.

Cobnut Cobnuts, which grow in Britain, are a type of hazelnut. You may be able to buy fresh nuts, particularly native cobnuts, still in their husks in season (early autumn) but most are sold dried and processed.

Coburg cakes Small cakes containing syrup and flavoured with spices.

Coca cola Trade name for a cola drink.

Coca leaves From the S. American plant, Erythroxylon coca; they contain the narcotic alkaloid cocaine, and are traditionally chewed by the natives of Peru as a stimulant. Originally the beverage Coca Cola contained coca leaf extract, although this was removed from the formulation many years ago.

Cocarboxylase An obsolete name for thiamin diphosphate, the metabolically active coenzyme form of vitamin B1.

Co-Carcinogen A chemical substance that enhances the action of a carcinogen but does not itself initiate cancer.

Cochineal A water-soluble red colour obtained from the female conchilla, Dactilopius coccus (Coccus cactus), an insect found in Mexico, Central America, and the Caribbean: 1kg of the colour is obtained from about 150 000 insects. Legally permitted in foods in most countries (E-120). Contains carminic acid (E-120). Cochineal red A is an alternative name for Ponceau 4R (E-124), often used to replace cochineal. Carmine is produced from cochineal.

Cochon de lati Translated from French to English, the word literally means, "pig in milk." To make this Cajun pig roast, use a suckling (young) pig to get the finest pork flavor. The Cajuns of southwest Louisiana have always enjoyed their pork, but consider a Cochon De Lait to be a special treat. Historically, men cooked the pig over an outdoor fire, while the women prepare other dishes inside the house. Many Cajuns consider the crackling skin the best part of the Cochon De Lait.

Cockles Several types of marine bivalve molluscs of genus Cardium, often sold preserved in brine or vinegar. A 50-g portion is a rich source of iron, iodine, and selenium; a source of protein and copper; contains 0.2 g of fat of which 33% is saturated; supplies 25 kcal.

Cocktail Mixed alcoholic drink; there are many recipes based on a wide variety of spirits and liqueurs, with fruit juice, milk, or coconut milk, normally shaken with crushed ice.

Cocoa Originally known as cacao, introduced into Europe from Mexico by the Spaniards in the early sixteenth century. The powder prepared from the seed embedded in the fruit of the cocoa plant, Theobroma cacao, also a milk drink prepared with cocoa powder. Used to prepare chocolate. Contains the alkaloid theobromine; caffiene is trimethylxanthine.

Cocoa butter The fat from the cocoa bean, used in chocolate manufacture and in pharmaceuticals; it has a low sharp melting point, between 31 and 35 °C, so it melts in the mouth; mostly 2-oleopalmitostearin.

Cocoa nibs Seeds of the fruit of the cocoa plant, Theobroma cacao, are left to ferment, which modifies the bitterness, and their colour darkens. They are then roasted and separated from the husks as two halves of the seed known as cocoa nibs. They contain about 50% fat, part of which is removed in the preparation of chocolate and cocoa for beverages.

Cocolait A form of coconut 'milk' made by applying high pressure to coconuts and homogenizing the oil and water emulsion plus coconut water (coconut milk) obtained. Bottled and used (e.g. in the Philippines) in place of cow's milk.

Coconut In Thailand they are called a maprao. They are thought to be native to Indonesia or Malaysia, but they now grow freely in all the tropical regions of the world. They are used for coconut juice when young and coconut cream when mature. Coconuts are green when young and brown with the hard inner nut when ripe.

They are the stones of the fruit and have a hard inner shell, which includes coconut milk surrounded by a bright, white, crunchy flesh.

Coconut cream The rich, solid milk found at the top of a can of coconut milk. If a recipe calls for coconut cream, simply scoop out the top solid portion. Each 14-ounce can of coconut milk contains approximately 3 to 4 ounces of coconut cream.

Coconut milk and cream Coconut milk isn't the liquid from inside the nut, but the extract of freshly grated coconut flesh. The flesh is first soaked in hot water, then allowed to cool, after which the liquid is strained off. It's available in tins from Asian and Caribbean stores and larger supermarkets. Coconut cream is sold in hard blocks. It can be diluted with hot water before using or added straight to the simmering liquid in the pan. Both give a distinctive taste and smoothness to curries, sauces and rice.

Cod A white fish, Gaddus morrhua and other species. The composition of all non-fatty fish, such as cod, hake, haddock, flatfish, is similar.

Cod liver oil The oil from codfish liver; the classic source of vitamins A and D, used for its medicinal properties long before the vitamins were discovered. An average sample contains 120-1200 µg vitamin A and 1-10 µg vitamin D per gram. British Pharmacopoeia standard: minimum 180 µg vitamin A and 2 µg vitamin D per gram.

Codes of practice In the area of food production. these refer to standards of procedure which cannot be covered by exact specifications and serve as agreed guidelines. They may originate from Government Departments, trade organizations, the Institute of Food Science and Technology, or individual companies.

Codex alimentarius A set of standards established by the WHO/FAO for the composition and labeling of foods including special dietary foods.

Coeliac disease (Celiac disease) Intolerance of the proteins of wheat, rye, and barley; specifically, the gliadin fraction of the protein gluten. The villi of the small intestine are severely affected and absorption of food is poor. Stools are bulky and fermenting from unabsorbed carbohydrate, and contain a large amount of unabsorbed fat (steatorrhoea). As a result of the malabsorption, affected people are malnourished and children suffer from growth retardation. Treatment is by exclusion of wheat, rye, and barley proteins (the starches are tolerated); rice, oats, and maize are generally tolerated. Manufactured foods that are free from gluten, and hence suitable for consumption by people with coeliac disease are usually labelled as 'gluten-free'. Also known as gluten-induced enteropathy, and sometimes as non-tropical sprue.

Coenzyme Coenzymes are a small organic non-protein molecules that carry chemical groups between enzymes. Many coenzymes are phosphorylated water-soluble vitamins. However, nonvitamins may also be coenzymes, such as ATP, the biochemical carrier of phosphate groups.Coenzymes are used up in the reactions in which they assist, (for example: NADH coenzyme is converted to NAD+ by oxidoreductses). Coenzymes are however regenerated and their concentration maintained at a steady level in the cell.A special subset of coenzymes are prosthetic groups. These have more in common with cofactors since they are tightly bound to enzymes and are not released as part of the reaction. Prosthetic groups include molybdopterin, lipoamide and biotin.

Coffee The coffee (coffea) plant in the Rubiacee family, to which belongs also, for example, the gardenia. Coffee beans are roasted to varying degree of darkness and can have a wide array of flavors. Additives to the beans, such as vanilla or hazelnut are popular in America. Coffee can be drunk black, or sweetened with sugar or honey, and lightened with milk or cream. The first definite dates go back to 800 B.C.; but already Homer, and many Arabian legends, tells the story of a mysterious black and bitter beverage with powers of stimulation. B the end of the 9th Century an Arab drink known as qahwa, literally meaning, "that which prevents sleep" was being made by boiling the beans. Its introduction to Europeans came through the Arab pilgrimages. The government forbade transportation of the plant out of the Moslem nations. Coffee beans were not allowed to be taken out of the country unless they had first been dried in sunlight or boiled in water to kill the seed-germ The actual spread of coffee was started illegally by either being smuggled or inadvertently taken by groups of pilgrims on their annual travels to Mecca. Venice, the key port of Europe, started the coffee drinking trend in Europe. The first coffee house was opened in 1640, and by 1763 Venice numbered no less than 218 coffee houses.

Non-caffeinated coffee In 1903, Ludwig Roselius, a German coffee importer, in an attempt to rescue a batch of ruined coffee beans, perfected the process of removing caffeine from the beans without destroying the flavor. He markets it under the brand name "Sanka." Sanka is introduced to the United States in 1923.

Instant coffee In 1906, George Constant Washington, an English chemist living in Guatemala, notices a powdery condensation forming on the spout of his silver coffee carafe. After experimentation, he creates the first mass-produced instant coffee (his brand is called Red E Coffee).

Coffee Cabinet When ice cream is added, Coffee Milk is called a "Coffee Cabinet" or "Coffee Cab." In other words, a "cabinet" is a local term for a "frappe" which is a regional term for an ice cream milk shake. It is though to be called a "cabinet" because it unknown originator kept his blender in a kitchen cabinet. Also mixers were often stored in square wooden cabinets.

Coffee contains caffeine. Decaffeinated coffee is coffee beans (or instant coffee) from which the caffeine has been extracted with solvent (e.g. methylene or ethylene chloride), carbon dioxide under pressure (supercritical CO_2), or water. Coffee decaffeinated by water extraction is sometimes labelled as 'naturally' decaffeinated.

Coffee Milk A lot like chocolate milk but with coffee-flavored syrup. It is milk with sweet coffee syrup added (two tablespoons of coffee syrup to 8 ounces of milk). The drink is served either by the glass or the half-ping (in a waxed-cardboard carton). In 1993, after much political debate, it was made "The Official State Drink of Rhode Island," Rhode Island is the only place in the world where you can get this drink. If you travel more than ten miles from the state border, no one will know what you're talking about. In Rhode Island, a milk shake is just what it says: milk to which you add flavoring and then shake. In most of American, if you order a milk shake, you get ice cream blended with milk. In Rhode Island and most of New England, you would get chocolate powder or syrup stirred into milk without ice cream. The Coffee Milk was first introduced to Rhode Islanders in the early 1920s. Two companies, Autocrat and Eclipse) used to vie for the chocolate syrup business. Their rivalry ended in 1991, when Autocrat bought the Eclipse brand name and secret formula. Both labels are now produced by Autocrat and are available in stores.

Cognac Brandy made in the Charentes region of north-west France, around the town of Cognac, from special varieties of grape grown on shallow soil and claimed to be distilled only in pot, not continuous, stills. Sometimes used (incorrectly) as a general name for brandy. See also armagnac.

Cognitive ability Knowledge, perception.

Cohort or follow-up study A study design in which data on exposures to possible risk factors for disease are collected from a group of people (cohort) who do not have the disease under investigation. The subjects are then followed for a period of time to see whether the later development of disease is related to the factors that were measured.

Complement The word complement (with an e in the second syllable, not to be confused with a different word, compliment with an i) has a number of uses. Generally a complement of X is something that together with X makes a complete whole; that supplies what X lacks. The first e in complete and the first e in complement are etymological cognates of each other (from the Latin word complere—to fill up—according to the Oxford English Dictionary). That fact can serve as a mnemonic for remembering that this is not compliment with an i.

Cohort A group of people who are followed in a scientific study.

Cohort study An observational study in which outcomes in a group of patients that received an intervention are compared with outcomes in a similar group i.e., the cohort, either contemporary or historical, of patients that did not receive the intervention.

Cointreau It is colourless, orange-flavored liquor from France.

Cola drinks Carbonated drinks containing extract of cola bean, the seed of the tree Cola acuminata, and a variety of other flavouring ingredients. Cola seed contains caffeine, and the drink contains 10-15 mg caffeine/100 mL; decaffeinated or caffeine-free varieties are also made.

Colby cheese It is a hard cheese that is similar to cheddar cheese, although it is softer with a more open texture, It may be made from either raw or pasteurized milk. It is made in the same way as cheddar cheese except that the curd is not matted and milled.

Colby jack It is a combination of Monterey Jack and colby cheeses.

Colcannon Colcannon is a famous Irish dish using mashed potatoes and cabbage that is served in a fluffy pile with a well in the centre filled with melted butter, so that you can dip each forkful into the butter before eating it. It gets its name from the old name "cole" for cabbage, which we still use in the term cole slaw or cabbage salad. In most Irish cookbooks, kale is used instead of cabbage. Also known as Kale Cannon or Kailkenny. In Scotland this dish is also known as Rumbledethumps. Traditionally eaten at Lughnasa or Samhain, the Irish version of Thanksgiving. Colcannon is a national Irish dish of sorts and it is traditional to put coins in the Colcannon (kids absolutely love this tradition). In England, this dish is called Bubble and Squeak. The dish is composed of potatoes mashed up with peas and cabbage and fried. Usually it's eaten for breakfast and is made by frying on both sides in bacon fat until crisp and brown. The dish originally contained beef along with the leftover cooked potatoes and cabbage, though today people don't generally bother with the meat. The name is apparently due to the sounds that are emitted during cooking, the vegetables bubble as they are boiled and then squeak in the frying pan.

Colchicine An alkaloid isolated from the meadow saffron, or autumn crocus (Colchicum spp.). It is an old remedy for gout. It inhibits cell division, and is used in experimental horticulture to produce plants with abnormal numbers of genes.

Cold charlottes They are made in a ladyfinger-lined mold and filled with a Bavarian cream. For frozen charlottes, a frozen souffle or mousse replaces the Bavarian cream.

Cold-shortening When the temperature of muscle is reduced below 10 °C while the pH remains above 6-6.2 (early in the post-mortem conversion of glycogen to lactic acid) the muscle contracts in reaction to cold and, when cooked, the meat is tough.

Cold-smoking Curing meat (hams, sausages, bacon, fish) in the smoke of smoldering wood or corncobs at temperatures from 60 to 100 degrees F.

Coleslaw A cold salad made with shredded cabbage mixed with mayonnaise as well as a variety of ingredients. The term coleslaw is a late 19th century term, which originated in the United States. Cole slaw (cold slaw) got it's name from the Dutch "kool sla"- the word "kool" means cabbage and "sla" is salad - meaning simply, cabbage salad. In English, that became "cole slaw" and eventually "cold slaw." The original Dutch "kool sla" was most likely served hot.

Coliform bacteria A group of aerobic, lactose-fermenting bacteria, of which Escherichia coli is the most important member. Many coliforms are not harmful, but since they arise from faeces, they are useful as a test of faecal contamination, and particularly as a test for water pollution. Some strains of E. coli produce toxins, or are otherwise pathogenic, and are associated with food poisoning.

Colitis Inflammation of the large intestine, with pain, diarrhoea, and weight loss; there may be ulceration of the large intestine (ulcerative colitis). See also Crohn's disease; gastro-intestinal tract; irritable bowel syndrome.

Collagen An insoluble fibrous protein found extensively in the connective tissue of skin, tendons, and bone. The polypeptide chains of collagen (containing the amino acids glycine and proline predominantly) form triple-stranded helical coils that are bound together to form fibrils, which have great strength and limited elasticity. Collagen accounts for over 30% of the total body protein of mammals.

Collagen hydrolysate A functional component of gelatin which may help improve some symptoms associated with osteoarthritis.

Collar A cut of pork from the neck of the animal. It's used for a number of different cuts such as spare ribs, chops, boneless steaks, diced pork and mince. The common feature of all the meat is that it's slightly fatty and therefore doesn't dry out when cooked for a long time. The cost of collar cuts is relatively low compared with other pork cuts and is particularly good for long, gentle cooking, such as in casseroles and stews.

Collard American name for varieties of cabbage (Brassica oleracea) which do not form a compact head. Generally known in the UK as greens or spring greens.

Collard, collards, or collard greens Any sort of cabbage in which the green leaves do not form a compact "head." They are mostly large "kales." Reaction to the smell of cooking collards separates true Southern eaters from the wannabes, as no kitchen odor is more distinctive than that of a pot of greens as they come to a boil. In the South, a large quantity of greens to serve a family is commonly referred to as a "mess o' greens." The traditional southern way to cook collards is to boil them with a piece of salt pork or ham hock slowly for a long time (the longer the better) until they are very soft. The typical way to serve greens is with freshly baked corn bread to dip into the "Pot-Likker." Pot likker is the highly concentrated and vitamin-filled broth that results from the long boil of the greens, It is, in other words, the "liquor" left in the pot.

Colloid Particles (the disperse phase) suspended in a second medium (the dispersion medium); can be solid, liquid, or gas suspended in a solid, liquid, or gas. Examples of gas-in-liquid colloids are beaten egg-white and whipped cream; of liquid-in-liquid colloids, emulsions such as milk and salad cream. See also emulsifying agents; stabilizers.

Colon Also known as the large intestine or bowel, consisting of three anatomical regions: the ascending, the transverse, and the descending colon. The colon normally has a considerable population of bacteria, while it is rare to find a significant bacterial population in the small intestine. The colon terminates at the rectum, where faeces are compacted and stored before voiding.

Colonic inertia Delayed colonic action. Symptoms include long delays in the passage of stool accompanied by lack of urgency to move the bowels

Colonoscopy Colonoscopy is a fiberoptic (endoscopic) procedure in which a thin, flexible, lighted viewing tube (a colonoscope) is threaded up through the rectum for the purpose of inspecting the entire colon and rectum and, if there is an abnormality, taking a tissue sample of it (biopsy) for examination under a microscope, or removing it.

Colostomy Surgical creation of an artificial conduit on the abdominal wall for voiding of intestinal contents following surgical removal of much of the colon and/or rectum. See also gastro-intestinal tract.

Colostrum Colostrum, which is also called first milk, is one of the oldest and most exceptional foods that can be found in nature. It is as old as motherhood itself, for colostrum is milk of any mammalian in the first 24 hours after birth. The effective substances that are present in the first milk are found nowhere else in nature in such high, perfectly balanced concentrations as only nature can do. Colostrum is important for the nutrition, growth and development of newborn infants and contributes to the immunologic defense of the neonates.

Colours Widely used in foods to increase their aesthetic appeal; may be natural, nature-identical, or synthetic. Natural colours include carotenoids (yellow to orange-red in apricots, carrots, maize, tomatoes), some of which are vitamin precursors. Chlorophylls are the green pigments in all leaves and stems. Anthocyanins are the red, blue, and violet pigments in beetroots, raspberries, and red cabbage. Flavones are yellow pigments in most leaves and flowers. There are twenty permitted synthetic colours (mainly azo dyes). Caramel is used for both flavour and as a brown colour made by heating sugar.

In addition to all these there are various ingredients such as paprika, saffron, and turmeric that also provide colour. See Appendix VIII.

COMA Committee on Medical Aspects of Food Policy; permanent Advisory Committee to the UK Department of Health.

Comminuted Finely divided; used with reference to minced meat products and fruit drinks made from crushed whole fruit including the peel.

Commodity foods As a result of federal surplus-removal and price-support programs, the USDA purchases excess food produced by American farmers. The USDA utilizes a number of commodity distribution and nutrition programs to provide these excess commodities to low-income Americans.

Community food projects grants program A grants program administered by CSREES to help communities become more self reliant at maintaining their food systems while addressing food, nutrition, and farm issues. Grants are awarded on a one-time basis to eligible private nonprofit entities. Community Food Projects grants have been used to establish Farm to School programs.

Community food security Defined as a situation in which all community residents obtain a safe, culturally acceptable, nutritionally adequate diet through a sustainable food system that maximizes community self-reliance and social justice.

Community garden A garden developed and maintained by members of a community. Community gardens are often established to serve as a catalyst for neighborhood development, beautification, recreation, therapy, and food production. In low-income communities, community gardens can provide fresh produce and serve as a source for youth programming.

Community kitchen A community organization that prepares meals for low-income clients. In some cases, meals prepared by a community kitchen are eaten onsite. These specific types of organizations are also known as Emergency Kitchens or Soup Kitchens. Community kitchen can also refer to an organization that rescues prepared and perishable surplus food from the retail and foodservice industries and then redistributes the food to non-profit community service agencies such as homeless shelters, afterschool programs, and senior centres. This second type of community kitchen often operates a job-training program to help low-income individuals obtain the skill necessary to find and maintain employment in the food service industry.

Competitive foods In schools, competitive foods refers to food and beverages available other than those served through the federally-reimbursed child nutrition programs, including food and beverages available through ΰ la carte lines, vending machines, snack bars, student stores and through fundraisers.

Complementary foods Any food, whether manufactured or locally prepared, that is suitable to use as a complement to breast-milk or to infant formula, when either becomes insufficient to satisfy the nutritional requirements of the infant. Such food is also commonly referred to as "weaning food" or "breast-milk supplement." Complementary foods are not covered under the WHO Code.

Complementary os transition foods Those offered to the child between 4-6 months of age as a complementary to mother's milk, beginning with pureed foods and gradually offering foods of greater consistency until the child can consume tha regular family diet in addition to mother's milk. Currently, the term "weaning diet" is not used, to avoid giving the idea that introducing solid foods implies the suspension of breastfeeding.

Complementation This term is used with respect to proteins when a relative deficiency of an amino acid in one is compensated by a relative surplus from another protein consumed at the same time. The protein quality is not the average of the separate values, but higher.

Compote A classic dish of fresh or dried fruits, simmered or baked in a light syrup. The fruit can be cooked whole or cut into pieces and almost anything can be used - limes, figs, apricots, rhubarb, berries. It's good to use seasonal fruits to get the best flavour. A savoury compote made with tomatoes or shallots is a tasty accompaniment to barbecued meat or fish.

Comsomme Madrilene It is a beef consomme with cubes of beef or chicken and vegetables julienne.

Conalbumin One of the proteins of egg-white, comprising 12% of the total solids. It binds iron in a pink-coloured complex; this accounts for the pinkish colour resulting when eggs are stored in rusty containers.

Concasse, concasser A French term for rough chopping of a food/foods with a knife or for breaking by pounding in a mortar. The term is frequently used to refer to coarsely chopped fresh tomatoes (peeled, seeded and chopped). It is often used in Italian-style pasta dishes.

Conde Dessert of creamed rice with fruit and red jam sauce. Also the name of a type of patisserie. condiment Seasoning added to flavour foods, such as salt, or herbs and spices such as mustard, ginger, curry, pepper, etc. Although some are relatively rich in nutrients, they are generally used in such small quantities that they make a negligible contribution to the diet (but see curry).

Condensed milk Condensed Milk is pure cow's milk properly combined with unadulterated cane sugar. The waster content of the milk is evaporated. Gail Borden (1801–1874), American dairyman, surveyor, and inventor, came up with the idea during a transatlantic trip on board a ship in 1852 when the cows in the hold became too seasick to be milked during the long trip, and an immigrant infant died from lack of milk. He was granted a patent for sweetened condensed in 1856. Condensed milk was not successfully canned until 1885. Condensed milk, initially sold from handcarts in New York City, became an immediate success in urban areas where fresh milk was difficult to distribute and store. Condensed milk was very popular during World War II in England because of how well is kept.

Condiment A spice, seasoning, or sauce that is used to give relish or to enhance meat or other foods, and to gratify the taste. Condiments usually supply little nourishment but add flavor to foods. Ketchup, butter, mustard, salt, mayonnaise, hot sauce, etc. are considered as condiments. The word is derived from the Latin word "condire," meaning to preserve or pickle.

Conduction In the process of conduction, heat is transferred directly from one molecule to another (for example, the hot coils from your stove element heat the cast-iron frying pan, which then transfers heat to the cheese sandwich being grilled). Conduction is not a speedy method of cooking, but it does do a good job. The time cooking takes will depend upon how well your pan conducts heat. Various materials conduct heat differently, so the material from which cooking utensils are made, makes a difference to how quickly, and how well, food cooks by conduction. Conduction also takes place as heat moves through the food itself, cooking it from the outside first and then moving through the food to the inside

Confectioners' sugar Also called powdered sugar. It is granulated sugar ground to a powder and sifted. Always sift it before using. In Britain it is called icing sugar and in France sucre glace. See Sugar.

Confectionery Delicacies made with sweet ingredients. Confectioneries sweetened with honey were made in Egypt at least 3,000 years ago. In the Middle Ages the Persians developed confectionery made with refined cane sugar, and during the 18th century in Europe, machinery for confectionery manufacture was first developed. Boiled or hard sweets such as fruit drops and clear mints are made by boiling a flavoured solution of sugar and corn syrup until the sugar concentration reaches a high level. On cooling, a hard, glassy product is formed. Caramels and toffees are manufactured in a similar way, but the mixture includes condensed or evaporated milk. Fondant, the basis for the 'soft centres' of many chocolates, is made by rapidly beating a hot, concentrated sugar mixture so that minute crystals are formed: fudge can be made by similarly beating hot caramel. Agar, pectin, or gelatine is added to sugar syrup to form jellies and Turkish delight, while gums and pastilles are made by dissolving gum arabic in sugar syrup.

Confidence Interval for the Mean The confidence intervals for the mean give us a range of values around the mean where we expect the "true" (population) mean is located (with a given level of certainty, see also Elementary Concepts). In some statistics or math software packages (e.g., in STATISTICA) you can request confidence intervals for any p-level; for example, if the mean in your sample is 23, and the lower and upper limits of the p=.05 confidence interval are 19 and 27 respectively, then you can conclude that there is a 95% probability that the population mean is greater than 19 and lower than 27. If you set the p-level to a smaller value, then the interval would become wider thereby increasing the "certainty" of the estimate, and vice versa; as we all know from the weather forecast, the more "vague" the prediction (i.e., wider the confidence interval), the more likely it will materialize. Note that the width of the confidence interval depends on the sample size and on the variation of data values. The calculation of confidence intervals is based on the assumption that the variable is normally distributed in the population. This estimate may not be valid if this assumption is not met, unless the sample size is large, say n = 100 or more.

Confidence interval In statistics, a confidence interval (CI) for a population parameter is an interval between two numbers with an associated probability p which is generated from a random sample of an underlying population, such that if the sampling was repeated numerous times and the confidence interval recalculated from each sample according to the same method, a proportion p of the confidence intervals would contain the population parameter in question. Confidence intervals are the most prevalent form of interval estimation.

Confit It is French term used to describe a way of preserving meat (usually pork, goose or duck). It is derived from an ancient method of preserving meat whereby it is salted and slowly cooked in its own fat. The meat or poultry is salted first and then slowly cooked in its own rendered fat. The resulting confit is then packed in crocks and sealed with more fat. Confit can be refrigerated up to 6 months. Confit d'oie and confit de canard are preserved goose and preserved duck, respectively. You can eat it cold, thinly sliced, in salads, or use it to add to hot dishes such as the French specialty "cassoulet".

Confounding factors Factors that distort an association because they are associated with an exposure as well as a disease or other outcome.

Congestive heart failure Congestive heart failure (CHF), also called congestive cardiac failure (CCF) or just heart failure, is a condition that can result from any structural or functional cardiac disorder that impairs the ability of the heart to fill with or pump a sufficient amount of blood throughout the body. It is not to be confused with "cessation of heartbeat", which is known as asystole, or with cardiac arrest, which is the cessation of normal cardiac function in the face of heart disease. Because not all patients have volume overload at the time of initial or subsequent evaluation, the term "heart failure" is preferred over the older term "congestive heart failure". Congestive heart failure is often undiagnosed due to a lack of a universally agreed definition and difficulties in diagnosis, particularly when the condition is considered "mild".

Confounding variable or confounding factor A "hidden" variable that may cause an association which the researcher attributes to other variables.

Congee Chinese soft rice soup or gruel; may be sweet or savoury. Commonly eaten for breakfast.

Congeners Flavour substances in alcoholic spirits that distil over with the alcohol; chemically a mixture of higher alcohols and esters. Said to be responsible for many of the symptoms of hangover after excessive consumption. See also fusel oil.

Congie The water from cooking rice, which contains much of the thiamin and niacin from the rice; used as a drink.

Congregate meal program A program which serves meals at a community location, such as a senior centre, where seniors can come and eat in the company of others. Congregate meal programs are often supported by the Elderly Nutrition Program. Some states also use funds from the Social Services Block Grant to support congregate meal programs.

Congress tart Small pastry case filled with ground almonds, sugar, and egg.

Congris Caribbean (Cuban); casseroled red beans served with rice.

Conjugated linoleic acid (CLA) A type of fatty acid found in cheeses and some meat products which may provide the health benefits of improving body composition and decreasing the risk of certain cancers.

Connective tissue Consists of the protein collagen which in fish is found between the muscle segments (myotomes); in meat it is spread through the muscle, uniting the muscle fibres into bundles and supporting the blood vessels (a kind of soft skeleton), and consists of both collagen and elastin.

A high content of connective tissue results in tougher meat.

Collagen is insoluble; it is converted to soluble gelatine by moist heat, so making the food more tender. Tough meat is softened to some extent by stewing, but roasting or frying has little effect. Elastin is unaffected by heating, and remains tough, elastic, and insoluble.

Consomme It is from the Latin word "consummare" meaning to "finish perfectly" and "raise to the highest point of achievement." Consomme is considered one of the finest of soups. It is a clear soup and it is essential to use stock made from raw meat, which has been clarified by the addition of beaten egg white and clean eggshells.

Constipation Difficulty in passing stools or infrequent passage of hard stools. In the absence of intestinal disease, frequently a result of a diet low in non-starch polysaccharide, and treated by increasing the intake of fruits, vegetables, and especially wholegrain cereal products.

Contaminants Undesirable compounds found in foods, the result of residues of agricultural chemicals (pesticides, fungicides, herbicides, fertilizers, etc.), through the manufacturing process or as a result of pollution. For many such compounds there are limits to the amount that may legally be present in the food. See also Acceptable Daily Intake.

Continuing Survey of Food Intake of Individuals (CSFII) A part of the National Nutrition Monitoring System which was the first nationwide dietary intake survey designed to be conducted annually. The survey is conducted by the USDA.

Contractures Static muscle shortening resulting from tonic spasm or fibrosis; frequently seen in individuals with cerebral palsy

Contrast radiology A test in which a contrast material (i.e., Barium) is used to coat the rectum, colon, and lower part of the small intestine so they show up on an x-ray.

Control A standard of comparison which can be a conventional practice, a placebo, or no intervention.

Control group The group of subjects in a study to whom a comparison is made in order to determine whether an observation or treatment has an effect. In an experimental study it is the group that does not receive a treatment. Subjects are as similar as possible to those in the test or treatment group.

Control of coexisting illnesses Measures to prevent and cure the occurrence of illnesses that aggravate the nutritionl state.

Controlled experiment In this type of research, study subjects (whether animal or human) are selected according to relevant characteristics, and then randomly assigned to either an experimental group, or a control group. Random assignment ensures that factors known as variables, which may affect the outcome of the study, are distributed equally among the groups and therefore could not lead to differences in the effect of the treatment under study. The experimental group is then given a treatment (sometimes called an intervention), and the results are compared to the control group, which does not receive treatment. A placebo, or false treatment, may be administered to the control group. With all other variables controlled, differences between the experimental and control groups may be attributed to the treatment under study.

Convection It is the spread of heat by a flow of hot air, steam, or liquid. This flow may be either natural or mechanical. In a pot of liquid, the liquid closest to the fire is heated first. As it is heated, it becomes lighter and rises to the top. The cooler, heavier liquid sinks down, becomes heated in turn, and rises. Therefore, a naturally circulating current of hot liquid is sent up throughout the pot.

Convection oven Convection ovens are simply traditional gas or electric ovens equipped with a fan, which circulates the hot oven air around the food. Foods cook more evenly and faster with this type of oven.

Convenience foods Processed foods in which a considerable amount of the preparation has already been carried out by the manufacturer, e.g. cooked meats, canned foods, baked foods, breakfast cereals, frozen foods.

Cookie In America, a cookie is described as a thin, sweet, usually small cake; in Australia and the UK it is called a biscuit. There are hundreds upon hundreds of cookie recipes in the United States. No one book could hold the recipes for all of the various types of cookies.

Bar cookies These cookies are baked in sheets and then cut into squares or bars. They are a softer type of cookie (more like a cake).

Drop cookies Cookies that are dropped from a spoon. Almost any cookie dough can be baked as a drop cookie (if additional liquid is added to the batter).

Molded cookies Molded cookies can be shaped by hand, stamped with a pattern before baking or baked directly in a mold.

Pressed cookies These cookies are formed by pressing dough through a cookie press (or pastry bag with a decorative tip) to form fancy shapes and designs.

Refrigerator cookies - Cookie dough is shaped into logs and is refrigerated until firm. They are then sliced and baked.

Rolled cookies - Rolled or crisp cookies are made from a stiff (or chilled) dough, which is rolled and cut into shapes with sharp cookie cutters, a knife, or a pastry wheel. They should be thin and crisp.

Cooking Required to make food more palatable, more digestible, and safer. There is breakdown of the connective tissue in meat, softening of the cellulose in plant tissues, and proteins are denatured by heating, so increasing their digestibility.

Cooking spray Aerosol cans sold in grocery stores containing vegetable or olive oil, which can be sprayed in a fine mist. This spray is used for "oiling" cooking pans so food does not stick. One of the benefits of using cooking spray is that fewer calories are added than if the pan is coated in oil.

Cooking, loss of nutrients In general, water-soluble vitamins and minerals are lost in the cooking water, the amount depending on the surface area to volume ratio, i.e. greater losses take place from finely cut or minced foods. Fat-soluble vitamins are little affected except at frying temperatures. Proteins suffer reduction of available lysine when they are heated in the presence of reducing substances, and further loss under extreme conditions of temperature. Dry heat, as in baking, results in some loss of vitamin B 1 and available lysine. The most sensitive nutrient by far is vitamin C, with vitamin B 1 next. Average losses from cereals are: boiling, 40% vitamins B1, B2, B6, niacin, biotin, and pantothenic acid; 50% total folate; baking, 5% niacin, 15% vitamin B2; 25% vitamins B1, B6, and pantothenic acid; 50% folate; with biotin being stable. In meat, losses are approximately 20% of all the vitamins for roasting, frying, and grilling and 20-60% for stewing and boiling.

Copha Copha is a solid fat that is derived from the coconut. It is used primarily in recipes where it is melted and combined with other ingredients and left to set.

Copper A dietary essential trace metal, which forms the prosthetic group of a number of enzymes. The Reference Nutrient Intake is 1.2 mg/day. Toxic in excess, and it is recommended that not more than 2-10 mg/day should be consumed habitually. Rich sources include: meat, poultry, game, fish and shellfish, avocado, nuts, pulses, bread, chocolate, beer, cider, coconut, mushrooms.

Copra Dried coconut 'meat' used for production of coconut oil for margarine and soap manufacture.

Coprophagy Eating of faeces. Since B vitamins are synthesized by intestinal bacteria, animals that eat their faeces can make use of these vitamins, which are not absorbed from the large intestine, the site of bacterial action.

Coquille St. Jacques Coquille is the French word for "shell." Translated, the name means "Shell of St. James." Coquilles St. Jacques are scallops cooked in white wine with a little salt, peppercorn, parsley, bay leaf, chopped shallots, and water. A sauce of fish stock, butter, flour, milk, egg yolks, and cream accompanies them. In the 12th century, the scallop was around the necks, worn on the robes, and on the hats of pilgrims traveling to the Spanish shrine of St. James the Apostle (St. Jacques in French) in Campostello, Spain. Galicians who would accept passing pilgrims into their homes also hung scallop shells over their doors. The shrine of St James ranked with Rome and the Holy Land as a destination for pilgrims. Pilgrimages were undertaken as a penance for grievous sins such as murder or adultery, to seek help with health problems, or simply as an act of worship. The scallop symbol identified them as harmless pilgrims and allowed them to move unmolested through wars and civil unrest.

Coral The ovaries of female lobsters, used as the basis for sauces; red-coloured when cooked.

Cordial, fruit Originally a fruit liqueur, and still used in this sense in the USA; in the UK a cordial is now used to mean any fruit drink, usually a concentrate to be diluted.

Cordials A sweet alcoholic beverage made from an infusion of flavoring ingredients and a spirit. Today cordials are usually served at room temperature in small glasses.

Cordon bleu It is French for "blue ribbon" or "cord." 1. The term is now used to mean "an exceptional cook." By the eighteenth century, the term Cordon-bleu was applied to anyone who excelled in a particular field. The term became chiefly associated with fine cooks.

2. There is a cooking school in Paris, established in 1895, called the Cordon Bleu. The "Grand Diplome" of the Cordon Bleu Cooking School is the highest credential a chef can have. It is considered to be one of the greatest references a chef can have.

3. The term is also applied to outstanding foods prepared to a very high standard, such as a chicken or veal dish stuffed with cheese and ham.

Coriander Coriander is related to the parsley family and native to the Mediterranean and the Orient. It represents a seeds, a leaf, and a powder used in cooking. Coriander, the leaf, is also known as cilantro and Chinese parsley. The flavors of the seeds and the leaves bear no resemblance to each other. The tiny (1/8-inch), yellow-tan seeds are lightly ridged. They are mildly fragrant and have an aromatic flavor akin to a combination of lemon, sage, and, caraway. Whole coriander seeds are used in pickling and for special drinks, such as mulled wine. Ground coriander seed is also called cumin.

Corn 1. The word "corn" is sometimes used to denote grains in general. Corn was the term used for whatever grain was the primary crop in a given place. Therefore, corn in one area might be barley, while in another area it might be wheat.

2. In the U.S., it applies to "maize" or "Indian corn" which was used for food by the earliest natives of the Western Hemisphere. Corn had an important part in early tribal ceremonies and celebrations.

Corn oil It is made from the germ of the corn kernel. Corn oil is almost tasteless and is excellent for cooking because it can withstand high temperatures without smoking. It is high in polyunsaturated fat and is used to make margarine, salad dressings, and mayonnaise.

Corn salad It is a salad green (not actually corn), having small, white to pale bluish flowers and edible young leaves. Mache leaves are tender, velvety green with either a mild or sweet, nutty flavor. It is also sometimes called mache, field salad, field lettuce, feldsalat, lamb's tongue, and lamb's lettuce. It is considered a gourmet green and usually is expensive and harc to find. This plant grows wild in Europe and is used as a forage crop for sheep. It is a pest in wheat and cornfields. Chefs, who love these early spring greens, desire it. Mache is very perishable, so use immediately. Cook it like spinach, or use it in fruit and vegetable dishes.

Corn syrup A common ingredient in the US made by adding enzymes to corn starch, turning it into a thick syrup of dextrose, maltose and/or glucose. It comes in two styles - dark and light. Light corn syrup is very sweet, like golden syrup while dark corn syrup has a molasses flavour. It's used widely in the food industry for sweetening soft drinks, alcohol, ketchup and pickles. The light version is available in the UK in larger supermarkets, but the dark molasses type is harder to find.

Corn, flour Flour corn is a variety of maize with large, soft grains and very friable endosperm, making it easy to grind to flour.

Cornbread A type of bread made from cornmeal flour. Maize (corn) is a major crop in the US and the southern states in particular use cornmeal (which is the product of ground, dried maize) to make a wide variety of dishes, including cornbread. Cornbread can include various flavourings such as cheese, spring onions or bacon and is usually baked in a rectangular pan cooked either thin and crisp or thick, light and airy. It's served with all kinds of dishes, such as deep-fried chicken or bowls of chilli, and can be used as the basis for stuffing for turkey. In Italy the same golden cornmeal is known as polenta.

Corned beef A beef brisket (a fibrous, tough muscle located in the belly between the animal's front legs) is considered the meat of choice, though a bottom round can also be used. The meat was preserved in brine using a salt so coarse that it was the size of corn kernels. The traditional corning mix also used saltpeter and spices. Thus, the term "to corn" was coined, and it refers to the process of making the brine for preserving the meat for several weeks. Corned beef is of British origin. Corning was a preservation method much used by their military. It was also found well suited to the rigors of colonial life, as few communities had butchers. Although the word "corn" is now used as a verb, it originally was a noun, describing small grains and other, particles. Corned beef was heavily salted and spiced with ingredients in particulate form. Corned beef was originally made with a cut known as "silverside" (part of the round).

Cornflakes Breakfast cereal made from maize, often enriched with vitamins. A 40-g portion of enriched cornflakes is a rich source of vitamins B 2, B 6, B 12, niacin, and folate; a good ource of vitamin B 1 and iron; provides 4.4 g of dietary fibre; supplies 145 kcal.

Cornflour Cornflour - or cornstarch as it's known in the US - is the finely powdered white starch extracted from maize kernels, which are soaked and ground to separate the germ and the bran. It's virtually tasteless and is used as a thickening agent. It cuts down the need for fat as, unlike other flours, it blends to a smooth cream with liquid.

However, it will form lumps if added directly to hot liquid so to use, blend with double the amount of cold liquid to cornflour and stir into the sauce to be thickened. Keep stirring while the sauce comes to the boil, and it will gradually thicken. It's best to cook the sauce for a few minutes to remove the slightly floury taste. Cornflour also makes a good coating for fish or meat, can be used to produce a light tempura batter and is also used to make certain cakes and biscuits.

Cornmeal In Italy, it is known as polenta. Made from ground corn, fresh ground cornmeal is excellent flour for baking. It is similar to semolina in texture. Tortillas and cornbread are two of the most common cornmeal based foods. Cornmeal is versatile enough to be used in both sweet and savory dishes.

Steel-ground cornmeal The husk and germ have been almost completely removed from the corn's hull. Because of this, it can be stored almost indefinitely in an airtight container in a cool, dark place.

Stone- or water-ground cornmeal This cornmeal retains some of the corn's hull and germ. Because of the fat in the germ, it is more perishable, Store in an airtight container in the refrigerator for up to four months.

Cornstarch A white, dense, powdery thickener that is finer than flour. It is extracted from the starch (endosperm) of the wheat of corn. It must be dissolved in a cold liquid before it is added to a hot mixture or it will lump. It results in a glazy opaque finish.

Coronary heart disease Coronary heart disease (CHD), also called coronary artery disease (CAD) and atherosclerotic heart disease, is the end result of the accumulation of atheromatous plaques within the walls of the arteries that supply the myocardium (the muscle of the heart). While the symptoms and signs of coronary heart disease are noted in the advanced state of disease, most individuals with coronary heart disease show no evidence of disease for decades as the disease progresses before the first onset of symptoms, often a "sudden" heart attack, finally arise. After decades of progression, some of these atheromatous plaques may rupture and (along with the activation of the blood clotting system) start limiting blood flow to the heart muscle. The disease is the most common cause of sudden death.

Correlation An association, or when one phenomenon is found to be accompanied by another. A correlation does not prove cause and effect. Correlation may also be defined statistically.

Cottage cheese Cottage cheese, as we know, is a soft, lumpy cheese, made from drained and pressed milk curds. It is a soft, uncured cheese made from skim milk or from reconstituted concentrated skim milk or nonfat dry milk solids. If the cheese contains 4% or more of fat, it is called creamed cottage cheese. It has also been known, at various times in various places, in various name such as pot cheese, smearcase, bonnyclabber, farmer cheese, sour-milk cheese, and curd cheese. For centuries the standard type of cheese was cottage cheese, made by souring milk. The technique of using rennet (a substance taken from the stomach lining of calves) to hard cheese first appeared in Switzerland around the 15th century. Since such cheese could be stored for lengthy periods, it soon became part of the basic food of travelers. The Gaelic term bonnyclabber (bainne clabhair), clabber cheese or clabbered milk dates back to at least 1631, while the name "cottage cheese" only shows up in 1850 or so. In the early part of the 19th century, the name for such cheese was "pot cheese," which is pretty much synonymous with cottage cheese today. By the 1820s, the German communities of American used the term "smear case" from Schmierkase. Other names are "farmer cheese," "sour-milk cheese," and "curd cheese."

Cotton candy Also known as candy flosh, spun sugar, and sugar cotton wool. A fluffy confection that is made from long spun sugar threads. Traditionally made by melting sugar and flossine together in a centrifuge. These resulting strands become long thread that collect on the sides of the centrifuge.

Cottonseed oil A clear yellow oil with almost no taste. It is produced from the seeds of the cotton plant and it is primarily used for commercial margarine and salad dressings.

Cottonseed Seed of Gossypium spp.; of double use in the food field since the oil is valuable as cooking oil, or for margarine manufacture when hardened, and the protein residue is a valuable animal feed. The oil is 25% saturated and 50% polyunsaturated.

Coulis 1. A French culinary term. It is a type of a sauce, usually a thick one, which derives its body (either entirely or in part), from pureed fruits or vegetables. A sauce of cooked down tomatoes can be a tomato coulis as can a puree of strained blackberries.

2. Today coulis also denotes some thick soups made with crayfish, lobster, prawns, and other crustaceans, the word being employed where bisque has formerly been used.

Country captain chicken A curried chicken dish. The chicken is browned and then stewed in a sauce of tomatoes, onion, garlic, and curry powder. At the end, golden raisins are added. The dish is served over rice sprinkled with toasted almonds. As with all chicken recipes in the South, Country Captain Chicken varies with the cook. Some recipes call for a long cooking time and other use quick-cooking chicken breasts. One thing is always certain about this dish; it is perfumed and slightly spiced with curry.

Court bouillon It is a French term that means, "short broth." It is used in place of water when boiling various types of food (mostly used for poaching fish or as a base for fish soups). The broth is made of wine, water, herbs, and spices.

It usually is also flavored with onions, celery, carrots and cloves.

Couscous Couscous is a small granular type of pasta which is made by sprinkling durum or hard wheat semolina grains with cold salted water and rolling and coating them in fine wheat flour. It's a staple ingredient in North Africa. Couscous is also the name of a dish in which the grains are steamed over a spiced stew of vegetables and/ or meat or chicken. Traditional couscous can be bought in the UK, but needs presoaking and takes a long time to cook - it's usually steamed. The quick-cook couscous is more convenient and involves just soaking or simmering the couscous in boiling water for about ten minutes to rehydrate it. You can buy flavoured couscous but it's usually better to add your own ingredients during cooking.

Couscous can be used hot or cold either as a main dish or as an accompaniment. Stir cooked vegetables into it (try roasted peppers and mushrooms) or toss with chopped nuts and dried fruits and flavour with a pinch of your favourite spice. Use it for stuffing vegetables or serve it sweetened with cinnamon and sugar as a dessert.

Couscousier This is the traditional pot in which couscous is cooked. It looks like an enormous double boiler with a deep bottom and a perforated top in which the couscous grain is steamed over an aromatic spicy stew.

Cover charge A fee levied by restaurante "to cover" the cost of tablecloths, napkins, cutlery, glasses, etc. It has also become the custom for nightclubs, which offer entertainment as well as food and drink, to levy a cover charge of these professional services.

Cow-heel Dish made from heel of ox or cow, stewed to a jelly; also known as neat's-foot.

Crab apple The small, sour fruit of the wild apple tree. Crab apples are generally too tart to eat raw and are more commonly used to make a sweet jelly for scones and brioches, or as a condiment for roasted meats and game. They're also used to make crab apple wine. As they're not grown commercially they're not readily available to buy. You're more likely to find them at farmers' markets or farm shops and pick-your-own farms.

Crab boil It is a phrase that describes a mixture of dried herbs and spices that are added to water in which crab, shrimp, or lobster is cooked (it's strong, pungent and spicy). They come either in a flow-through packet, in dry powdered form, or as a liquid concentrate. The blend is sold packaged in supermarkets or specialty stores. Crab boil includes some or all of the following: whole allspice, bay leaves, hot chiles, cloves, ginger, mustard seeds, and peppercorns.

Crab Louie Salad This famous west coast salad is also called "King of Salads," and is sometimes written as Crab Louis Salad. Today there are as many versions of this famous salad as there are cooks.

Crab Shellfish; Cancer and Carcinus spp.; king crab is Limulus polyphemus. A 100-g portion (500 g with shell) is a rich source of protein, niacin, zinc, copper, and selenium; a good source of iron; a source of vitamins B2 and B6; contains 400 mg of sodium and 5 g of fat of which 13% is saturated; supplies 130 kcal (545 kJ).

Crackers Plain, thin biscuits such as water biscuits, cream crackers, and wholemeal crackers, made from wheat flour, fat, and bicarbonate as a raising agent. A 40-g portion (5 biscuits) contains 3-6 g of fat; provides 1-2 g of dietary fibre and 160-280 mg of sodium; supplies 170 kcal (715 kJ).

Cracklin, cracklings Also called gratons or grattons by the Cajuns. Cracklings are bits of roasted or deep-fried pork skins. You can make your own, or you may be able to find them at small Mom & Pop groceries.

Cracknel 1. Plain biscuit made with paste which is boiled before baking so that it puffs up.

2. Brittle toffee filling for chocolates.

Cran A traditional measure for herrings containing 37½ gallons (167 L) or about 800 fish.

Cranberry As cranberries bounce when they're ripe, they are also called bounceberries. Also since their blossom resembles the neck of a sand hill crane, thus another name, "crane-berries." Gradually, this word became "cranberry," the name we use today. These berries, blueberries and Concord grapes are North America's only true native fruits. They are grown in huge, sandy bogs on low, trailing vines across northern North America. Cranberries are usually harvested in September and October. Although, they can be hand-scooped (dry-harvested), most are mechanically harvested while the bogs are flooded. The cranberry helped sustain Americans for hundreds of years. Native Americans used cranberries in a variety of foods. They also used it as a medicine to treat arrow wounds and as a dye for rugs and blankets. Ripe berries were mixed with fat and meat to make pemmican. Native Americans taught the Pilgrims how to use cranberries. The Pilgrims considered cranberries such a delicacy that in 1677 the Plymouth colonists sent 10 barrels of them to King Charles II. The tart fruit did not impress him. Cultivation of the cranberry began around 1810. Captain Henry Hall (a veteran of the Revolutionary War), of Dennis, Massachusetts, made an accidental discovery that led to their commercial cultivation. He noticed that the wild cranberries in his bogs grew better when sand blew over them. Captain Hall began transplanting his cranberry vines, fencing them in, and spreading sand on them himself

Crawfish boil A traditional event or party where friends and family gather to feast on pounds of steaming, boiled crawfish that are highly seasoned with a secret blend of Cajun spices, and served with boiled skin-on potatoes, whole onions, and corn-on-the-cob. In the Spring, whole families will go out fishing on the bayous or crawfish farms in an age-old tradition that thrives to this day. Boiling crawfish is an art and every cook seems to have their own recipe and opinions about what should and should not go into the pot.

Crawfish Sometimes it is also spelled crayfish but the word is always pronounced crawfish. Crawfish resemble tiny lobsters, but are also know in the South as mudbugs because they live in the mud of freshwater bayous. They are more tender than lobster, more delicate than shrimp, and has a unique flavor all its own. These delicious crustaceans are now raised commercially and are an important Louisiana industry. Louisiana is famous for its Cajun cuisine of which crawfish is a traditional element. The local Indians are credited with harvesting and consuming crawfish even before the Cajuns arrived. They would bait reeds with venison, stock them in the water, and then pick up the reeds with the crawfish attached to the bait. By using this method, the Indians would catch bushels of crawfish for their consumption. By the 1930s, nets were substituted, and by the 1950s, the crawfish trap was used. Crawfish have become synonymous with the hardy pioneers that settled there after being forced to leave their homes in Nova Scotia, but up until 40 years ago crawfish were used mainly as bait; it took too much effort to remove the meat from the tiny crustacean.

Cream 1. To work one or more foods until smooth and creamy with a spoon or spatula, rubbing the food against the sides of the mixing bowl until of the consistency of cream. See creaming.

2. A rich filling for cakes, eclairs, cream puffs, flans, or fancy tarts. It is somewhat similar to custard filling.

3. The rich, fatty, aggregation of oil globules found in milk.

Half and half cream It is a blending of heavy cream and milk and has about 12% butterfat, 7% milk solids, and 51% water.

Heavy cream Also called whipping cream. It contains about 40% butterfat, 5% milk solids, and over 50% water.

Light cream It contains about 20% butterfat and 7% milk solids; the rest is water.

Cream cheese It is a soft, white, smooth, cheese that melts quickly and should not be frozen. It is similar to unripe Neufchatel cheese but has a higher fat content. It is one of the most popular soft cheeses in the United States.

Cream line index The cream line or layer usually forms about 6% of the total depth of milk. The cream line index is the ratio between the percentage cream layer and the percentage of fat in the milk; in ordinary bulk pasteurized milk it is about 1.7.

Cream of tartar Cream of tartar (potassium hydrogen tartrate) is a component of baking powder. (Baking powder comprises baking soda and cream of tartar.) Cream of tartar is a by-product of winemaking; it's derived from refined tartaric acid, which forms on the inside of wine barrels, or from the whitish crystals (known as 'white diamonds') that precipitate out of some wines. It's used in baking and in making desserts. It gives a creamy texture to icings and is used to stabilise and increase the volume of beaten egg whites, so is often used in making meringues.

Cream puff A very light, delicate, hollow pastry puff made from choux pastry. It is usually filled with a sweetened whipped cream or custard. Sometimes they are filled with savory fillings (such as chicken salad). See pate a choux.

Creaming Creaming incorporates air into the butter, margarine, or vegetable shortening to give the cake a light, fine-grained texture. When creaming butter and sugar together, beat sugar gradually into room temperature butter to be sure it is absorbed. If you use an electric mixer to cream, use medium speed. Excessive speed can damage the air bubbles and melt the butter, resulting in a loss of volume and a cake that's too dense.

Creatine In 1832 the French scientist Chevreul discovered a new ingredient of meat to which he gave the name Creatine, according to the source from which it was extracted (Kreas Greek for flesh). The German scientist Justus von Liebig confirmed that Creatine is a regular constituent of flesh. Creatine levels in wild animals were 10 times higher compared to captive animals suggesting that physical activity might have an influence on the amount of Creatine present in flesh. A meat extract (Liebigs Fleischextrakt) was the only source for Creatine supplementation over the next century.

Anecdotal reports in the early 1990's suggested that Creatine Monohydrate supplementation might improve sport performance. British track and field 1992 Olympic champions Linford Christie (100 m dash) and Sally Gunnell (400m hurdles) reportedly used Creatine Monohydrate, as did the Cambridge University rowing team in training for three months before defeating the heavily favoured Oxford. Numerous controlled clinical trials followed in the upcoming years proving the benefits of Creatine supplementation in different sports.

Many celebrated professional athletes and Olympic champions acknowledge Creatine use and estimated 80% of the athletes at the 1996 Summer Olympics in Atlanta used Creatine. Mark McGwire, one of major league baseball's greatest sluggers, used Creatine during the 1998 season and his legendary race to set the single season home run record, making Creatine Monohydrate the most popular sports nutrition in the US. Creatine supplementation has become a common practice among professional, elite, collegiate and amateur athletes to enhance exercise performance.

Today, Creatine Monohydrate is one of the best-studied supplements in the field of sports nutrition and its proven efficacy as an ergogenic substance was reviewed and accepted by numerous authorities

Creme brulee It is simple custard of nothing more than cream, eggs, sugar, and vanilla that is topped with a caramelized topping. The origins of this custard are very much in contention, with the English, Spanish, and French all staking claim. 1. The Spanish have taken credit for this dessert as Crema Catalana since the 18th century.

2. The English claim it originated in the 1860s at Trinity College, Cambridge. It is said that it was born when an English chef accidentally burned custard he had sprinkled with sugar. The chef then passed it off as an original creation calling it burnt cream. It is also called Trinity Cream and Cambridge Burnt Cream.

Around the end of the 19th century, the French translation came into vogue. It is thought that Thomas Jefferson, who loved the dish, may have influenced the dish to be called creme brulee. The theory is that Jefferson always referred to this dish by its French name and before long, American and English people were doing the same. Whatever its origins, creme brulee came to the U.S. sometime in the 19th century in New Orleans. It wasn't until the 1980s that creme brulee gained popularity after being introduced by Chef Alain Sailhac of New York's Le Cirque restaurant.

Creme de menthe It is the most popular of liqueurs and it tastes of fresh mint. It comes in green and white colours. It is commonly served after dinner.

Creme fraiche It is a matured, thickened cream that has a slightly tangy, nutty flavor and velvety rich texture. The thickness can range from that of commercial sour cream to almost as solid as room temperature margarine. In France, the cream is unpasteurized and therefore contains the bacteria necessary to thicken it naturally. In America, where all commercial cream is pasteurized, the fermenting agents necessary can be obtained by adding buttermilk or sour cream. To make creme fraiche, combine 1 cup whipping cream and 2 tablespoons buttermilk in a glass container. Cover and let stand at room temperature from 8 to 24 hours, or until very thick. Stir well before covering and refrigerate up to 10 days. It is an ideal addition for sauces or soups because it can be boiled without curdling. It is also delicious spooned over fresh fruit or other desserts such as warm cobblers or puddings.

Creole cuisine 1. The word originally described people of mixed French and Spanish blood who migrated from Europe or were born in southeast Louisiana.

2. It is also a local term used in the New Orleans area meaning the finest regionally raised products (such as Creole garlic, Creole tomatoes, etc).

3. Today the term has expanded and now embraces a type of cuisine. Creole cuisine uses more spices than Cajun cuisine and is considered more sophisticated and complex. Cajun cooking is "city cooking." New Orleans, the capital of Creole cuisine, had established a culinary reputation by early 19th century.

The Creoles were the European born aristocrats, wooed by the Spanish to establish New Orleans in the 1690's. Second born sons, who could not own land or titles in their native countries, were offered the opportunity to live and prosper in their family traditions here in the New World. They brought with them not only their wealth and education, but also their chefs and cooks. With these chefs came the knowledge of the grand cuisines of Europe. The influences of classical and regional French, Spanish, German and Italian cooking are readily apparent in Creole cuisine. The terminologies, precepts, sauces, and major dishes carried over, some with more evolution than others, and provided a solid base or foundation for Creole cooking.

Creole cooking is based upon French stews and soups, and is influenced by Spanish, African, Native American, and other Anglo Southern groups. The Spanish brought into the cuisine the use of cooked onions, green peppers, tomatoes, and garlic. African chefs brought with them the skill of spices and introduced okra. Native foodstuffs, such as crawfish, shrimp, oysters, crabs, and pecans found their way into both Cajun and Creole cuisine. From the Choctaw Indians came the use of file, a powdered herb from sassafras leaves, to thicken gumbo. One factor typically overlooked in the development of Creole-style cooking was that it was food prepared for affluent whites by their black slaves and servants. So often the emergence of a new dish was the result of creative chefs intermingling their cooking experience and heritage with the tastes of their employers.

Crepe Thin French pancake, served with sweet or savoury fillings or toppings. The best known is crкpes Suzette, which are crкpes served with a sauce made from fresh orange juice, orange zest, sugar, butter and Grand Marnier, flamed at the table before serving. If you invest in a proper crкpe pan it can make life easier - it's a short-sided frying pan about 20cm/8in across. The non-stick versions are best.

Crepes can be served as soon as they're made but they can be pre-made. Layer each crкpe between a sheet of greaseproof paper then wrap them in cling film and either store them in the fridge for use the next day. They freeze well, too, for up to a month.

Crepes Suzettes Probably the most famous crepe dish in the world. In a restaurant, a crepe suzette is often prepared in a chafing dish in full view of the guests. They are served hot with a sauce of sugar, orange juice, and liqueur (usually Grand Marnier). Brandy is poured over the crepes and then lit.

Crespolini Italian; pancakes filled with spinach, cream cheese, and chicken liver, baked in bichamel sauce.

Cretinism Mental retardation resulting from the adverse action of iodine deficiency on the maturation of the child's nervous system.

Crimp 1. To seal a double crusted pie by pinching the edges together.

2. To gash a freshly caught fish on both sides of the body at intervals of about one and one-half inches. The fish is then plunged into ice-cold water for about one hour. This is done to keep the flesh firm and to retain the original flavor.

Crimping 1. Slashing a large fish at intervals before cooking, to make it easier for the heat to penetrate the flesh.

2. Trimming cucumber or similar foods in such a way that the slices appear to be 'deckled'.

3. Decorating the double edge of a pie or tart or the edge of shortbread by pinching it at regular intervals with the fingers, giving a fluted effect.

criolla The traditional cuisine of the Spanish-speaking Caribbean and Latin America; derived from French, Spanish, African, and American cookery. See also crиole.

Crisp 1. To make crisp by immersing in cold water or refrigerating. This is used particularly with greens.

2. To crisp foods by heating in the oven.

3. A crisp is fruit topped with a crumbly mixture of butter, sugar, flour and, sometimes, nuts. Other crisp toppings include oatmeal, buttered breadcrumbs, cookie crumbs, graham cracker crumbs, and cake crumbs.

Crochette This is the Italian croquette. Its main ingredients are bound with a bechamel sauce.

Crohn's disease Chronic inflammatory disease of the bowel, of unknown origin, treated with antibiotics to prevent infection and with anti-inflammatory agents. Sufferers may be malnourished as a result of both loss of appetite due to illness and also malabsorption. Also known as regional enteritis, since only some regions of the gut are affected. See also gastro-intestinal tract.

Croissant Croissant is the French word for "crescent-shaped." Originally the croissant was made from rich bread dough but is now usually made with dough similar to puff pastry. Layers of dough are separated by butter creating a flaky, moist, richly flavored pastry. They can also be served stuffed. It originated in 1686, in Budapest, when the attacking Turks were defeated thanks to the bakers (during their night baking, detected the enemy's approach and gave the alarm in time). The bakers were granted the privilege of making a special pastry, which they shaped into crescents like the crescent moon on the Turkish flag. They called them "gipfel".

When Marie Antoinette became the Queen of Louis XVI, she brought the recipe with her to France. The French bakers enriched the dough and developed the process of refrigerating the dough after each butter application and of folding and refolding the dough.

Crop residues Plant materials remaining from the former crop that are left on the soil surface after planting form crop residues. Crop residues reduce soil erosion, air and surface water pollution, conserve soil moisture, and improve the soil by adding organic matter.

Croquembouche The word can also be written croque-en-bouche. It derives from the French word croquer meaning to "munch or crunch" or "crisp-in-the-mouth." The term applies to foods that are glazed with sugar. A croquembouche consists of balls of baked choux pastry (called profiteroles and cream puffs) stacked in a pyramid (cone shape). The pastry is covered with spun caramelized sugar. It is considered the traditional French "wedding cake" and when featured as a wedding centerpiece, it is known as a "piece monte." It also plays an important role at French baptisms, christenings, and other French gatherings.

Croquette Croquette is derived from the French word "croquer" meaning to "crunch or munch." Ette is a suffix meaning "small." It literally means "a small crunchy morsel." Croquettes come in various shapes such as balls, pear-shaped, and barrel-shaped. They are made from a wide variety of ingredients, such as minced meat, fish or poultry, mashed potatoes, rice, tapioca, and semolina. The main ingredient is bound with egg yolk or a mixture of butter, egg, flour, and milk. It is fried in hot oil until golden brown and crispy.

Cross-sectional A study in which a group (or groups) of individuals are composed into one large sample and studied at only a single point in time

Crostini Crostini means "little toasts" in Italian. Technically, the appetizer is named after the toast that makes up its base. They are small slices of bread, usually brushed with olive oil or butter, then toasted. They are then topped with a variety of savory toppings. They are the Italian version of canapıs. A long thin loaf (such as a baguette bread) will work well. Slice it on a diagonal into half-inch slices. The topping should be spread about a quarter-inch thick. In addition to bread, you can also use polenta squares, cut to the same size and fried for a few minutes, or until crisp and golden, in hot oil.

Croute In French the word means "crust." 1. It is the French culinary name for round or oval pieces of stale bread fried in butter (or any other fat). They are used as a foundation upon which all manner of fish, meat, and vegetables preparations are served either as hors d' oeuvres, canapıs, or for garnishings.

2. Also the name of thin slices of stale crusty bread, toasted or not, which are added to some soups at the time of serving.

Croutons Small cubes of bread that have been fried and then drained and cooled. As they cool, they develop a crisp texture and are used as a garnish for soups or in salads such as Caesar salad or fattoush. In salads, add them at the last minute to prevent them from going soggy, and leave them out if the salad is served with a starchy meal such as pasta, potatoes or rice. They can also be used for stuffings.

Crowdie Scottish; soft cheese made from buttermilk or soured milk curd, also a dish of buttermilk and oatmeal.

Crown roast A crown roast is made from either lamb or pork. It is made from the rib chops, using enough ribs (two racks or parts of two), to make a handsome crown. After it is cooked, the tips of the bone are often covered with paper frills.

Crown-rump length Length between a child's head and buttocks, sometimes used as an estimator of length

Cruciferae Family of plants with flowers with four equal petals; most vegetables in this family belong to the genus Brassica.

Crudites Pieces of crisp raw vegetables, eg. cucumber, celery, radishes.

Cruller American; deep-fried bun made from baking powder dough. Similar to a doughnut.

Crumb Small particle of bread, cake, or biscuit, as broken off by rubbing. crumble Flour, fat, and sugar (a rubbed-in plain cake mix) baked as a topping over fruit instead of pastry. For savoury crumble the sugar is omitted and cheese and seasoning are added.

Crumb softeners Derivatives of monoglycerides added to bread as emulsifiers to give a softer crumb and retard staling. There are several of these compounds which are combinations of different monoglycerides, E-430-436; also called polysorbates. See also superglycinerated fats.

Crumpet Crumpets are British griddlecakes. A cross between a pancake and an American-style English muffin, the crumpet is a soft yeast-raised bread that is poured into special rings about the size of a small pancake (flat discs about three inches across and an inch or so deep), then baked on a stovetop. They are similar to an English muffin (one side is smooth, the other full of tiny holes) but flatter. You don't slice a crumpet and it is best toasted. Some, especially in the north of England, call crumpets muffins, while others, particularly in the Midlands call them pikelets (a much thinner and bigger version of a crumpet).

Crust The crisp outer part of a loaf of bread; also used for the sediment thrown off as wines mature.

Crustacea Zoological class of hard-shelled marine arthropods (shellfish) including crabs, crayfish, lobster, prawns, scampi, shrimps.

Crustacean Crustacean derives from the Latin word "crusta" meaning "crust, shell, or hard surface." "Cean" is the Latin suffix indicating "belonging to." The word came to mean a class of animals, mainly sea animals, with hard shells (edible shellfish with shells, such as crabs, crawfish, lobster, langoustine, mussels, scallops, scampi, and shrimp).

Cryogenic freezing Freezing with extremely cold freezants such as liquid nitrogen or solid carbon dioxide.

Cryovac Trade name of thermoplastic resin wrapping film which can be heat-shrunk onto foods.

Cryptoxanthin Yellow carotenoid in a few foods such as yellow maize and the seeds of Physalis, the Cape gooseberry. A hydroxylated derivative of carotene which is a source of vitamin A in the body.

Crystal boiling Chinese method of cooking; food is heated in a pan of boiling water, then removed from the heat and cooking continued by the retained heat.

CSFP Commodity Supplemental Food Program. CSFP is a USDA program that makes commodity foods available to low-income pregnant women, new mothers, infants, children up to age six, and the elderly. The USDA makes the commodities available to state agencies, which then distribute them to public and non-profit local agencies that serve these populations. This program does not operate in all states.

CSM Corn-soya-milk; a protein-rich baby food (20% protein) made in the USA from 68% pre-cooked maize (corn), 25% defatted soya flour, and 5% skim milk powder, with added vitamins and calcium carbonate.

CSREES Cooperative, State, Research, Education, and Extension Service. The agency within the USDA that supports research, education and extension programs in the Land-Grant University System. Related to hunger and nutrition, CSREES administers the Expanded Food and Nutrition Education Program.

CTC machine A device consisting of two contra-rotating toothed rollers that rotate at different speeds and provide a crushing, tearing, and curling action: used in breaking up leaves of tea to form small particles.

Cuaranta y tres Spanish; liqueur flavoured with herbs and spices; the name means 'forty-three'.

Cube Cut into small, straight-sided cubes. The size is specified if it is critical to the recipe. Larger cubes are often called chunks.

Cuccia It is the Italian word for "cooking" or "kitchen."

Cucumber Fruit of Cucumis sativus, a member of the gourd family, eaten as a salad vegetable; it is 95% water; a 50-g portion provides 0.3 g of dietary fibre and supplies 5 kcal (20 kJ). See also gherkin.

Cucurbit A term used for vegetables of the family Cucurbitaceae, or gourds.

Cuisine bourgeoise A French cooking style that varies from region to region, based solely on local ingredients. Can best be described as high quality home cooking

Cuisine Francasise Literally means the "new French cooking." This movement was started in 1974. It avoids rich, flour-thickened sauces in favour of reduced stocks and it placed strong emphasis on the ingredient's freshness, lightness of texture, clear flavors, simplicity, and aesthetic presentation

Cuisine naturelle This was a movement in the 1970s and 1980s which emphasized natural products in all dishes and avoided the use of cream, butter, oil, fat, lard, and used very little sugar.

Cuisine The work cuisine has come to mean the "art of cooking" or "cookery" in France and throughout the world. It derives from the Latin word coquina meaning, "cooking" and from the word coquere meaning "to cook."

Cuisson Cooking juices from meat, poultry, or fish. cullis See coulis.

Cuitlacoche Also called huitlacoche, corn mushroom, maize mushroom, Mexican truffle, and corn smut or smut corn. It is a costly and much-coveted corn fungus or parasite that occasionally balloons on sweet corn causing kernels swell to 10 times their normal size during the rainy season. It is very popular Mexican delicacy and considered a gourmet rage in the United States. It is often compared to caviar or truffles (not so much in terms of taste but cost and delicacy). Its earthy, smoke-like flavor is reminiscent of mushrooms. It is sold canned and frozen in gourmet markets. It's used in a variety of dishes—typically appropriate for dishes that call for cooked mushrooms.

Culinary Comes from the Latin word "culina" which means a kitchen. Today the word means anything to do with cooking.

Cultural controls An integrated pest management method which includes annual crop rotation to discourage pests and weed production.

Cultured butter It is made from cream to which lactic acid cultures have been added. The mild fermentation that results produces a richer, more developed flavor.

Cumberland sauce Sauce made from redcurrant jelly, orange, lemon, and port, served with ham, venison, and lamb. cumin (cummin) Pungent herb, the crescent-shaped seed of Cuminum cyminum (parsley family); used in curry powder and for flavouring cordials. Black cumin is the seed of Nigella sativa (fennel flower) and sweet cumin is anise (Pimpinella anisum).

Cumin Same as ground coriander seed that is produced by the cilantro plant at full maturity. Also see coriander. Cumin is native to countries that border the Mediterranean Sea; the ancient Persians, the Egyptians, and the Hebrews used cumin. During ancient Roman times, when pepper was hard to get, cooks substituted cumin seed for the pepper.

Cup North American and Australian measure for ingredients in cooking; the standard American cup contains 250 mL (8 fl oz).

Cup cake Small individual cake or bun, typically baked in a paper case and topped with icing. Also known as fairy cake.

Curacao A liqueur made from the rind of Seville oranges and brandy or gin; 30% alcohol, 30% sugar; 300 kcal (1260 kJ)/100 mL.

Curd tension A measure of the toughness of the curd formed from milk by the digestive enzymes, and used as an index of the digestibility of the milk.

Curdle The undesirable effect of overcooking. When a food (usually a dairy product based sauce or custard) becomes lumpy or separated and forms curds.

Curdling Milk and Cheese Products Curdling can be due to heat coagulation, which may occur more readily with homogenized than with non-homogenized milk. This is because homogenization apparently decreases the stability of the protein in the milk. This is especially evident in making scalloped potatoes. White sauces or gravies made of homogenized milk may appear curdled because the added fat does not combine well with that of the homogenized milk. Another factor that contributes to curdling is acid. Adding an acid product, like tomatoes when making tomato soup, or using older milk, which has become more acid can cause curdling.

Salt will also contribute to curdling. Add salt last, if possible. Adding ham to scalloped potatoes may cause curdling, due to the high salt content.

Curds Clotted protein formed when fresh milk is treated with rennet; the fluid left is whey.

Curing of meat A method of preservation by treating with salt and sodium nitrate (and nitrite), which serves to inhibit the growth of pathogenic organisms while salt-tolerant bacteria develop. During the pickling process the nitrate is converted into nitrite, which combines with the muscle pigment, myoglobin, to form the red-coloured nitrosomyoglobin which is characteristic of pickled meat products.

Currant This fruit gets its name from Corinth, a once famous city of ancient Greece, where currants were cultivated and exported in considerable quantities. It is related to the gooseberry and there are black, red, and white currents. The black ones are generally used for preserves, syrups, and liqueurs (such as cassis), while the red and white berries are usually eaten raw. Currant can also refer to a small Zante grape that originated in Greece that is used for baking.

Curry A curry is basically a sort of stew containing vegetables, spices, and usually some kind of meat often served over rice. It is the mainstay of Indian cuisine. While we usually think of curry as a very spicy dish, there are also many subtle and mild curries. The origin of word is rather straightforward: it comes from Tamil, a language found primarily in Southeastern India and Sri Lanka. The Tamil word kari means "sauce or relish for rice." Subsequent forms included "carree," "carrye" and "kerry" before our modern spelling "curry" became current in the 18th century

Curry ingredients Curry powder originated from India. Today, curry is categorized as mild, hot, and very hot. A standard curry powder would include turmeric, coriander, cumin, pepper (essential), cloves, cardamom, ginger, nutmeg, tamarind, and chili pepper. It may be further seasoned with fennel, caraway, ajowan, ginseng, dried basil, mustard seeds, and cinnamon.

Curry powder The spices for curry powder have varied for thousands of years. The word curry comes from the South Indian word kari, which means "sauce." Curry powder is not one single spice (it actually is a blend of many spices). Curry powder should not be confused with curry leaves, which are obtained from a native tree of India. Curry powder, as we know it in the United States, simply does not exist in Indian cooking. Spices should be bought whole and ground and blended as needed. This way the flavors are truly aromatic and blends are tailor-made to suit individual recipes and personal taste. There are a lot of variations in curry powder blends. As a general rule, a curry powder blend will contain six or more of the following items: cumin, coriander, fenugreek, turmeric, ginger, pepper, dill, mace, cardamon, and cloves.

Custard Custard is a combination of eggs and milk, which may be sweetened or unsweetened, cooked in a double boiler (as soft custard), or baked (which gives it a jelly-like consistency). Custards require slow cooking and gentle heat in order to prevent separation (curdling).

Custard apple The fruit of one of a number of species of tropical American trees of the family Anonaceae. Sour sop, Anona muricata, has white fibrous flesh and is less sweet than the others; the fruit may weigh up to 4 kg (8 lb). The sweet sop (A. squamosa) is also known as the 'true' custard apple, and is especially popular in the West Indies. The bullock's heart (A. reticulata) has buff-coloured flesh. A 100-g portion is a rich source of vitamin C and supplies 90 kcal.

Cut An area of severed skin. Wash a cut or scrape it with soap and water, and keep it clean and dry. Putting alcohol, hydrogen peroxide, or iodine into a wound can delay healing, and should be avoided. Seek medical care if you think you might need stitches, as delay can increase the rate of wound infection. If the cut results from a puncture wound through the shoe, there is a high risk of infection, and you should see your healthcare professional. Redness, swelling, increased pain, and pus draining from the wound also indicate an infection that requires professional care.

Cut in To work with a pastry blender or two knives until sold fat and dry ingredients are evenly and finely divided, especially in making dough.

Cutting-in Combining the fat with other ingredients in a mixture by cutting with a knife.

CVA Cerebrovascular accident.

Cyanogen(et)ic glycosides Organic compounds of cyanide found in a variety of plants; chemically cyanhydrins linked by glycoside linkage to one or more sugars. Toxic through liberation of the cyanide when the plants are cut or chewed. See also almond; amygdalin.

Cyclamate A sweetener which is 30 times sweeter than sucrose, calorie free and heat stable and works synergistically with other sweeteners. It is approved for tabletop use in Canada and more than 50 countries in Europe, Asia, South America and Africa. Since 1970, however, the use of cyclamate has been banned in the United States on the basis of a study that suggested that cyclamates may be related to the development of bladder tumors in rats. Although 75 subsequent studies have failed to show that cyclamate is carcinogenic, the sweetener has yet to be reapproved for use in the United States.

Cymogran Trade name for a protein-rich food which is low in phenylalanine for feeding patients with phenylketonuria.

Cystathioninuria A genetic disease affecting the metabolism of the amino acid methionine and its conversion to cysteine. May result in mental retardation if untreated. Treatment is by feeding a diet low in methionine and supplemented with cysteine, or, in some cases, by administration of high intakes of vitamin B 6 (about 100-500 times the normal requirement).

Cysteine A non-essential amino acid, but nutritionally important since it spares the essential amino acid methionine. In addition to its role in protein synthesis, cysteine is important as the precursor of taurine, in formation of coenzyme A from the vitamin pantothenic acid and in formation of the tripeptide glutathione. It is used as a dough 'improver' in baking. See also cystine.

Cystic fibrosis (CF) An inherited disorder of the exocrine glands, primarily the pancreas, pulmonary system and sweat glands, characterized by abnormally thick luminal secretions

Cysticercosis Infection by the larval stage of tapeworms caused by ingestion of their eggs in food and water contaminated by human faeces. Normally the larval form develops in the animal host, and human beings are infected with the adult form by eating undercooked infected meat.

Cystine The dimer of cysteine produced when its sulphydryl group (—SH) is oxidized forming a disulphide (—S—S—) bridge. Such disulphide bridges are especially important in maintaining the structure of proteins, and also in the rτle of the tripeptide glutathione as an antioxidant. Hair protein (keratin) is especially rich in cystine, which accounts for about 12% of its total amino acid content.

Cystinuria A genetic disease in which there is abnormally high excretion of the amino acids cysteine and cystine, resulting in the formation of kidney stones. Treatment is by feeding a diet low in the sulphur amino acids methionine, cysteine, and cystine.

Cytochrome P 450 A family of cytochromes which are involved in the detoxication system of the body. They act on a wide variety of (potentially toxic) compounds, both endogenous metabolites and foreign compounds (xenobiotics), rendering them more water-soluble, and more readily conjugated for excretion in the urine. cytochromes Haem-containing proteins present in every type of living cell (except the strictly anaerobic bacteria). Some cytochromes react with oxygen directly; others are intermediates in the oxidation of reduced coenzymes. Unlike haemoglobin, the iron in the haem of cytochromes undergoes oxidation and reduction.

Cytokines A type of protein released by cells of the immune system, which act through specific cell receptors to regulate immune responses

Cytokinins Substances that stimulate cell division (cytokinesis) and control the development of plants; found in seed embryos, developing fruits, and buds. They are derivatives of the purine adenine.

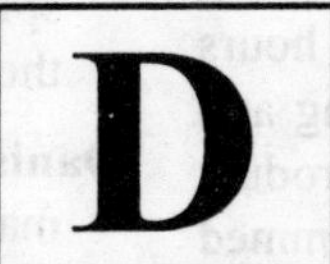

D and l An obsolete way of indicating dextrorotatory and laevorotatory optical activity, now replaced by (+) and(–).

D-, L-, and DL- Prefixes to chemical names for compounds that have a centre of asymmetry in the molecule, and which can therefore have two forms (isomers).

Most naturally occurring sugars have the D-conformation; apart from a few microbial proteins and some invertebrate peptides, all the naturally occurring amino acids have the L-configuration. Chemical synthesis yields a mixture of the D- and L-isomers (the racemic mixture), generally shown as DL-. See also R-.

Dagwood It is a multi-layered sandwich with a variety of fillings. Used to denote a sandwich put together so as to attain such a tremendous size and infinite variety of contents as to stun the imagination, sight, and stomach of all but the original maker.

Daikon A long, white vegetable of the radish family, also known as mooli. It's crunchy, with a mild peppery flavour, similar to watercress. Unlike other radishes it's as good cooked as it is raw. In Chinese and Japanese cookery it's used for vegetable carving as well as cooking. Daikon is sometimes available in larger supermarkets, but you're more likely to find it in Asian or Caribbean food shops.

Daikon radish The word Daikon actually comes from two Japanese words: dai (meaning large) and kon (meaning root). Daikon is a root vegetable said to have originated in the Mediterranean and brought to China for cultivation around 500 B.C. Roots are large, often 2 to 4 inches in diameter and 6 to 20 inches long. There are three distinct shapes - spherical, oblong and cylindrical. Radishes have been developed in the Orient which develop very large roots, reportedly up to 40 or 50 pounds, and with leaf top spreads of more than 2 feet (they require a long growing season for such development. These types are grown in the U.S., mainly by Orientals for use in oriental dishes). Most of the commonly available Chinese radishes are white, but some are yellowish, green or black.

Daily value DV, a term on food labels based on the RDA (Recommended Dietary Allowance) designed to help consumers use food label information to plan a healthy diet.

Daiquiri Correctly a trade name for rum; commonly used for a mixture of rum and fresh lime juice, or other fruit juice.

Dairy products Foods and other products derived from the processing of milk. Separation of milk by centrifugation yields skimmed milk and cream. Churning the cream disrupts the fat globules, removes water, and produces butter, containing over 80% fat, and buttermilk. Cream is retailed in various stages of concentration, for example single cream and double cream; other less concentrated forms include evaporated milk (containing about 65% water) and condensed milk (about 26% water). Yogurt (or yoghurt) is produced by inoculating whole milk with bacteria, principally of the genera Streptococcus and Lactobacillus. The acid they produce during incubation at about 43°C for four to five hours coagulates the milk, to which sweetening and flavouring may be added. Whey is a by-product of cheese manufacture and, as with skimmed milk, may be dried to a powder form for use in the food industry or fed to farm animals in the fresh liquid state.

Daltose Trade name for a carbohydrate preparation consisting of maltose, glucose and dextrin for infant feeding.

Damascene Original name for damson.

Damson Small dark purple plum (Prunus damascena); very acid and mainly used to make jam. An 80-g portion provides 2.4 g of dietary fibre and supplies 30 kcal.

Dandelion Commonly considered a weed, dandelions provide excellent salad leaves when they're young (larger, older leaves become bitter). They grow wild all over Europe, the US and Asia. If you pick your own, do so early in the year - in the spring when the leaves are small and sweet, before the flower forms. Take care though, because they may have been chemically sprayed and if so should be avoided. Also avoid picking dandelions by the roadside as they will have absorbed petrol fumes. In some parts of Europe, cultivated varieties are available that have longer, more tender leaves. These are available from specialist herb growers in the UK.

Dandelion The leaves of the weed Taraxacum officinale may be eaten as a salad or cooked. In France dandelion greens are known as pis- en-lit because of their diuretic action. A 50-g portion of the leaves is a good source of vitamins C and A (4000 μg carotene); a source of calcium and iron; supplies 25 kcal (105 kJ). The root can be cooked as a vegetable, or may be roasted and used as a substitute for coffee.

Dandelion green A dark green, thick, jagged-edged leaf from the dandelion plant. Dandelion greens have a slightly bitter flavor with a bite, which intensifies as the greens age. The leaves may be served raw, in a mixed salad, or cooked like spinach. If you pick your own, make sure that they are chemical free.

Danish blue After World War II, Danish cheese makers created a new blue cheese. By using Bleu d'Auvergen and Bleu des Causses as models, they began making a cheese that we know today as Danish Blue. It is made with large machinery and modern technology. It is a flawless blue cheese but it is considered uninteresting and with a predominant flavor of salt.

Danish pastry Rich, sweet, yeast pastry confection filled with fruit or nuts. Originally Viennese, not Danish; indeed in Danish it is known as Wienerbrod.

Dariole Also known as a madeleine tin, this is a small steep-sided metal mould about 8cm (3.2in) tall, with flared sides (narrower at the bottom than at the top). It's used for individual servings of all kinds of sweet or savoury dishes including pastries, mousses, jellies, timbales or portions of rice or potatoes. Castle pudding is a classic dessert that's always made in a dariole mould.

Dark adaptation In the eye, the visual pigment rhodopsin is formed by reaction between vitamin A aldehyde and the protein opsin, and is bleached by exposure to light, stimulating a nerve impulse (this is the basis of vision). At an early stage of vitamin A deficiency it takes considerably longer than normal to adapt to see in dim light after exposure to normal bright light, because of the limitation of the amount of rhodopsin that can be reformed. Measuring the time taken to adapt to dim light (the dark adaptation time) thus provides a sensitive index of early vitamin A deficiency. More severe vitamin A deficiency results in night blindness, and eventually complete blindness.

Dartois (d'Artois) Small light pastry, filled and flavoured (either sweet or savoury) served as an hors d'oeuvre or dessert.

Dash A measuring term referring to a very small amount of seasoning added to food. In general, a dash can be considered to be somewhere between 1/16 and a scant 1/8 teaspoon.

Date Widely grown in Arab countries, the date is the fruit of the date palm. Dates are sweet and rich with a chewy, sticky texture. Fresh dates are plump and dark brown with a glossy sheen. Dried dates look very similar and it can be hard to tell the difference if you buy them packaged. Dried dates are often coated in syrup to keep them soft and sticky. As dates are harvested in late autumn and early winter, this is when the best selection is available in the shops and they're more likely to be fresh. Fresh or dried, they keep really well - for at least a few months in a cool, dark cupboard. They also freeze well.

There are hundreds of varieties, but degelt noor from North Africa and the Middle East is the most plentiful. Medjool are large, deep-red coloured dates, usually from Jordan or California. They're expensive but worth it for their delicious toffee-like taste. You can buy clusters of dates still on the stem or packaged in boxes - stoned or with the stones still in. Buy stone-in dates for the best flavour.

Eat them as a sweet snack, or chop them up and scatter them on your cereal in place of sugar or honey. Chopped up they can also be added to cakes, biscuits and desserts. They're delicious served with cheese or as an after-dinner treat. North African cuisine makes varied use of dates, notably in tagines and sweet couscous dishes.

Date marking On packaged foods, 'Best before' is the date up until the food will remain in optimum condition, i.e. will not be stale. Foods with a shelf life of up to 12 weeks are marked 'best before day, month, year'; foods with a longer shelf life are marked 'best before end of month, year'. Perishable foods with a shelf life of less than a month may have a 'sell-by' date instead. 'Use by' date is given for foods that are microbiologically highly perishable and could become a danger to health; it is the date up to and including which the food may be safely used if stored properly.

Frozen foods and ice cream carry star markings which correspond to the star marking on freezers and frozen food compartments of refrigerators. Food in a 1-star rated compartment (-4 °C, 25 °F) will keep for one week; 2-star rated (-11 °C, 12 °F), 1 month; 3-star rated (-18 °C, 0 °F), 3 months. Corresponding times for ice cream are 1 day, 1 week, 1 month (after such times they are still fit to eat but the texture changes).

DATEM Diacetyl tartaric esters of mono- and diglycerides used as emulsifiers to strengthen bread doughs and delay staling of the bread (E-472(e)).

Dates One of the earliest fruits know to man, dates were grown in Mesopotamia (now Iraq) and in Egypt more than 5,000 years ago. Called "the candy that grows on trees," they served as food for camel caravans making treks across the dessert.

Daube A classic French method of cooking a type of stew, usually using a single joint of meat braised in red-wine stock, with vegetables and herbs. Once the meat is cooked, the braising liquid is thickened, then reduced and served with the meat and vegetables. A daube usually refers to a piece of beef cooked this way.

Dauphinoise To cook something 'ŏ la Dauphinoise' means to bake it in a slow oven with cream and garlic. A gratin dauphinoise is a classic dish of thinly sliced potatoes cooked in this way - with garlic, cream, milk, butter and often gruyθre cheese - rich, but very delicious! Serve it as an accompaniment to meat or vegetable dishes.

Defecography A test that uses x-rays to look at the behaviour of the rectum and anus during attempts to defecate.

Deglaze To deglaze is to add wine, stock or other liquid to a hot pan or roasting tin in which food has been roasted or sautied. Use a wooden spatula to scrape all the tasty bits sticking to the bottom and sides of the pan and stir them into the juices. Reduce the liquid slightly and serve it with the food as a sauce or gravy.

Deionized water Water that has had the cations and anions removed by passing it over a bed of ion-exchange resins.

Delange syndrome A congenital syndrome characterized by short stature, microcephaly, delayed development and mental retardation, a number of distinct facial features, and upper limb anomalies; also called Cornelia deLange syndrome and Brachmann-deLange syndrome

Delicata squash It is a winter squash that grows only 6 to 9 inches long and 2 to 3 inches in diameter. It has a small seed cavity yielding lots of edible flesh. The skin is also edible. It ranges in colour from cream to yellow with green stripes.

Delmonico steak The meaning of a Delmonico steak has changed over the years and from place to place. Depending on the place, the name today is regularly used as a synonym for a club steak, a New York strip steak, a boneless rib-eye steak, and several other cuts, as described below. This is unfortunate because the name originally applied to a very rare, tender and tasty steak that became world-famous in the 19th Century.

Demerara sugar This pale-coloured and mild-tasting raw cane sugar is named after its place of origin - Demerara, in Guyana - but it's now imported from various other places such as Jamaica, Malawi and Mauritius. It has large sparkling golden crystals and a crunchy texture. Traditionally used to sweeten coffee, it's perfect for sprinkling but can also be used for baking, particularly in things that need extra crunchiness such as crumbles, cheesecake bases, flapjacks and biscuits. You can also buy fine demerara sugar, which is better for cake baking. Keep it stored in an airtight container somewhere cool and dry to prevent the crystals from going hard.

Demersal fish Those fish found living on or near the bottom of the sea, including cod, haddock, whiting, and halibut. They contain little oil (1-4%). See white fish.

Demi-glace French word meaning "half-glaze." A mixture of equal proportions of brown stock and brown sauce that has been reduced by half until it can coat a spoon. See Espagnole sauce (brown sauce) for more information.

Demi-glace sauce Demi-glace sauce is a rich brown sauce often used by chefs. It's made from a reduction of clear stock and sauce espagnole - stock that has been thickened with a roux, diced vegetables and tomato purie - and is the basis for classic sauces such as Madeira, Diane and reform sauce. As an easier alternative for home cooking, you could use a good quality homemade beef stock that has been boiled and then reduced. Add a splash of Madeira or sherry for flavour.

Demineralized water Water that has had all the minerals and impurities removed by passing it over a bed of ion-exchange resins.

Denaturation, protein A change in the structure of protein by heat, acid, alkali, or other agents which results in loss of solubility and coagulation (as in boiled egg). It is normally irreversible. Denatured proteins lose their biological activity (e.g. as enzymes), but not their nutritional value. Indeed, their digestibility is improved compared with the original structures, which are relatively resistant to enzymic hydrolysis.

Dendritic salt A form of ordinary table salt, sodium, chloride, with the crystals branched or star-like (dendritic) instead of the normal cubes. This is claimed to have a number of advantages: lower bulk density, more rapid solution, and an unusually high capacity to absorb moisture before becoming wet.

Dental caries 1. A disease affecting the hard tissues of the teeth resulting in progressive decay.

Bacteria that accumulate in a dense mass known as plaque on the surface of the teeth ferment dietary carbohydrates (see fermentation) to form acids that de-mineralise the hard tissues underneath. Hence, cariogenicity refers to the capacity of a food or drink to lead to caries in those who consume it. Periodontal disease is a related bacterial infection that affects the softer supporting tissues of the teeth.

2. Dental caries, also known as tooth decay or dental cavities, are holes that damage the structure of teeth. The occurrence of dental caries is globally widespread, and the disease can lead to pain, tooth loss, infection, and, in severe cases, death. An estimated 90% of schoolchildren worldwide and most adults have experienced dental caries, with the disease being more severe in Asian and Latin American countries and least in African countries. In the United States, dental caries is the most common chronic childhood disease; at least five times more common than asthma. It is the most important cause of tooth loss in children.

Depectinization The removal of pectins from fruit juice to produce a clear, thin juice instead of a viscous, cloudy liquid, by the use of enzymes which hydrolyse pectins to smaller, soluble compounds.

Dermatitis A lesion or inflammation of the skin; many nutritional deficiency diseases include more or less specific skin lesions (e.g. ariboflavinosis kwashiorkor, pellagra, scurvy), but most cases of dermatitis are not associated with nutritional deficiency, and do not respond to nutritional supplements.

Descaling fish Removing the scales from a fish is best done by first cutting off the fins and then holding on to the tail and scraping away the scales the 'wrong' way - from tail to head with a large knife. This tends to be a messy job because the scales often fly about, so it's best to do it in a carrier bag. Or easier still, buy your fish from a good fishmonger and they'll do it for you!

Descriptive epidemiology The study of variations in the occurrence of disease in terms of person, place and time, without the purpose of establishing causal inference.

Desmosine The compound that forms the cross-linkage between chains of the connective tissue protein elastin.

Dessert Meaning a usually sweet food served as the final course of a meal. The word was first recorded in 1600 and it derives from a French word meaning, "to clear the table." This etymology is still reflected in current table service, where it is customary to remove everything from the table that's not being used (salt/pepper shakers, breadbaskets, sometimes even flowers) before serving dessert.

Detoxication The metabolism of (potentially) toxic compounds to yield less toxic derivatives which are more soluble in water and can be excreted in the urine or bile. A wide variety of 'foreign compounds' (i.e. compounds that are not normal metabolites in the body), sometimes referred to as xenobiotics, and some hormones and other normal body metabolites, are metabolized in the same way.

Developmental delay A term referring to a disorder in an individual who is not developing according to the expected time frame; often used in place of the term mental retardation in children younger than 5 years of age

Developmental disability A disability that begins during the developmental period (before age 22 years); federal legislation defines developmental disability in the Developmental Disabilities Assistance and Bill of Rights Act Amendments of 2000 (PL 106-402)

Devil's Food Cake A light-textured chocolate layer-type cake with a deep reddish brown colour. The cake generally has more baking soda, a stronger flavor, and a darker colour than regular chocolate cake. Devil's food cake was the favourite dessert of the early 1900s.

Deviled A term describing food that is dark, rich, chocolate, spicily piquant or stimulating it is "deviled." Means a highly seasoned, chopped, ground, or whole mixture that is served hot or cold. Many foods, including eggs and crab, are served "deviled."

Devonshire cream Originally from Devonshire County, England, it is a thick, buttery cream often used as a topping for desserts. It is still a specialty of Devon, Cornwall, and Somerset, as this is where the right breed of cattle is raised with a high enough cream content to produce clotted cream. It is also known as Devon cream and clotted cream. Clotted cream has a consistency similar to soft butter. Before the days of pasteurization, the milk from the cows was left to stand for several hours so that the cream would rise to the top. Then this cream was skimmed and put into big pans. The pans were then floated in trays of constantly boiling water in a process known as scalding. The cream would then become much thicker and develop a golden crust, which is similar to butter. Today however, the cream is extracted by a separator, which extracts the cream as it is pumped from the dairy to the holding tank. The separator is a type of centrifuge, which extracts the surplus cream at the correct quantity so that the milk will still have enough cream to be classified as milk.

Dewberry A hybrid fruit, a large variety of blackberry; rather than climbing, the plant trails on the ground.

Dexedrine Anorectic (appetite suppressing) drug used in the treatment of obesity.

Dexfenfluramine Anorectic (appetite suppressing) drug used in the treatment of obesity.

Dextran A polysaccharide composed of linked fructose units, produced by the action of Betacoccus arabinosus on sugar. It can cause problems in sugar factories, but is clinically useful as a plasma extender for transfusion.

Dextrins A mixture of soluble compounds formed by the partial breakdown of starch by heat, acid or enzymes (amylases). Formed when bread is toasted. Nutritionally equivalent to starch; industrially used as adhesives, in the sizing of paper and textiles, and as gums.

Dextrose Alternative name for glucose. Commercially the term 'glucose' is often used to mean corn syrup (a mixture of glucose with other sugars and dextrins) and pure glucose is called dextrose.

Dextrose equivalent value (DE) A term used to indicate the degree of hydrolysis of starch into glucose syrup. It is the percentage of the total solids that have been converted to reducing sugars: the higher the DE, the more sugars and less dextrins are present.

Liquid glucoses are commercially available ranging from 2 DE to 65 DE. A complete acid hydrolysis converts all the starch into glucose but produces bitter degradation products. Glucose syrups above 55 DE are termed 'high conversion' (of starch); of 35-55 DE, regular conversion; below 20 DE the products of hydrolysis are maltins or maltodextrins

DFD meat Stands for 'dark, firm, dry'; the condition of meat when the pH remains high through lack of glycogen (which would form lactic acid). It poses a microbiological hazard. See also meat conditioning; rigor mortis.

Diabetes Diabetes is the name for a group of medical disorders characterized by high blood sugar levels. Normally when people eat, food is digested and much of it is converted to glucose—a simple sugar—which the body uses for energy. The blood carries the glucose to cells where it is absorbed with the help of the hormone insulin. For those with diabetes, however, the body does not make enough insulin, or cannot properly use the insulin it does make. Without insulin, glucose accumulates in the blood rather than moving into the cells. High blood sugar levels result.

Diabetes mellitus A chronic condition associated with abnormally high levels of sugar (glucose) in the blood.. Absence or insufficient production of insulin (which is produced by the pancreas and lowers blood glucose) causes diabetes. The two types of diabetes are referred to as insulin dependent (type I) and non-insulin dependent (type II). Symptoms of diabetes include increased urine output and appetite as well as fatigue. Diabetes mellitus is diagnosed by blood sugar (glucose) testing. The major complications of diabetes mellitus include dangerously elevated blood sugar, abnormally low blood sugar due to diabetes medications, and disease of the blood vessels which can damage the eye, kidneys, nerves, and heart. Treatment depends on the type of the diabetes.

Diabetic foods Loose term for foods that are specially formulated to be suitable for consumption by people with diabetes mellitus; generally low in carbohydrate (and especially sugar), and frequently containing sorbitol, xylulose, or sugar derivatives that are slowly or incompletely absorbed.

Diacetyl The main flavour and aroma agent in butter, formed during the ripening stage by the organism Streptococcus lactis cremoris. Synthetic diacetyl is added to margarine as 'butter flavour'. Chemically it is CH 3.CO.CO.CH3.

O CH3 C—C H3C O

Fig. Diacetyl

Diallyl sulfide A type of sulfide/thoil found in onions, garlic, olives, leeks and scallions which may provide the health benefits of lowering LDL cholesterol and of maintaining a healthy immune system.

Diarrhea Passing frequent and loose stools that can be watery. Acute diarrhea goes away in a few weeks, and becomes chronic when it lasts longer than 4 weeks.

Diarrhoea Frequent passage of loose watery stools, commonly the result of intestinal infection; rarely as a result of adverse reaction to foods or disaccharide intolerance. Severe diarrhoea in children can lead to dehydration and death; it is treated by feeding a solution of salt and sugar to replace fluid and electrolyte losses.

Osmotic diarrhoea is diarrhoea associated with retention of water in the bowel as a result of an accumulation of non-absorbable water-soluble compounds; especially associated with excessive intake of sorbitol and mannitol. Also occurs in disaccharide intolerance.

Diastatic activity of flour A measure of the ability of flour to produce maltose from its own starch by the action of its own maltase (diastase). This sugar is needed for the growth of the yeast during fermentation. See also amylograph.

Diet Strictly, a diet is simply the pattern of foods eaten; the normal or habitual intake of food of an individual or population. Commonly used to mean a modified pattern of food consumption for some special purpose, e.g. a slimming, therapeutic, or low-salt diet (see salt-free diets) and sometimes named for the person who originated it.

Diet history A method of dietary assessment in which subjects are asked open-ended questions about their usual dietary intakes.

Dietary fibre Material mostly derived from plant cell walls which is not digested by human digestive enzymes but is partially broken down by intestinal bacteria to volatile fatty acids that can be used as a source of energy. A large proportion consists of non-starch polysaccharides (NSP); these include soluble fibre that reduces levels of blood cholesterol and increases the viscosity of the intestinal contents: and insoluble fibre (cellulose and cell walls) that acts as a laxative. Earlier known as roughage or bulk.

Dietary Guidelines for Americans Issued by the United States Department of Agriculture and the Department of Health and Human Services (USDA/DHHS) every five years, the Dietary Guidelines are based on scientific consensus and form the cornerstone of federal nutrition policy. The fifth edition, issued in 2000, contains ten guidelines. Its message, built around three actions "Aim, Build and Choose," strives to motivate Americans with the following advice 1. Aim for Fitness

2. Build a Healthy Base and

3. Choose sensibly. This revised set of guidelines is the first to recommend daily physical activity and the first to include a guideline specific to food safety.

Dietary orientation recommendations for the choice, preparation, domestic conservation and consumption of foods, by way of criteria which consider their nutritional values and specific indications according to physiological conditions (growth, pregnancy, lactation), pathologies (obesity, diabetes, nutrient deprivation) and, also, their socio-economic justification (nutritive value x cost). See healthy dietary practices.

Dietary recall A method of dietary assessment in which subjects are asked to recall their food consumption over a specific period of time.

Dose-response assessment 1. Estimating the potency of a chemical.

2. In exposure assessment, the process of determining the relationship between the dose of a stressor and a specific biological response. 3. Evaluating the quantitative relationship between dose and toxicological responses.

Dietary reference values A UK set of standards of the amounts of each nutrient needed to maintain good health. People differ in the daily amounts of nutrients they need; for most nutrients the measured average need plus 20% (statistically 2 standard deviations) takes care of the needs of nearly everyone and in the UK this is termed Reference Nutrient Intake, elsewhere known as Recommended Daily Allowances or Intakes (RDA or RDI), or Population Reference Intake (PRI). This figure is used to calculate the needs of large groups of people in institutional or community planning. Obviously some people require less than the average (up to 20% or 2 standard deviations less). This lower level is termed the Lower Reference Nutrient Intake, LRNI (also known as the Minimum Safe Intake, MSI, or Lower Threshold Intake). This is an intake at or below which it is unlikely that normal health any nutrient at or below LRNI then detailed investigation of his/her nutritional status would be recommended.

For energy (total calorie) intake only a single Dietary Reference Value is used, the average (Estimated Average Requirement), because there is potential harm (of obesity) from ingesting too much. See also Energy balance, and Appendices II-VI.

Dietary traditions Refers to the slow or rapid changes that occur in the child's eating patterns as breastfeeding is being substituted by other products in preparation for consumption of the norml family diet. A critical period for nutritional risk.

Dietetics The study or prescription of diets under special circumstances (e.g. metabolic or other illness) and for special physiological needs such as pregnancy, growth, weight reduction. See also dietitian.

Dietetic foods Foods prepared to meet the particular nutritional needs of people whose assimilation and metabolism of foods are modified, or for whom a particular effect is obtained by a controlled intake of foods or individual nutrients. They may be formulated for people suffering from physiological disorders or for healthy people with additional needs. See also PARNUTS.

Diethylpropion Anorectic (appetite suppressing) drug used in the treatment of obesity.

Dietic products Drinks or processed foods with characteristics such as low-calorie or reduced fat content, destined to the treatment of particular situation of medical or nutritional interest.

Diet-induced thermogenesis The increase in heat production by the body after eating. It is due to both the metabolic energy cost of digestion (the secretion of digestive enzymes, active transport of nutrients from the gut, and gut motility) and the energy cost of forming tissue reserves of fat, glycogen, and protein. It can be up to 10-15% of the energy intake. Also known as the specific dynamic action (SDA) or thermic effect of foods and luxus konsumption.

Dietitian A Registered Dietitian, designated by the letters RD, RDN, Pt.P and R.Dt., is an authority on healthy eating, food and nutrition. She/He has a Bachelor's degree specializing in food and nutrition, has completed an internship or graduate degree, and is a member of a provincial College of Dietitians. The title "dietitian" is protected and can only be used by individuals who meet these high educational standards. The term "Nutritionist" is not protected and may be used by people with different levels of education and knowledge.

Dietitian, dietician According to the US Department of Labor, Dictionary of Occupational Titles, one who applies the principles of nutrition to the feeding of individuals and groups; plans menus and special diets; supervises the preparation and serving of meals; instructs in the principles of nutrition as applied to selection of foods. In the UK the training and state registration of dietitians (i.e. legal permission to practice) is controlled by law. See also nutritionist.

Digestibility The proportion of a foodstuff absorbed from the digestive tract into the bloodstream, normally 90-95%. It is measured as the difference between intake and faecal output, with allowance being made for that part of the faeces that is not derived from undigested food residues (such as shed cells of the intestinal tract, bacteria, residues of digestive juices). Digestibility measured in this way is referred to as 'true digestibility', as distinct from the approximate measure, 'apparent digestibility', which is simply the difference between intake and output.

Digestion The breakdown of a complex compound into its constituent parts, achieved either chemically or enzymically. Most frequently refers to the digestion of food, which means breakdown by the digestive enzymes of proteins to amino acids, starch to glucose, fats to glycerol and fatty acids. These breakdown products are then absorbed into the bloodstream. See also gastro-intestinal tract.

Digezyme A multi-enzyme complex consisting mainly of amylase starch hydrolyzing enzyme), protease (protein hydrolyzing enzyme)and lipase (fat hydrolyzing enzymes). In addition to these, it also contains cellulase (that hydrolyzes cellulose) and lactase (that hydrolyzes lactose). The enzymes in this complex are of microbial origin (fungal amylase, lipase, lactase, cellulase; and a bacterial neutral protease). The product is therefore entirely of non-animal origin.

Dijon mustard "Dijon" is the general term of a style of mustard produced in Dijon, France, and only mustard made there may label itself as such. Grey Poupon mustard is the only exception. They have been licensed to produce it in the U.S. Dijon and Dijon-style mustard is made from husked and ground mustard seeds, white wine, vinegar, and spices.

Dill The aromatic herb Anethum graveolens (a member of the parsley family). The dried ripe seeds are used in pickles, sauces, etc. The young leaves are also used, fresh, dried, or frozen (dill weed) to flavour fish and other dishes. Dill pepper is a mixture of dill seed, dill weed, and ground black pepper, used as a condiment, especially with salmon.

Dim sum In Cantonese, Dim Sum means "the heart's delight" or "touch the heart." They are also know as Yam Cha. Dim Sum is Cantonese cuisine that comes mainly in the form of steamed and fried dumplings containing a wide array of fillings. They are usually served in tiers of bamboo steamers or small to medium-sized plates (so that many different varieties can be sampled) or they are served like "dessert carts". That is a cart filled with several different types for people to pick and choose from. Long before the Spanish created tapas and the Americans discovered finger foods, the southern Chinese were gathering for yum cha (tea) and sampling savory morsels known as dim sum.

Diphenyl Also known as biphenyl (E-230), one of two compounds (the other is orthophenylphenol, OPP, E-231) used for the treatment of fruit after harvesting to prevent the growth of mould. For making marmalade, citrus fruits that have not been treated with diphenyl are available.

Direct-certification A process by which categorically eligible children are automatically certified to receive free meals and snacks through the child nutrition programs. With direct certification families do not have to submit an application to the child nutrition programs. Rather, the state agency responsible for child nutrition programs coordinates with other state administering agencies to obtain the names of children whose families participate in designated programs such as Food Stamps, Food Distribution Program on Indian Reservations (FDPIR), TANF, and Medicaid. The Child Nutrition and WIC Reauthorization Act of 2004 mandated phased-in direct certification between the school meals programs and the Food Stamp Program. Direct certification via FDPIR, TANF, and Medicaid is optional.

Dirty rice Dirty rice is a Cajun (South Louisiana) specialty. Dirty Rice gets its name from the appearance of the finished dish. The chopped up meats that are added gives it the appearance of "dirt" mixed in with the rice. It is white rice cooked with chopped or ground chicken livers and gizzards, onions and seasonings. The ground giblets give the rice a 'dirty' appearance, but an excellent flavor. You can use your favourite meat, poultry or sausage.

Disaccharide intolerance Impaired ability to digest lactose, maltose, or sucrose, due to lack of lactase, maltase, or sucrase in the small intestinal mucosa. The undigested sugars remain in the intestinal contents, and are fermented by bacteria in the large intestine, resulting in painful, explosive, watery diarrhoea. Treatment is by omitting the offending sugar from the diet.

Lack of all three enzymes is generally caused by intestinal infections, and the enzymes gradually recover after the infection has been cured. Lack of just one of the enzymes, and hence intolerance of just one of the disaccharides, is normally an inherited condition.

Lactose intolerance due to loss of lactase is normal in most ethnic groups after puberty; it is only among people of northern ethnic origin that lactose persists into adult life.

Disaccharide Sugars composed of two monosaccharide units; the nutritionally important disaccharides are sucrose, lactose, and maltose. See carbohydrate.

Disc mill One or more revolving circular plates between which substances are ground; the discs are separated by projecting teeth or pins. Used to grind grain, fruit, sugar, chocolate, pastes, etc.

Disease Illness or sickness often characterized by typical patient problems (symptoms) and physical findings (signs). Disruption sequence The events that occur when a fetus that is developing normally is subjected to a destructive agent such as the rubella (German measles) virus.

Disjoint To separate joints of poultry or break into pieces.

Dislipidemias Term that refers to alterations, nearly always due t excesses, in the levels of lipids or fats, such as cholesterol an triglycerides, in the blood.

Disomy Inheritance of both copies of a chromosome from the same parent

Disorder A disturbance in regular or normal function. An abnormal condition.

Dissolve To stir a solid food and a liquid food together to form a mixture in which none of the solid remains. Sometimes heat is needed to form the mixture.

Distention An uncomfortable swelling in the intestines.

Distilled water Water that has had all the minerals and impurities removed through distillation; it is generally used for pharmaceutical purposes.

Diuretics Substances that increase the production and excretion of urine. They may be either compounds that occur naturally in foods (including caffeine and alcohol), or drugs used medically to reduce the volume of body fluid (e.g. in the treatment of hypertension and oedema).

Diverticular disease Diverticulosis is the presence of pouch-like hernias (diverticula) through the muscle layer of the colon, associated with a low intake of dietary fibre and high intestinal pressure due to straining during defecation. Faecal matter can be trapped in these diverticula, causing them to become inflamed, causing pain and diarrhoea, the condition of diverticulitis. See also gastro-intestinal tract.

Diverticulosis A condition of having multiple diverticulum in the walls of the colon. Also called uncomplicated diverticular disease. [See Diverticula, Diverticulosis, Diverticulitis What's the Difference?

Divinity A delicate, soft-textured candy that is made by slowly beating hot, cooked sugar syrup into beaten egg whites. Chopped nuts or candied fruit and food colouring can be added.

Djenkolic acid A sulphur-containing amino acid found in the djenkol bean, Pithecolobium lobatum, which grows in parts of Sumatra. It is a derivative of cysteine, and is metabolized but, being relatively insoluble, any djenkolic acid that escapes metabolism can crystallize in the kidney tubules and cause damage.

DNA Also known as Deoxyribonucleic acid. This is the molecule that carries the genetic information for most living systems. The DNA molecule consists of four bases (adenine, cytosine, guanine and thymine) and a sugar phosphate backbone, arranged in two connected strands to form its characteristic double helix.

Docosanoids Long-chain polyunsaturated (essential) fatty acids with 22 carbon atoms.

Dogfish A cartilaginous fish, Scilliorinus caniculum, or Squalis acanthias, related to the sharks; sometimes called rock salmon or rock eel.

Dollop To place a scoop or spoonful of a semi-liquid food, such as whipped cream, on top of another food. The term also refers to the scoop or spoonful of food, as in "a dollop of whipped cream."

Do-maker process For continuous bread making. Ingredients are automatically fed into a continuous dough mixer, the yeast suspension being added in a very active state.

Doner kebab Middle-Eastern, Greek, and Turkish (showarma in Arabic). Slices of lamb, highly flavoured with herbs and spices, wound around a revolving spit, cooked in front of a vertical charcoal (or sometimes gas) fire. See also kebab.

Double blind placebo controlled study Considered the "gold standard" of clinical research studies, the double blind placebo controlled study provides dependable findings that are free of bias introduced by either the subject or the researcher. In this type of study, neither the subject nor the researcher conducting the study know whether the test substance or a placebo has been administered. For the results to be valid and to ensure that the subject cannot violate the "blindness," the placebo and the test substance must be virtually identical (i.e., look, smell and taste similar). The "blindness" of the study is crucial. It eliminates the possibility that a participant's personal beliefs will undermine the study's validity. It also prevents the researcher's expectations from influencing the test results.

Double blinding A process in a clinical study that conceals the treatment from both the patient and the investigator.

Double-blind food challenge Food challenge test where neither the patient nor the clinical investigator knows the identity of the administered substance.

Double-blind placebo-controlled study Considered the "gold standard" of clinical research studies, the double-blind placebo-controlled study provides dependable findings that are free of bias introduced by either the subject or the researcher. In this type of study, neither the subject nor the researcher conducting the study know whether the test substance or a placebo has been administered. For the results to be valid and to ensure that the subject cannot violate the "blindness," the placebo and the test substance must be virtually identical (i.e., look, smell and taste similar). The "blindness" of the study is crucial. It eliminates the possibility that a participant's personal beliefs will undermine the study's validity. It also prevents the researcher's expectations from influencing the test results.

Dough Mixture of flour and liquid (water or milk) used to make bread and pastry. May contain yeast or baking powder as leavening agent.

Dough cakes A general term to include crumpets, muffins, and pikelets, all made from flour, water and milk. The batter is raised with yeast and baked on a hot plate or griddle (hence sometimes known as griddle cakes). Crumpets have sodium bicarbonate added to the batter; muffins are thick and well aerated, less tough than crumpets; pikelets are made from crumpet batter that has been thinned down.

Doughnut Cake made from fried, sweetened dough leavened with yeast or baking powder; may be filled with jam or cream.

Douglas bag An inflatable bag for collecting expired air to measure the consumption of oxygen and production of carbon dioxide, for the measurement of energy expenditure by indirect calorimetry.

Down syndrome Trisomy 21; a genetic disorder in which an individual has an extra 21st chromosome, typically characterized by low muscle tone, cardiac problems, GI malformations and a distinct facial appearance

Dragree They are tiny round, hard candies used for decorating cakes, cookies, and other baked goods. They come in a variety of sizes (from pinhead to 1/4-inch) and colours, including silver. They are not edible and can be found at any specialty party store. Dragrees can also be almonds with a hard sugar coating that are edible and probably can be found at your local pastry shop.

Drambuie Scottish liqueur based on malt whisky, sweetened with heather honey, and flavoured with herbs.

Drawn butter An American term for butter that has been defatted and cleared of all cloudy residue and impurities.

Dredge To lightly coat food that is going to be fried with flour, breadcrumbs, or cornmeal. The coating helps to brown the food and provides a crunchy surface. Dredged foods need to be cooked immediately. Breaded foods (those dredged in flour, dipped in egg then dredged again in breading) can be prepared and held before cooking.

Dredging Sprinkling food with flour, sugar, etc. Fish and meat are often dredged with flour before frying, while cakes and biscuits are dredged with fine sugar as a decoration.

Dressing food To prepare food for cooking or serving in such a way that it looks as attractive as possible. Sometimes denotes a special method of preparation, as in dressed crab. See also salad dressing.

DRI A joint collaboration with Canada and the US, DRIs are revised recommendations for vitamins and minerals from the Institute of Medicine, an arm of the National Academy of Sciences, which will gradually replace the Recommended Dietary Allowances or RDA guidelines. DRIs are being developed for vitamins and minerals that currently have no RDAs.

Dried fruits Dried currants, dates, figs, prunes, raisins, and sultanas all have similar analyses; a 100-g portion is a source of iron and supplies 250 kcal.

Dried, milk Milk that has been evaporated to dryness, usually by spray- or roller-drying. May be whole (full-cream) milk (26% fat), three-quarter cream (not less than 20% fat), half-cream (not less than 14% fat), quarter-cream (not less than 8% fat), or skim milk (1% fat).

Drinking water Water that comes from a government-approved source and has undergone some treatment and filtration; it can be bottled or available on tap and used for drinking and general culinary purposes.

Drug-nutrient interactions Deficiency caused by effects of drugs on the absorption or metabolism of vitamins or minerals. Sometimes this is the mode of action of the drug in treating the disease; in other cases it is an undesirable side-effect.

Drunken foods Chinese; meat or fish is highly seasoned and marinated, then steamed or lightly simmered. After draining it is steeped in wine for several days before serving.

Drupe Botanical term for a fleshy fruit with a single stone enclosing the seed that does not split along defined lines to liberate the seed, e.g. apricot, cherry, date, mango, olive, peach, plum.

Dry-blanch-dry process A method of drying fruit so as to retain the colour and flavour; it is faster than drying in the sun and preserves flavour and colour better than hot air drying. The material is dried to 50% water at about 82°C, blanched for a few minutes, then dried at 68°C over a period of 6-24 h to 15-20% water content.

Drying Method of preserving food by removing most of the water, so as to prevent bacterial and mould growth. Freeze-drying is evaporation of the water from a frozen food, so retaining textural properties and nutrients.

Drying oil Any highly unsaturated oil that absorbs oxygen and, when in thin films, polymerizes to form a skin. Linseed and tung oil are examples of drying oils used in paints and in the manufacture of linoleum, etc. Nutritionally they are similar to edible oils, but when polymerized, are toxic. See also iodine value.

Dublin bay prawn Scampi or Norway lobster; a shellfish, Nephrops norvegicus, see lobster.

Duchenne muscular dystrophy The most common of several childhood muscular dystrophies, it is an inherited disorder (X-linked recessive) with progressive degeneration of muscle, onset is generally before age 6 years

Dulcin A synthetic material (p-phenetylurea or p-phenetolcarbamide, discovered in 1883) which is 250 times as sweet as sugar but is not permitted in foods. Also called sucrol and valzin.

Dulcitol A six-carbon sugar alcohol which occurs in some plants and is formed by the reduction of galactose; also known as melampyrin, dulcite, or galacticol.

Dulse Edible purplish-brown seaweeds, Rhodymenia palmata and Dilsea carnosa, used in soups and jellies.

Dumpling A ball of dough, usually boiled, but may be baked. Generally served with soups and stews.

Dun Brown discolouration in salted fish caused by mould growth.

Dunaliella bardawil A red marine alga discovered in 1980 in Israel, which is extremely rich in U+0B2-carotene, containing 100 times more than most other natural sources.

Dundee cake Rich fruit cake decorated with split almonds.

Dunst Very fine semolina (starch from the endosperm of the wheat grain) approaching the fineness of flour. Also called break middlings (not to be confused with middlings, which is branny offal).

Duodenum First part of the small intestine, between the stomach and the jejunum; the major site of digestion. Pancreatic juice and bile are secreted into the duodenum. So called because it is about twelve fingerbreadths in length. See also gastro-intestinal tract.

Durum wheat A hard type of wheat of the species Triticum durum (most bread wheats are Triticum vulgare); largely used for the production of semolina intended for the preparation of pasta.

Dutch oven A semicircular metal shield which may be placed close to an open fire; fitted with shelves on which food is roasted. It may also be clamped to the fire bars.

Duxelle Finely chopped mushrooms that are cooked in butter with shallots and wine. When cooked dry, duxelle make a good filling for omelets, fish, and meat. They may also be moistened with wine or broth and served as a sauce. Duxelle are also flavored with fresh herbs and brandy or Madeira wine. This is the creation of La Varenne, the great chef employed by the Marquis d'Uxelles in 1650. La Varenne is said to have been the first great French cook of modern time. His cookbook, called "Le Cuisinier Francois," published in 1650 is considered to be a primer of the French cuisine.

Dyox Trade name for chlorine dioxide used to treat flour.

Dysmotility Abnormal contractions, of varying frequency and severity, of the muscles in the gastrointestinal tract, which may or may not be associated with symptoms. They differ from functional gastrointestinal disorders, which are defined by symptoms that may or may not have dysmotility, but which are also associated with low pain thresholds (visceral hypersensitivity). When occurring in the stomach or small intestine, dysmotility can result in disorders like gastroparesis or pseudo-obstruction with or without symptoms such as bloating, pain, nausea, and vomiting due to either disorganized contractions, or weak contractions. When occurring in the large intestine, dysmotility can result in disorders like Hirschsprung's disease or colonic inertia that can produce symptoms of constipation, or other conditions that cause diarrhea. The abnormal motility involves changes in the contractions that either move or hold back stool. Abnormalities of "dysmotility" can be measured with special motility testing.

Dyspepsia Any pain or discomfort associated with eating. Dyspepsia may be a symptom of gastritis, peptic ulcer, gall-bladder disease, etc., or, if there is no structural change in the intestinal tract, it is called 'functional dyspepsia'. Treatment includes a bland diet. See also indigestion.

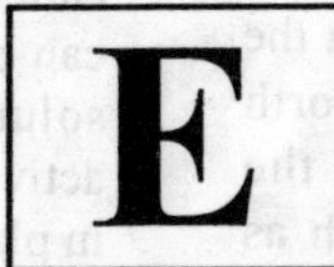

E. coli O157:H7 The bacteria Escherichia coli O157:H7 is a type of E. coli associated with foodborne illness. Healthy cattle and humans can carry the bacteria. It can be transferred from animal to animal and animal to human, and from animal to human on food. Transmission from person to person through close contact is a potential problem, especially among young children in daycare.

Early intervention services Established by Part H of PL 97-457 of 1986 (now Part C of the IDEA of 1997); community-based therapeutic and educational services for infants and children under 3 years of age with developmental delays

Earth-nut The small edible tuber of the umbellifer Conopodium denudatum, or C. majus, also called pignut or fairy potato. Also another name for the peanut.

Easter soup (Mayieritsa) Greek soup traditionally prepared to celebrate the end of the Lenten fast, made from the pluck (i.e. tripe, intestines, heart, and liver) and feet of a lamb.

Eating disorders Impacting both physical and mental health, people develop eating disorders as a way of dealing with the conflicts, pressures and stresses of life. Left untreated, they can be fatal. Their eating disorder may be used as a way to express control when the rest of their life seems chaotic. Common eating disorders include Anorexia, Binge Eating and Bulimia.

Eau de framboise A raspberry spirit. Eau de framboise is often used in cooking to flavour sweet and savoury dishes. It can also be drunk as a digestif or aperitif.

Eau de vie Translated from the French, eau-de-vie means "water of life." It is an alcohol distillate that is rich with taste, flavor, and aroma. The French use the expression "eau-de-vie" as a generic term for all brandies. It is unlikely, however, that you will hear Cognac and Armagnac ordered in this manner.

EBT Electronic Benefits Transfer. EBT is the method by which food stamp and other benefits are distributed via an electronic debit card. Some states also use EBT to distribute benefits under WIC and some other programs.

Eccles cake Pastry filled with dried fruit, melted butter, and sugar. Named originally for the town of Eccles in greater Manchester.

Eclair Small finger-shaped cake prepared from choux pastry, filled with cream or confectioner's custard, coated with chocolate or coffeeflavoured icing.

Ecologist An individual who studies the interrelationships between organisms and their environment.

Ectomorph Description given to a tall, thin person, possibly with underdeveloped muscles. See also endomorph; mesomorph.

Ecuelle A device for obtaining peel oil from citrus fruit. It consists of a shallow funnel lined with spikes on which the fruit is rolled by hand. As the oil glands are pierced, the oil and cell sap collect in the bottom of the funnel.

Edam cheese Edam cheese was first made in the vicinity of Edam in the Province of North Holland, Netherlands. It is known in the Netherlands by various local names, such as manbollen, katzenkopf, and tete de maure. Like gouda, it is a semi-firm to hard, sweet-curd cheese made from cow's milk. Originally it was made from whole milk, but now the fat content of the milk is usually reduced to about 2.5%. Edam cheese is also made in the U.S. It is usually shaped like a flattened ball, but in the U.S., it is made also in a loaf shape. It is coated in a red wax with a creamy yellow, semi soft to hard interior. It melts quickly under heat when shredded.

Edible flowers Squash and pumpkin blossoms are edible. Prepare the blossoms by washing and trimming the stems and removing the stamens. One cooking method is to dip in tempura batter and quickly deep fry. Other uses include as a garnish and as a last minute addition to clear soups. Other edible flowers include anise hyssop, basil flowers, bee balm, borage, chamomile, chive blossoms, chrysanthemum, ciary, dandelion, day lilies, fuchsia, scented flower of juda, marigold, mustard flower, nasturtiums, oregano, pansy, pineapple sage, roquette, rose, rosemary flower, savory flower, violas, and violet.

Do not eat flowers that were purchased from a florist or any other source where you do not know whether or not they were sprayed with pesticides. Also, do not eat home grown flowers that were treated with chemicals. If you don't know whether the plant has been treated with chemicals, do not eat it.

Do not use the popular "crystallized" flower recipes where flowers are dipped in egg white then sugar. The raw egg white dip may contain salmonella bacteria that can result in foodborne illness.

EDTA Ethylene diamine tetra-acetic acid, a compound that forms stable chemical complexes with metal ions (i.e. a chelating agent). Also called versene, sequestrol, and sequestrene. It can be used both to remove metal ions from a solution (or at least to remove them from activity) and also to add metal ions, for example in plant fertilizers.

Eel A long thin fish, Anguilla anguilia; the conger eel is Conger myriaster. Eels live in rivers but go to sea to breed. A 100-g portion is a rich source of protein, niacin, and vitamins A, D, and B12; a good source of niacin and vitamin B2; a source of vitamins B1, and B6; contains 20g of fat and supplies 300 kcal.

Efferent nerves Nerve fibers that carry impulses away from the brain and spinal cord (central nervous system), which cause a muscle or gland to contract, or which modify or inhibit its contraction.

Efficacy The extent to which an intervention improves the outcome for people under ideal circumstances. Testing efficacy means finding out whether something is capable of causing an effect at all.

Egg Hens' eggs are sold by size (EU); size 0 (weighs 75 g or more); size 1: 70g; size 2: 65 g; size 3: 60 g; size 4: 55 g; size 5: 50-55 g (weighed with shell which is about 10% of the total weight). Useful in food preparation to thicken sauces and custard, as an emulsifier, to hold air in meringues and sponges, and as a binder in croquettes.

Average portion of two eggs is a rich source of vitamins D and B12; a good source of protein, niacin, and vitamins A and B2; a source of zinc; contains 170 mg of sodium; 13 g of fat, of which 35% is saturated and 50% mono-unsaturated; supplies 175 kcal. The egg-white is 60% of the whole and the yolk 30%.

Duck eggs weigh about 85 g of which 10% is shell. One egg is a rich source of vitamins A, D, and B12; a good source of protein and vitamin B2; contains 90 mg of sodium and 9 g of fat of which 30% is saturated and 20% polyunsaturated; supplies 120 kcal.

Egg cream Despite it name, the Egg Cream contains no eggs or cream. The basic ingredients are milk, seltzer, and chocolate syrup. Egg Cream will lose its head and turn flat if not drunk immediately or within three minutes. It is perfectly proper to "gulp" an Egg Cream. Soda fountains all over New York City have their own version and the Egg Cream has become a New York institution. For many years, the Egg Cream remained a product sold only through New York soda fountains. It is being bottled now by a couple of small companies. True New Yorkers insist that it is not a classic Egg Cream without Fox's U-Bet Chocolate Syrup.

Egg proteins What is generally referred to as egg protein is a mixture of individual proteins, including ovalbumin, ovomucoid, ovoglobulin, conalbumin, vitellin, and vitellenin. Egg-white contains 10.9% protein, mostly ovalbumin; yolk contains 16% protein, mainly two phosphoproteins, vitellin and vitellenin.

Egg wash Beaten raw egg, sometimes mixed with water and a little salt, used for glazing pastry or bread to give it a shine when baked. Useful for blind baking because it seals the pastry base, ensuring it won't absorb moisture, and also gives the pastry a good golden colour.

Egg white The white of an egg is in three layers: an outer layer of thin white, a layer of thick white, richer in ovomucin, and an inner layer of thin white surrounding the yolk. The ratio of thick to thin white varies, depending on the individual hen. A higher proportion of thick white is desirable for frying and poaching, since it helps the egg to coagulate into a small firm mass instead of spreading; thin white produces a larger volume of froth when beaten than does thick.

Eggnog A chilled Christmas beverage that consists of a blend of milk or cream, beaten eggs, sugar, nutmeg, and usually liquor of some kind (rum, brandy, or whiskey). The recipe for eggnog has changed very little in the last 150 years.

Eggplant, Aubergine - A member of the nightshade family, the eggplant is related to the potato, tomato, and pepper and has its origins in India and Southeast Asia. Arab and Asian traders brought eggplant to the Middle East, North Africa, and finally Europe. The first eggplants were small, round, egg-shaped and white (that's how this vegetable got its name). The prime eggplant season is July through October, but the purple variety is available all year long. Learn more about the Eggplant.

Eggs Benedict A breakfast or brunch specialty consisting of two toasted English muffin halves, each topped with a slice of ham or Canadian bacon, a poached egg, and some Hollandaise sauce.

Eggs Sardou This is one of New Orleans' grand egg dishes, created, as were so many classic dishes, at the famous Antoine's Restaurant. It consists of poached eggs, topped with creamed spinach, artichoke hearts, and hollandaise sauce. Legend has it that Antoine Alciatore (18224-1877) created this dish especially for French playwright Victorien Sardou (1831-1908) on the occasion of a dinner he hosted for the playwright. During the 19th century, Sardou produced light comedies, satiric tragedies, and historical dramas such as La Tosca. Sardou is considered one of the greatest figures of the Art Nouveau culture and his plays were popular in America.

Eggs–Shell Colour Some people prefer brown eggs to white, or vice versa. The only difference is in the breed of the hen. If hens have the same type of feed ration, the eggs will be nutritionally equivalent, regardless of shell colour. They also have the same flavor, keeping quality, and whipping and cooking characteristics.

Egg-white The white of an egg is in three layers: an outer layer of thin white, a layer of thick white, richer in ovomucin, and an inner layer of thin white surrounding the yolk. The ratio of thick to thin white varies, depending on the individual hen. A higher proportion of thick white is desirable for frying and poaching, since it helps the egg to coagulate into a small firm mass instead of spreading; thin white produces a larger volume of froth when beaten than does thick.

Eicosanoids Compounds formed in the body from long-chain polyunsaturated fatty acids (eicosenoic acids), including the prostaglandins, prostacyclins, thromboxanes, and leukotrienes, all of which act as local hormones and are involved in wound healing, inflammation, platelet aggregation, and a variety of other functions.

Einkorn A type of wheat, the wild form of which, Triticum boeoticum, was probably one of the ancestors of all cultivated wheats. Still grown in some parts of southern Europe and the Middle East, usually for animal feed. The name means 'one seed', from the single seed found in each spikelet.

Eiswein Wine made from grapes that have frozen on the vine, picked and processed while still frozen, so that the juice is highly concentrated and very sweet. Similar Canadian wines are known as ice wine. See wine classification, Germany.

EITC Earned Income Tax Credit. EITC is a tax benefit for low- to moderate-income working families. Workers who qualify for the EITC and file a federal income tax return can receive a refund, making this an important program to support low-income families. Partnering with EITC outreach campaigns is one way of conducting multi-benefit outreach for food and nutrition programs.

Elastin A fibrous protein that is the major constituent of the yellow elastic fibres of connective tissue. It is rich in glycine, alanine, proline, and other nonpolar amino acids that are cross-linked, making the protein relatively insoluble. Elastic fibres can stretch to several times their length and then return to their original size. Elastin is particularly abundant in elastic cartilage, blood-vessel walls, ligaments, and the heart.

Elastin insoluble protein in connective tissue, which is not changed by cooking, and hence is the cause of tough meat.

Elder A common hedgerow bush (Sambucus nigra); the flowers are used to flavour cordials, syrups, fruit jellies, and elderflower wine. The fruit is used for making jelly and wine (elderberry wine).

Elderberry The purple/black fruit of the elder tree, elderberries can be eaten raw but are quite sour and tart. They are better used to make jams, pies, and homemade wine. The creamy white elderberry flowers can be added to salads or batter-dipped and fried like fritters.

Elderly nutrition program Administered through the Administration on Aging at HHS, this program provides grants and meal subsidies to state agencies to support meals for the elderly in group settings and meals delivered to participants' homes. The program does not include means testing, but it targets its services to elderly with the greatest economic or social need. In addition to providing meals, the program also has a goal of increasing socialization of its participants. At the state level, this program is administered through the State Agency on Aging or Indian Tribal Organizations.

Election cake The cake is actually a classic English fruitcake or plum cake. The original cakes included molasses, spice, raisins, and currants were used in this cake. Later brandy was added.

Electrolyte An electrolyte is a substance containing free ions which behaves as an electrically conductive medium. Because they generally consist of ions in solution, electrolytes are also known as ionic solutions, but molten electrolytes and solid electrolytes are also possible. They are sometimes referred to in abbreviated jargon as lytes.

Elixir Alcoholic extract (tincture) of a naturally occurring substance; originally devised by medieval alchemists (the elixir of life), now used for a variety of medicines, liqueurs, and bitters.

Ellagic acid A natural cancer fighting agent found in strawberries.

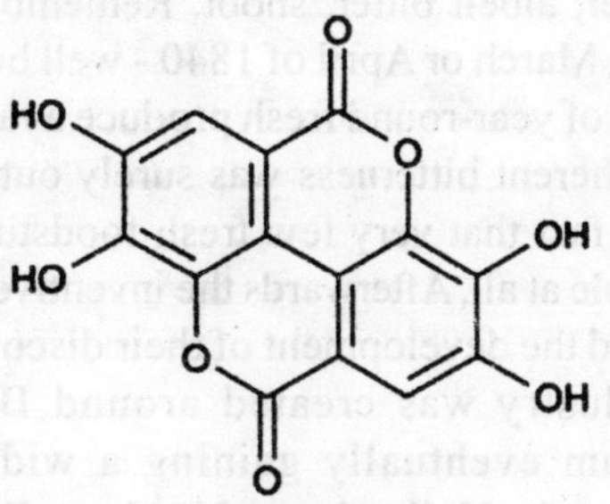

Fig. Ellagic acid

Elute To wash off or remove. Rather specifically applied to removal of adsorbed chemicals from the substance that adsorbed them, as in chromatography. See also ion exchange resins.

Emaciation Extreme thinness and wasting, caused by disease or undernutrition. See also cachexia; Protein-energy malnutrition.

Emblic Berry of the South-East Asian malacca tree, Emblica officinalis, similar in appearance to the gooseberry. Also known as the Indian gooseberry. An exceptionally rich source of vitamin C: 600 mg per 100 g.

Embolism Blockage of a blood vessel caused by a foreign object (embolus) such as a quantity of air or gas, a piece of tissue or tumour, a blood clot (thrombus), or fatty tissue derived from atheroma, in the circulation.

Emergency food providers Private, nonprofit organizations that provide food to individuals and households in need. Emergency food providers obtain most food through bulk purchasing and donations; however, the federal TEFAP program also makes excess commodities available to the emergency food network.

Emince French; a dish of meat cut into thin slices, covered with sauce, and baked in an earthenware dish.

Emmental Semi-hard cow's milk cheese originally from Switzerland; has large round holes formed by gases from bacterial fermentation during ripening.

Emmer A type of wheat known to have been used more than 8000 years ago. Wild emmer is Triticum dicoccoides and true emmer is T. dicoccum. Nowadays grown mainly for animal feed.

Empanada Flaky meat pies made from olive-oil pastry and served as tapas in Spain and as a popular snack in Latin America. Meat filling is most common but they can be filled with anything - fish, vegetables, cheese, even fruit. The classic empanada comes from Galicia in north-west Spain and is made with chicken, onions and peppers.

Emprote Trade name for a dried milk and cereal preparation consumed as a beverage, containing 33% protein.

Emulsifiers A food additive consisting of a substance that enables nonmiscible liquids (such as oil and water) to maintain a stable emulsion, as in mayonnaise, margarine, and peanut butter. Natural emulsifying agents, such as egg yolk, agar, and lecithin, have now been largely replaced by synthetic chemical emulsifiers.

Emulsify An emulsion is a stable suspension of fat and another liquid. To emulsify is to combine fats (such as butter or oil) with a liquid (such as vinegar or citric juices) into a smooth and even blend using an emulsifier (such as an egg yolk) which binds to each set of ingredients and prevents them from separating. Hollandaise is a classic emulsified sauce.

Emulsifying agents Substances that are soluble in both fat and water and enable fat to be uniformly dispersed in water as an emulsion. Foods that consist of such emulsions include butter, margarine, salad dressings, mayonnaise, and ice cream. Stabilizers maintain emulsions in a stable form. Emulsifying agents are also used in baking to aid the smooth incorporation of fat into the dough and to keep the crumb soft. Emulsifying agents used in foods include agar, albumin, alginates, casein, egg yolk, glycerol monostearate, gums, Irish moss, lecithin, soaps.

Emulsifying salts Sodium citrate, sodium phosphates, and sodium tartrate, used in the manufacture of milk powder, evaporated milk, sterilized cream, and processed cheese.

Emulsion An intimate mixture of two immiscible liquids (for example oil and water), one being dispersed in the other in the form of fine droplets. They will stay mixed only as long as they are stirred together, unless an emulsifying agent is added.

En papillote A French word meaning "in a paper bag." En papilotte is a cooking process that cooks foods in their own juices in a bag (sealing foods to cook in their own juices, rather than adding water as in steaming, re-enforces flavors rather than diluting them). Traditionally the food is enclosed with parchment paper, but today is also cooked enclosed in aluminum-foil bags. Pastry is also used in the same way, such as pasties. The bag is slit open tableside so that thc diner can enjoy the escaping aroma.

Endemic deprivation Deprivation illnesses such as iron-deprivation anemia, energy-protein malnutrition and goiter, that appear with a regular and practically constant frequency, and a prevalence above the "normal" limits of tolerance.

Endive Also known as Belgaina endive, French endive, and witloof chicory. Endive is the blanched shoots of the chicory root. To produce blanched (white) shoot, the roots are dug up and stored in a cool, darkened location or in forcing beds, when they are covered with sand. They are harvested when they are 4 to 6 inches long and about 1 1/2 inches wide. It can be eaten raw as a salad green or braised in butter or cream sauce as a side dish.

The local tale around Brussels, Belgium places a farmer in the period around 1840 that had placed some chicory roots in a cellar for future transformation into a coffee substitute. Whether he forgot them in his cellar, or hid them there to avoid a purported chicory root tax, is not well documented. Nonetheless upon discovering them in the spring he found that the roots have sprouted in their dark, damp environs producing a tender, albeit bitter, shoot. Remember we're talking March or April of 1840 - well before the advent of year-round fresh produce availability. The inherent bitterness was surely outweighed by the fact that very few fresh foodstuffs were available at all. Afterwards the inventive farmers pursued the development of their discovery and an industry was created around Brussels, Belgium eventually gaining a widespread presence in Holland and Northern France as well. Today we know that endive is grown to some extent on virtually every continent.

Endocrine disruption Not considered as an adverse endpoint per se but as a step or mechanism that could lead to toxic outcomes, such as cancer or adverse reproductive effects.

Endocrine glands Those (ductless) glands that produce and secrete hormones, including the thyroid gland (secreting thyroxine and triiodothyronine), pancreas (insulin and glucagon), adrenal glands (adrenaline, noradrenaline, glucocorticoids, mineralocorticoids), ovary and testes (sex steroids). Some endocrine glands respond directly to chemical changes in the bloodstream; others are controlled by hormones secreted by the pituitary gland, under the control of the hypothalamus.

Endogenous Produced inside an organism or cell. The opposite is external (exogenous) production.

Energy density Energy density is the amount of energy stored in a given system or region of space per unit volume or per unit mass, depending on the context. In some cases it is obvious from context which quantity is most useful: for example, in rocketry, energy per unit mass is the most important parameter, but when studying pressurized gas or magnetohydrodynamics the energy per unit volume is more appropriate. In a few applications (comparing, for example, the effectiveness of hydrogen fuel to gasoline) both figures are appropriate and should be called out explicitly (hydrogen has a higher energy density per unit mass than does gasoline, but a much lower energy density per unit volume in most applications).

Endopeptidases Enzymes that hydrolyse proteins (i.e. proteinases or peptidases), by cleaving peptide bonds inside protein molecules, as opposed to exopeptidases, which remove amino acids from the end of the protein chain. The main endopeptidases in digestion are chymotrypsin, elastase, pepsin, and trypsin.

Endoscopy A procedure that uses an endoscope to diagnose or treat a condition. There are many types of endoscopy; examples include colonoscopy, sigmoidoscopy, gas:roscopy, enteroscopy, and esophogealgastroduodenoscopy (EGD).

Endosperm The inner part of cereal grains; in wheat it comprises about 83% of the grain. Mainly starch, it is the source of semolina. Contains only about 10% of the vitamin B 1, 35% of the vitamin B 2, 40% of the niacin, and 50% of the vitamin B 6 and pantothenic acid of the whole grain. See also flour, extraction rate.

Endotoxins Toxins produced by bacteria as an integral part of the cell, so they cannot be separated by filtration; unlike exotoxins, they do not usually stimulate antitoxin formation but the antibodies that they induce act directly on the bacteria. They are relatively stable to heat compared with exotoxins.

Energy The ability to do work. The SI unit of energy is the joule, and nutritionally relevant amounts of energy are kilejoules (kj, 1000 J) and megajoules (MJ, 1,000,000 J). The calorie is still widely used in nutrition; 1 cal = 4.186 J (approximated to 4.2). While it is usual to speak of the calorie or joule content of a food it is more correct to refer to the energy content or yield. The total chemical energy in a food, as released by complete combustion (in the bomb calorimeter) is gross energy. Allowing for the losses of unabsorbed food in the faeces gives digestible energy. Allowing for loss in the urine due to incomplete combustion in the body (e.g. urea from the incomplete combustion of proteins) gives metabolizable energy. Allowing for the loss due to diet-induced thermogenesis gives net energy, i.e. the actual amount available for use in the body. See also energy conversion factors.

Energy balance The difference between intake of energy from foods and expenditure on basal metabolism and physical activity. Positive energy balance leads to increased body tissue, the normal process of growth. In adults positive energy balance leads to creation of body reserves of fat, resulting in overweight and obesity. Negative energy balance leads to utilization of body reserves of fat and protein, resulting in wasting and undernutrition.

Energy conversion factors Various factors are used to calculate the energy yields of foodstuffs. The complete heats of combus*ion (gross energy) as determined by calorimetry are: protein, 5.7 kcal (23.9 kJ); fat, 9.4 kcal (39.5 kJ); carbohydrate, 4.1 kcal (17.2 kJ)/gram. The Rubner conversion factors for metabolic energy yield are: protein, 4.1 kcal (17 kJ); fat, 9.3 kcal (39 kJ); carbohydrate, 4.1 kcal (17 kJ)/gram The Atwater factors also allow for losses in digestion and incomplete oxidation of the nitrogen of proteins: protein, 4 kcal (16.8 kJ); fat, 9 kcal (37.8 kJ); carbohydrate, 4 kcal (16.8 kJ)/gram. The following factors are used in general practice: carbohydrate 4 kcal (17 kJ); fat, 9 kcal (38 kJ); carbohydrate (as monosaccharides), 4 kcal (1.7 kJ); alcohol, 7 kcal (29 kJ); sugar alcohols, 2.4 kcal (10 kJ); organic acids, 3 kcal (13 kJ).

Energy expenditure Utilisation by the body of chemical energy from food components or body stores during the process of metabolism which is eventually dissipated as heat plus the heat generated by muscular activity, either in shivering or in physical activity. Usually used to mean the day's total energy (calorie) loss as heat.

Energy Intake The chemical energy in foods that can be metabolised to produce energy available to the body; usually used to mean the day's total energy (calories) supplied by all the food and drink consumed.

Energy metabolism The various reactions involved in the oxidation of metabolic fuels (mainly carbohydrates, fats, and proteins), to provide energy (linked to the formation of ATP (adenosine triphosphate) from ADP (adenosine diphosphate) and phosphate ions).

Energy-rich bonds An outdated and chemically incorrect concept in energy metabolism, which suggested that the bond between ADP and phosphate in ATP, and between creatine and phosphate in creatine phosphate, which have a high chemical free energy of hydrolysis, somehow differs from 'ordinary' chemical bonds.

Enfleurage A method of extracting essential oils from flowers by placing them on glass trays covered with purified lard or other fat, which eventually becomes saturated with the oil.

English Muffin A round (about 3 inches in diameter) muffin that is made from soft yeast dough and baked on a griddle. The origin of the English Muffin can be dated back to the 10th century in Wales. A yeast-leavened cake called Bara Maen was baked on hot stones in 10th century Wales. A similar cake or muffin baked on hot griddles was popular in 19th century England, where the hot, fresh muffins were peddled door to door by the "muffin man." The prominence of the muffin men in English society even became a popular children's nursery rhyme and song, "Have you seen the muffin man, the muffin man, the muffin man? Have you seen the muffin man, that lives in Drury Lane?"

Enocianina Desugared grape extract used to colour fruit flavours. Prepared by acid extraction of the skins of black grapes; it is blue in neutral conditions and turns red in acid.

Enriched foods Enriched foods are those that nutrients have been added to replace the nutrients which were lost during food processing. For example, B vitamins are lost in processing wheat to white flour and these are then added back to the flour.

Enrichment The addition of nutrients to foods. Although often used interchangeably, the term fortification is used of legally imposed additions, and enrichment means the addition of nutrients beyond the levels originally present. See also nutrification; restoration.

Enteral nutrition Tube feeding with a liquid diet directly into the stomach or small intestine. See also gastrostomy feeding; nasogastric tube; nutrient enemata; parenteral nutrition.

Enteric nervous system (ENS) Autonomic nervous system within the walls of the digestive tract. The ENS regulates digestion and the muscle contractions that eliminate solid waste.

Enteritis Inflammation of the mucosal lining of the small intestine, usually resulting from infection. Regional enteritis is Crohn's disease.

Enterocele The descent of loops of small intestine into the pelvis, that bulge into the vagina during straining. An enterocele may cause pain and/or obstructed defecation.

Enterocolitis Inflammation of the intestines ganglion A mass of nerve cells.

Enterocyte Enterocyte is a type of epithelial cell of the superficial layer of the small and large intestine tissue. These cells can help breaking up molecules and transport them into the tissue. Glucose, from the intestinal lumen, crosses the apical membrane of the enterocyte using the Na+ dependent glucose transporter; moves through the cytosol and exits the enterocyte via the basolateral membrane (into the blood capillary) using GLUT-2. Galactose uses the same transport system. Fructose, on the other hand, crosses the apical membrane of the enterocyte, using GLUT-5. It is thought to cross into the blood capillary using one of the other GLUT transporters.

Enterogastrone Hormone secreted by the small intestine which inhibits the activity of the stomach. Its secretion is stimulated by fat; hence, fat in the diet inhibits gastric activity.

Enterokinase Obsolete name for the intestinal enzyme enteropeptidase.

Enteropathy Any disease or disorder of the intestinal tract.

Enteropeptidase An enzyme secreted by the small intestinal mucosa which activates trypsinogen (from the pancreatic juice) to the active proteolytic enzyme trypsin. See also protein digestion.

Enteroscopy Examination of the inside of the small intestine using an endoscope.

Enterotoxin Substances more or less specifically toxic to the cells of the intestinal mucosa, normally produced by bacteria.

Enteroviruses Viruses that multiply mainly in the intestinal tract.

Entoleter A machine used to disinfest cereals and other foods. The material is fed to the centre of a high-speed rotating disc carrying studs so that it is thrown against the studs; the impact kills any insects and destroys their eggs.

Entrecote It is a beefsteak, which is cut from between the animal's ribs. It is often placed between sheets of oil paper and pounded until it is thinned. It is then grilled or sautted in butter for about one minute. A common name for entrecote is minute steak.

Entree A dressed savoury dish, served hot or cold, complete in its dish with the sauce. The term is used both for the main part of a meal (especially in France) and also to describe courses intermediate between hors d'oeuvre and main course.

Entremeses Spanish; mixed hors d'oeuvre dishes served as a prelude to a meal.

Entremets A French word that means "between dishes." Today, when one finds the term on a French menu, it refers to "desserts." The word originally once referred to foods or small side dishes that were served between courses of a grand dinner. Entrements were customarily served to royalty during the early 18th century when sometimes as many as thirty-two different courses were served.

E-numbers Within the EU food additives may be listed on labels either by name or by their number in the EU list of permitted additives.

Environmental Protection Agency (EPA) The EPA's mission is to protect human health and safeguard the natural environment—air, water and land—upon which life depends. Through regulation, EPA tries to ensure the human population and the environment are protected from environmental risks and exposures.

Enzyme Enzymes are proteins that accelerate, or catalyze, chemical reactions. In these reactions, the molecules at the beginning of the process are called substrates and the enzyme converts these into different molecules: the products. Almost all processes in the cell need enzymes in order to occur at significant rates. Consequently, since enzymes are extremely selective for their substrates and speed up only a few reactions from among many possibilities, the set of enzymes made in a cell determines which metabolic pathways occur in that cell.

Enzyme activation A number of compounds increase the activity of enzymes; sometimes this is a part of normal metabolic regulation and integration (e.g. the responses to hormones), and sometimes it is the action of drugs.

Enzyme activation assays Used to assess the nutritional status of an individual with respect to vitamins B1, B2, and B6. A sample of red blood cells in a test-tube is tested for activity of the relevant enzyme before and after adding extra vitamin; enhancement of the enzyme activity beyond a standard level serves as a biochemical index of a shortage of the vitamin in question. The enzymes involved are transketolase for vitamin B1, glutathione reductase for vitamin B2 and either aspartate or alanine aminotransferase for vitamin B6.

Enzyme induction Synthesis of new enzyme protein in response to some stimulus, normally a hormone, but sometimes a metabolic intermediate or other compound (e.g. a drug or food additive).

Enzyme inhibition A number of compounds reduce the activity of enzymes; sometimes this is a part of normal metabolic regulation and integration (e.g. the responses to hormones), and sometimes it is the action of drugs. Some inhibitors are reversible, others act irreversibly on the enzymes, and therefore have a longer duration of action (the activity of the enzyme remains low until more has been synthesized).

Enzyme repression Reduction in synthesis of enzyme protein in response to some stimulus such as a hormone or the presence of large amounts of the end-product of its activity.

Eosinophilic gastroenteritis A rare disease characterized by food-related reactions, infiltration of certain white blood cells (eosinophils) in the GI tract, and an increase in the number of eosinophils in the blood.

Epicure A person who enjoys and has a discriminating taste and appreciation for all fine food and drink. Term was named after the famous Greek philosopher Epicurus (342-270 B.C.).

Epidemiological transition Changes that occur in the morbidity-mortality profile of a population, describing the pyramid of demographic transition from a youthful population to one that is mature or elderly. The most characteristic epidemiological fact is the passage from tha malnutrition / infection pole to obesity / chronic degenerative disease pole.

Epidemiology Epidemiology is the scientific study of factors affecting the health and illness of individuals and populations, and serves as the foundation and logic of interventions made in the interest of public health and preventive medicine. It is considered a cornerstone methodology of public health research, and is highly regarded in evidence-based medicine for identifying risk factors for disease and determining optimal treatment approaches to clinical practice. The acting epidemiologist works on issues ranging from the practical, such as outbreak investigation, environmental exposure, and health promotion, to the theoretical, including the development of statistical, mathematical, philosophical, and biological theory. To this end, epidemiologists employ a range of study designs from the observational to experimental, with the purpose of revealing unbiased relationships between exposures such as nutrition, biological agents, stress, or chemicals to outcomes such as disease, wellness and health indicators. Defining the diseases, drawing disease causal chain / chains, and formulation of health strategy are important aspects of epidemiology. Modern epidemiologist use disease informatics as a tool.

Epigramme French; small pieces of neck or breast of lamb, cooked, then dipped in egg and breadcrumbs and grilled or fried.

Epinephrine An adrenal hormone that stimulates autonomic nerve reaction. It is used in the treatment of anaphylaxis to open airways and blood vessels.

Epithelial Tissue forming the outer layer of body surface.

Epithelium This article discusses the epithelium, an animal anatomical structure. For the fungal anatomical structure of the same name, see Pileipellis. In skinology epithelium is a tissue composed of a layer of cells. In humans, it is one of four primary body tissues. Epithelium lines both the outside (skin) and the inside cavities and lumen of bodies. The outermost layer of our skin is composed of dead stratified squamous epithelial cells, as are the mucous membranes lining the inside of mouths and body cavities. Other epithelial cells line the insides of the lungs, the gastrointestinal tract, the reproductive and urinary tracts, and make up the exocrine and endocrine glands.

Epsom salts Magnesium sulphate, originally found in a mineral spring in Epsom, Surrey, England; acts as a purgative because the osmotic pressure of the solution causes it to retain water in the intestine and so increase the bulk and moisture content of the faeces.

Equilibrium humidity The relative humidity of the atmosphere with which the substance under consideration is in equilibrium.

Erdbeergeist German spirit distilled from strawberries with added alcohol.

Erepsin Name given to a mixture of enzymes contained in intestinal juice, including aminopeptidases and dipeptidases.

Ergosterol A sterol isolated from yeast; when treated with ultra-violet light, it is converted to ercalciol (ergocalciferol, vitamin D2). This is the main source of manufactured vitamin D.

Ergot A fungus that grows on grasses and cereal grains; the ergot of medical importance is Claviceps purpurea, which grows on rye. The consumption of infected rye is harmful, causing the disease known as St Anthony's fire (ergotism), and can be fatal.

The active principles in ergot are alkaloids (ergotinine, ergotoxine, ergotamine, ergometrine, etc.), which yield lysergic acid on hydrolysis. This is believed to be the active component. Its effect is to increase the tone and contraction of smooth muscle, particularly of the pregnant uterus. For this reason ergot has been used in obstetrics, but pure ergonovine maleate and ergotonine tartrate are preferable.

Ergotism Poisoning due to an ergot infection of rye which occurs from time to time among people eating rye bread. The last outbreak in the UK was in Manchester in 1925, when there were 200 cases. Symptoms appear when as little as 1% of ergot-infected rye is included in the flour.

Eriodictin A flavonoid (flavonone) found in citrus pith, a constituent of what is sometimes called vitamin P.

ERS Economic Research Service. The research division within the USDA that conducts research on programs and issues under the USDA's jurisdiction. Related to hunger, ERS conducts research and analysis on food security levels and various aspects of administration and implementation of federal nutrition and commodity distribution programs.

Erucic acid A mono-unsaturated fatty acid, cis-13-docosenoic acid found in rape seed (Brassica napus) and mustard seed (B. junca and B. nigra) oils; it may constitute 30-50% of the oil in some varieties. It causes fatty infiltration of heart muscle in experimental animals, and the amount of ordinary rape seed oil used in margarines is consequently limited. Low erucic acid varieties of rape seed have been developed for food use.

Eructation The act of bringing up air from the stomach, with a characteristic sound. Also known as belching.

Erythorbic acid The D-isomer of ascorbic acid, also called Daraboascorbic acid and iso-ascorbic acid, with only slight vitamin C activity. It is as powerful an antioxidant as vitamin C and is used in foods for that purpose.

Erythroamylose An old name for amylopectin.

Erythropoiesis The formation and development of the red blood cells in the bone marrow.

Erythrosine BS Red colour permitted in foods in most countries (E-127, known as Red number 3 in USA). Used in preserved cherries, sausages, and meat and fish pastes; it is unstable to light and heat. Chemically the disodium or potassium salt of 2,4,5,7- tetraiodofluorescein.

Escabeche A spicy cold pickle or marinade made from herbs, spices, vinegar and olive oil that originated in Spain and was used mainly for preserving fish and other cooked foods. It's mostly used for small cooked fish, which are de-headed, fried or lightly browned and then marinated for 24 hours, but any firm-fleshed white fish works well. Simply coat the fish in seasoned flour, pan-fry in a little oil, then pour the marinade on top. Escaboche of fish are usually served as an hors d'oeuvre.

Escalope A thin slice of boneless meat, often beaten even thinner for quick cooking. It's cut from the leaner parts of certain animals, in particular veal, pork and turkey. It can also be used to refer to thick slices of fish with a strip of skin on one side. The classic method of preparing veal escalopes is to coat them with breadcrumbs before frying them.

Escargot The French word for "snail." They can be terrestrial, freshwater, or marine. Escargot is the common name for the land gastropod mollusk. The edible snails of France have a single shell that is tan and white, and 1 to 2 inches diameter.

Esophagitis An irritation of the esophagus, usually caused by acid that flows up from the stomach.

Espagnole or brown sauce Traditionally made from beef stock, aromatics, herbs and, sometimes, tomato paste. Brown sauce is the basis from which many other sauces are made. Brown sauce consists of a liquid thickened with a cooked mixture of butter and flour called a roux. The difference is that for a brown sauce, the roux is cooked much longer; it must be stirred over low heat until it acquires a nut-brown cast that intensifies the colour and flavor of the sauce. This lengthier cooking diminishes the thickening power of the starch, a factor that should be taken into consideration before you start cooking. To make a brown sauce of medium thickness, allow two tablespoons of both butter and flour for each cup of liquid.

Espresso Espresso is a process of extracting flavor from coffee beans. Served in very small cups, this is a dark, strong coffee made by forcing steam through finely ground, Italian-roast coffee. The literal meaning of the word espresso is, made on the spur of the moment or fast.

In 1901, Italian Luigi Bezzera invented and espresso and the first espresso machine that contained a boiler and four divisions. Each could take varying sized filters that contained the coffee. He patented his espresso machine on September 1, 1902, which he called the "Espresso Coffee Machine." According to historians, he was not happy because his employees were taking too long for their coffee breaks! If only he could shorten the brewing process used to make traditional coffee, his employees would take shorter breaks. Bezzera had an idea to introduce pressure to the coffee brewing process, reducing the time needed to brew. His marketing efforts were unsuccessful, and he became penniless.

In 1905, Desidero Pavoni purchased Bezzera's patent and began manufacturing machines based on the Bezzera style machine. In 1906 the original Espresso Coffee was presented to the world at an exhibition in Milano, Italy. They mass produced these machines and in 1927 the first espresso machine was installed in the United States at Regio's in New York. Regio's still displays the machine.

Essence or extract These are concentrated flavourings (for example from vanilla pods, almonds, anchovies or coffee beans) used to flavour and enhance foods, and can also refer to synthetic flavourings. They're usually sold in small bottles or jars.

Vanilla extract is extracted from pure vanilla pods whereas vanilla essence is made synthetically. The distinction between extract and essence isn't always so clear cut, however, so read the labels carefully. Commercial beef extracts include Bovril and Oxo. Marmite, for instance, is a commercial yeast extract.

Essential 1. Something that cannot be done without.

2. Required in the diet, because the body cannot make it. As in an essential amino acid or an essential fatty acid.

3. Idiopathic. As in essential hypertension. "Essential" is a hallowed term meaning "We don't know the cause."

Essential Amino Acids Nine amino acids that can not be synthesized by mammals and are therefore dietarily essential.

Essential Fatty Acids Make cell membranes, hormones, and prostaglandins. Vegetable oils such as canola, flaxseed, walnut, corn, soybean, and safflower oils, fish, and fish oil supplements.

Essential nutrient Those nutrients that are required by the body and cannot be synthesized in the body in adequate amounts to meet requirements, so must be provided by the diet: includes the essential amino acids and fatty acids, vitamins, and minerals. Really a tautology, since by definition nutrients are essential dietary constituents.

Ester Esters are usually encountered as sweet smelling organic compounds commonly produced by many plants and fruits. However, the most common esters found in nature are fats and vegetable oils, which are esters of glycerol and fatty acids.

Esters An organic compound produced by reaction between acid and alcohol.

Ethylene Ethene; a gas of the formula CH 2 =CH 2, produced by fruit as a hormone to speed ripening. This explains why some fruits ripen faster if they are stored in a plastic bag. It is used commercially in very small amounts to speed fruit ripening after harvesting.

Etouffee The term literally means, "smothered." It is a cooking method of cooking something smothered in a blanket of chopped vegetables over a low flame in a tightly covered pan. Crawfish and shrimp etoufees are delicious New Orleans specialties.

Evaporated milk Evaporated milk is pure cow's milk which has been concentrated to double richness. Nothing has been added to the original milk and nothing taken away except some of the water (60% of which has been removed by evaporation). In 1899, grocer E.A. Stuart and a fellow business partner founded the Pacific Coast Condensed Milk Company in Kent, Washington. It was based solely on the little-understood, relatively new process of evaporation. Evaporated milk even went to war over the years, as American soldiers carried cans of condensed milk into battle during World War I, World War II, and the Korean War. The inhospitable conditions in which these brave men and women often found themselves made a versatile food product like evaporated milk standard issue.

Executive Chef The term literally means "the chief' in French. Every kitchen has a chef or executive chef who is responsible for the operations of the entire kitchen. (A commonly misused term in English, not every cook is a chef.)

Exergonic Chemical reactions that proceed with the output of energy, usually as heat (then sometimes known as exothermic reactions) or light. The reactions involved in the oxidation of food-stuffs are generally exergonic.

Exotaxins Toxic substances produced by bacteria which diffuse out of the cells and stimulate the production of antibodies which specifically neutralize them (antitoxins), They are generally heat-labile and inactivated in about l hour at 60°C. Exotoxins include those produced by the organisms responsible for botulism, tetanus, and diphtheria.

Expansion rings In relation to cans, the concentric rings stamped into the ends of the can to allow bulging during heat processing without straining the seams unduly.

Expeller cake The residue from oilseeds after most of the oil has been removed by pressing; it is a valuable source of protein, especially for animal feeding.

Experimental design Nutrition science advances by observation (for example, nutritional epidemiologists observe statistical associations between what people eat and their patterns of health and disease) and by experiment, in which subjects are given specifically formulated diets and certain effects are noted. For example, to test the metabolic effects of components of diets, experiments are performed in which a diet containing the test substance (treatment) is compared against a reference diet (control) which, if possible, is the same in all respects other than the test substance and in which the test substance is substituted by a suitable placebo. Subjects should be allocated randomly to diets so that factors other than those tested, and which may otherwise confound the results, are equalised between treatments. Ideally, neither the subjects nor the experimenters should be aware of the identity of treatment and placebo groups (double-blind).

Experimental group The group of subjects in an experimental study which receives a treatment.

Exposure assessment Exposure assessment is a branch of environmental science that focuses on the processes that take place at the interface between the environment containing the contaminant(s) of interest and the organism(s) being considered.These are last steps in the path from realease of an environmental contaminant, through transport to its effect in a biological system. It tries to measure of much of a contaminant can be absorbed by an exposed target organism, in what form, at what rate and how much of the absorbed amount is actually available to produce a biological effect. Although the same general concepts apply to other organisms, the overwhelming majority of applications of exposure assessment are concerned with human health, making it an important tool in public health.

Extensograph An instrument for measuring the stretching strength of dough as an index of its baking quality.

External validity External Validity is a form of experimental validity [1]. An experiment is said to possess external validity if the experiment's results hold across different experimental settings, procedures and participants [2,3]. If a study possesses external validity, its results will generalize to the larger population.

Extracellular In cell biology, molecular biology and related fields, the word extracellular (or sometimes extracellular space) means "outside the cell". This space is usually taken to be outside the plasma membranes, and occupied by fluid. The term is used in contrast to intracellular (inside the cell).The cell membrane (and, in plants, the cell wall) is the barrier between the two, and chemical composition of intra- and extracellular milieu can be radically different. In most organisms, for example, a Na+/K+ ATPase pump maintains a high sodium level outside cells while keeping potassium low, leading to chemical excitability.

Extremophiles Micro-organisms that can grow under extreme conditions of heat (thermophiles) and extreme thermophiles, some of which live in hot-springs at 100 °C), or cold (pshyrophiles), in high concentrations of salt (halophiles), high pressure, or extremes of acid or alkali.

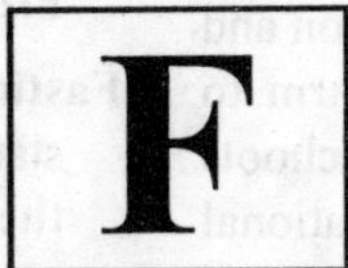

Faggot 1 Traditional British meatball made from pig offals and meat. A 150-g portion is an exceptionally rich source of iron and a rich source of vitamins B1, B2, and niacin; contains 28 g of fat; supplies 400 kcal (1680 kJ).

2 Bundle of herbs, bouquet garni.

Fajita The Spanish word for skirt steak. Most people associate the word fajita with strips of meat that go into the taco. Fajita is a highly flavorful cut of meat that comes from the outer covering of the breast near where the brisket comes from.

Falafel A Middle Eastern snack that is also known as ta'amica. It is considered the national dish of Egypt, but is popular throughout the Middle East. They are sold on every corner; from restaurants to side walk stands. A traditional falafel sandwich consists of six ground, deep-fried chickpea balls stuffed into pita bread along with finely cut up tomatoes, cucumbers, and tahini sauce.

Family 1. A group of individuals related by blood or marriage or by a feeling of closeness.

2. A biological classification of related plants or animals that is a division below the order and above the genus.

3. A group of genes related in structure and in function that descended from an ancestral gene.

4. A group of gene products similarly related in structure and function and of shared genetic descent.

5. Parents and their children. The most fundamental social group in humans.

FAO Food and Agriculture Organization of the United Nations, founded in 1943; headquarters in Rome. Its goal is to achieve freedom from hunger worldwide. According to its constitution the specific objectives are 'raising the levels of nutrition and standards of living... and securing improvements in the efficiency of production and distribution of all food and agricultural products'.

Farfalle Literally 'butterfly' in Italian, this is pasta shaped like little butterflies or bow-ties. It's very popular with children because of its novelty factor. Allow about 75g of pasta per person. If you can't find farfalle, fusilli is a good substitute. Certain pasta shapes hold different sauces better than others. Cheese or rich tomato sauces cling well to farfalle because it's a relatively small pasta shape with a large surface area.

Farina Farina is a coarsely ground endosperm of hard wheat. Farina is used in breakfast cereals.

Farm bill Authority for the Food Stamp Program is contained within the Farm Bill. This legislation can also affect commodity distribution programs such as TEFAP and CSFP and the child nutrition programs that receive commodity foods. In addition to nutrition programs, authority for many other USDA programs and activities is contained within the Farm Bill. The Farm Bill was most recently reauthorized by the Farm Security and Rural Investment Act of 2002, P.L. 107-171.

Farm to cafeteria Part of the Child Nutrition and WIC Reauthorization Act of 2004, Farm to Cafeteria projects link local farmers and schools to bring locally-grown food into the National School Lunch Program. Examples of Farm to Cafeteria projects include salad bars, seasonal items incorporated into lunch menus, and school gardens. Although currently no funds have been appropriated for the implementation of this program, schools in 17 states have started their own programs, sometimes referred to as Farm to School programs, with funding from community organizations and Community Food Projects Grants from the USDA.

Farmer's cheese Farmer's cheese is a fresh cheese that is a form of pressed cottage cheese. Most of the liquid is pressed out leaving a very dry, crumbly cheese that is often flavored with fruit or nuts. It is an all-purpose cheese good for eating or using in cooking. It is sliceable and also can be crumbled. It can be replaced, if necessary, with drained cottage cheese.

Farmers market A market where consumers can purchase fresh produce and other food items (such as meat, dairy products, and baked goods) directly from small to medium-sized farmers. Farmers markets are often located in urban settings, providing an important link between rural and urban communities. Some farmers markets also have the ability to accept EBT, allowing consumers to use their food stamp benefits to purchase food at these locations.

Fast food According to the Oxford English Dictionary, the first documented use of "fast food" in reference to a restaurant came in 1951 in an article in a trade journal called "Fountain and Fast Food Service." Fast food seems to have been originally applied to restaurants and catering businesses that served "steam table" delicacies, as well as to convenience foods a busy housewife could quickly whip up. The history of fast food started as neighborhood restaurants opened by idealistic young people in the 1950s - Carl's Jr., McDonald's, Dominoes Pizza, etc.

Fasting Going without food. The metabolic fasting state begins some 4 hours after a meal, when the digestion and absorption of food are complete and body reserves of fat and glycogen begin to be mobilized. In more prolonged fasting the blood concentration of ketone bodies rises, as they are exported from the liver for use by muscle and other tissues as a metabolic fuel.

FAT 1. Factory acceptance test (see Acceptance test), a software engineering conceptFar Eastern Air Transport, an airline of the Republic of China on TaiwanFile Allocation Table, a file system format used by Microsoft operating systems; and othersForces Armıes Tchadiennes, the Chad armed forces of the government of President Fllix Malloum Frente Autıntico del Trabajo, a Mexican labor confederationFresno Yosemite International Airport (IATA airport code)Fully Automatic Time, automatic-sensored method of recording race times during running events.

2. Fats consist of a wide group of compounds that are generally soluble in organic solvents and largely insoluble in water. Fats may be either solid or liquid at normal room temperature, depending on their structure and composition. Although the words "oils", "fats" and "lipids" are all used to refer to fats, "oils" is usually used to refer to fats that are liquids at normal room temperature, while "fats" is usually used to refer to fats that are solids at normal room temperature. "Lipids" is used to refer to both liquid and solid fats.

Fat replacers Fat replacers are developed to duplicate the taste and texture of fat, but contain fewer calories per gram than fat. Fat replacers generally fall into three categories carbohydrate, protein or fat based. The ingredients that are used to replace fat depend on how the food product will be eaten or prepared. For example, not all fat replacer ingredients are heat stable. Thus, the fat replacer that worked well in a salad dressing may not work well in a muffin mix.

Fat substitute Fat substitutes are substances that contribute a similar mouth feel, texture, or taste to a food product as normal fat. Some are as caloric as fats, but can be used in smaller amounts, while others are not metabolized and thus make a negligible contribution to the caloric content of the food.

Fats, dietary fats Fat provides 9 calories per gram. Fat is important to maintain cell walls, provide insulation and concentrated energy. Fat also carries the fat-soluble vitamins A, D, E and K through the body. Food sources of fat include meat, poultry, fish, eggs, nuts, butter, margarine, oil and some dairy products.

In food, there are two types of fat saturated and unsaturated. Saturated fats are solid at room temperature and come chiefly from animal food products. Examples are butter, lard, meat fat, solid shortening, palm oil, and coconut oil. Unsaturated fats, which include monounsaturated and polyunsaturated, are liquid at room temperature and come from plant oils such as olive, peanut, corn, cottonseed, sunflower, safflower, and soybean. Hydrogenated fats are unsaturated fats that have been processed (hyrdogenated) to make them more saturated, spreadable, and longer lasting. Hydrogenation produces trans-fatty acids, which may have health effects similar to those of saturated fatty acids. The most common sources of hydrogenated fats are stick or tub margarine, commercial baked goods, and fried foods from restaurants and fast-food chains.

Fat-soluble vitamins Vitamins - organic substances that cannot be produced in the body but are essential for cellular functions and must be obtained from the diet - carried in fat and usually acquired from fatty foods. Vitamins A, D, E and K are the fat-soluble vitamins.

Fatty acid Fatty acids are generally classified as saturated, monounsaturated or polyunsaturated. These terms refer to the number of hydrogen atoms attached to the carbon atoms of the fat molecule. In general, fats that contain a majority of saturated fatty acids are solid at room temperature, although some solid vegetable shortenings are up to 75 percent unsaturated. Fats containing mostly unsaturated fatty acids are usually liquid at room temperature and are called oils. Also, see "fats", or "hydrogenation."

Fatty liver Fatty liver or steatorrhoeic hepatosis is a reversible condition seen in chronic alcoholism and many other conditions, where large vacuoles of lipid accumulate in hepatocytes (the cells of the liver). Accumulation of fat in liver cells will cause the liver to enlarge. The lipid within the vacuoles is a particular type of lipid known as triglyceride. Triglyceride molecules consist of a glycerol backbone with three fatty acid molecules joined on.

Fatty streak Fatty streak, though not composed of fat, is the term generally given to the earliest stages of atheroma, as viewed at autopsy, looking at the inner surface of arteries, without magnification. It is not visible by current technologies in living humans, even by IVUS, the most advanced imaging technology for seeing artery walls.

Fava beans Fresh or dried broad beans (the term fava bean is used more frequently in the US). Fresh broad beans only have a short natural season during the summer and are often sold frozen or canned. They're sweet and delicious with a smooth creamy texture.

Fresh beans are more popular than the dried variety, which tend to be quite floury. Young thin beans are eaten pods and all, but larger, older broad beans need to have the tough pods removed. After boiling or steaming them (for about five minutes), peel away the thin, pale sheath covering the bean.

Dried broad beans don't hold their shape very well, so they're often used to make spreads or purees. They're also good for flavouring meat stews or lamb dishes. Egyptian ful medames is a dish of cooked broad beans (a small dried variety called 'ful') flavoured with garlic and lemon.

FDA The Food and Drug Administration, an agency within the U.S. Public Health Service, which is a part of the Department of Health and Human Services.

FDPIR Food Distribution Program on Indian Reservations. This USDA program provides commodity foods to low-income households, including the elderly, living on Indian reservations, and to Native American families residing in designated areas near reservations.

Federal poverty level (FPL) A measure used to determine the household income level for a family to be considered in poverty. The measurement was developed in 1965 by multiplying the USDA's economy food plan (predecessor to the Thrifty Food Plan) by three. The measurement is updated each year based on price increases reflected in the Consumer Price Index.

Feijoa A native to subtropical South America and commercially grown in New Zealand and Northern California. Feijoas are available during spring and early summer. They are also called pineapple guavas, describing the taste of the creamy, white, juicy, granular flesh. The taste is a combination of pineapple and guava or strawberry with a hint of spearmint. Ripe fruit should have a full rich aroma and should "give" or feel tender to the touch, like a ripe plum or pear. Feijoas can be ripened at room temperature by enclosing in a paper bag with an apple. Once they are ripened, the fruit can be stored in the refrigerator for about a week.

Feingold diet Exclusion of foods containing synthetic colours, flavours, and preservatives and limitation of intake of fruits and vegetables such as oranges, apricots, peaches, tomatoes, and cucumbers; intended to treat hyperactive children. There is little evidence either that these foods are a cause of hyperactivity or that the exclusion diet is beneficial.

Fennel There are two main types of this aromatic plant - the vegetable and the herb. Both have pale green, celery-like stems and bright green, feathery foliage. Florence fennel, also called finocchio or Italian fennel, has a broad, bulbous base with a mild aniseed flavour and is treated like a vegetable. Both the base and stems can be eaten raw in salads or cooked by braising or roasting. Look for small tender white bulbs - the darker green bulbs tend to be bitter. Cut off the root end and the leaves and peel the outer layer of skin away, then cut either downwards or across the bulb. To cook, just boil in salted water for about 15 minutes or until it's tender. The herb has greenish-brown seeds and feathery green leaves, both of which have a strong aniseed flavour that complements fish, especially oily varieties such as mackerel or herring.

Fermentation A form of anaerobic respiration occurring in certain microorganisms, e.g. yeasts. Alcoholic fermentation comprises a series of biochemical reactions by which pyruvate (the end product of glycolysis) is converted to ethanol and carbon dioxide. It is the basis of the baking and brewing industries (see baker's yeast). In lactic-acid fermentation, which occurs in many microorganisms and (when sugar is in short supply) in animal cells, the end product is lactic acid. Microorganisms display a range of fermentations, producing not only ethanol or lactic acid, but other products, such as propionic and butyric acids, acetate, and methane.

Fermented foods Foods that have been subjected to processing involving the action of yeasts or bacteria.

Fermentograph An instrument for measuring the gas-producing power of a dough.

Fernet Branca Italian; bitter digestif; herbs and spices steeped in white wine and brandy.

Ferric ammonium citrate The chemical form in which iron is sometimes added to foods. Occurs as brown-red scales (16.5-18.5% iron) and as green scales (14.5-16% iron).

Fertilizer Any organic or inorganic material, either natural or synthetic, used to supply elements (such as nitrogen, phosphate and potash) essential for plant growth. If used in excess or attached to eroding soil, fertilizers can become a source of water pollution.

Ferulic acid A type of phenol found in various fruits and vegetables and citrus fruits which has antioxidant like activities that may reduce the risk of degenerative diseases, heart disease and eye disease.

Feta cheese A classic Greek cheese usually made from goat's or sheep's milk. It is now also made from cow's milk. Salted and cured in a brine solution (which can be either water or whey) for a week to several months (this is why it is sometimes called a pickled cheese and has a sharp, salty taste. Feta dries out rapidly when removed from the brine. Feta cheese is white, usually formed into square cakes, and can range from soft to semi-hard, with a tangy, salty flavor that can range from mild to sharp. It has been and still remains a significant part of Greek diet and its name is often connected with the Greek history and tradition. Feta cheese is one of the oldest cheeses in the world. Without refrigeration cheese made as many as 6000 years ago, spoiled easily. One of the only ways to preserve cheese was to preserve cheese with salt. Greek mythology has it that the Cyclops Polyphemus raised plump sheep, using their rich milk to make a delicious cheese which Ulysses discovered during his interminable travels.

Fetal alcohol spectrum disorder Fetal alcohol spectrum disorder (FASD) describes a spectrum of permanent and often devastating birth-defect syndromes caused by maternal consumption of alcohol during pregnancy. The main effect of fetal alcohol exposure is brain damage. This can be caused during any trimester, because the fetus's brain continues to develop throughout the entire pregnancy. The brain damage is often accompanied by, and reflected in, distinctive facial stigmata, as seen in the photograph on the right.

Fetal alcohol syndrome A syndrome resulting from the teratogenic effects of alcohol during fetal development; possible symptoms include developmental delay, short stature, microcephaly and hyperactivity

Fettuccine Alfredo Fettuccine tossed with butter, heavy cream, and grated cheese. In 1908, Alfredo di Lelio, a small restaurateur and chef, living above his small Rome restaurant with his pregnant wife, created Fettuccine Alfredo to tempt the palate of his pregnant wife who had lost her appetite and was becoming weaker. Alfredo decided that he would invent a dish that his wife could not resist. His wife loved it and legend says she cleaned her plate and a short time later, Alfredo II was born to the music of customers downstairs in the restaurant, all crying for his new irresistible dish.

Fiber Dietary fiber generally refers to parts of fruits, vegetables, grains, nuts and legumes that can't be digested by humans. Meats and dairy products do not contain fiber. Studies indicate that high fiber diets can reduce the risks of heart disease and certain types of cancer. There are two basic types of fiber insoluble and soluble. Soluble fiber in cereals, oatmeal, beans and other foods has been found to lower blood cholesterol. Insoluble fiber in cauliflower, cabbage and other vegetables and fruits helps move foods through the stomach and intestine, thereby decreasing the risk of cancers of the colon and rectum.

Fibrin The blood protein formed from fibrinogen which is responsible for the clotting of blood.

Fibrinogen One of the proteins of the blood plasma which is responsible for the clotting of blood. When prothrombin is activated to thrombin in response to injury, it converts fibrinogen to fibrin, which is deposited as strands that trap the red cells and form the clot.

Fibrosis Fibrosis is the formation or development of excess fibrous connective tissue in an organ or tissue as a reparative or reactive process, as opposed to formation of fibrous tissue as a normal constituent of an organ or tissue. Fibrosis-related diseases:Cystic fibrosis of the pancreas and lungsEndomyocardial fibrosis, idiopathic myocardiopathyCirrhosis can result from fibrosis of the liverIdiopathic pulmonary fibrosis of the lungDiffuse parenchymal lung diseaseMediastinal fibrosisProgressive massive fibrosis, a complication of coal workers' pneumoconiosisProliferative fibrosis, neoplastic fibrosisTuberculosis (TB) can cause fibrosis of the lungs.

Fig Figs were probably one of the first fruits to be dried and stored by man. There was a fig tree in the Garden of Eden, and in fact, the fig is the most talked about fruit in the Bible. Whether a fig was the forbidden fruit is debatable, but it is definite that a fig tree provided the first clothing; "...the eyes of both of them were opened, and they knew that they were naked; and they sewed fig leaves together, and made themselves aprons." The ancient city of Attica was famous for its figs and they soon became a necessity for its citizens, rich or poor. Solon, the ruler of Attica (639-559 BC), actually made it illegal to export figs out of Greece, reserving them solely for his citizens. The Persian King Xerxes, after his defeat by the Greeks at Salamis in 480 BC, had figs from Attica served him at every meal to remind him that he did not possess the land where this fruit grew. The Spanish missionary fathers who first planted them at the San Diego Mission in 1759 brought figs to California. Fig trees were then planted at each succeeding mission, going North through California. Although considered a fruit, the fig is actually a flower that is inverted into it. The seeds are drupes (or the real fruit). Figs are the only fruit to fully ripen and semi-dry on the tree. They are generally available twice each year, in June and again in late August or September. Both crops are harvested from the same tree.

Figueredas Spanish (Valenciana); a spiced seafood dish similar to paella, but served on a bed of pasta rather than rice.

File Also called gumbo file powder. File powder, which is made from the ground dried leaves of the sassafras tree. File is a thickening agent that must be stirred in a dish after it is removed the heat to prevent a stringy or ropey texture from developing. It is used as a seasoning and primarily thickening agent in gumbo, and has a wonderfully pungent and aromatic flavor. File should never be added to a pot of gumbo while it's cooking, but rather added to individual servings (if cooked or reheated, it will turn stringy). It was introduced into Creole cooking by the Choctaw Indians of Louisiana. The Indians thought the sassafras tree had special healing powers. They combined the roots and leaves with water to make a healing tonic.

Filet Mignon The term "filet mignon" is a French derivative, the literal meaning is small (mignon) bone-less meat (filet). Cut from the small end of the beef tenderloin. Depending upon what part of the United States you're in, the tenderloin muscle of the cow or short loin, becomes Filet Mignon, Chateaubriand, Tournedos, Medallions, or Filet de Boeuf. Filet Mignon is also know as Tenderloin Steak (in fact most often I see it as Tenderloin Steak). Filet Mignon or Tenderloin Steak is a cut of meat that is considered the king of steaks because of its tender, melt in the mouth texture. It comes from the small end of the tenderloin (called the short loin), which is found on the back rib cage of the animal. Because this area of the animal is not weight-bearing, the connective tissue is not toughened by exercise resulting in extremely tender meat. Filet mignon slices found in the market are generally one to two inches thick and two to three inches in diameter, but true mignons are no more than one inch in diameter and are taken from the tail end.

Fillet The term used to describe a boneless, lean cut of meat, fish or poultry. Fillet of beef is a prime cut and different parts of it are called different names depending on which part of the fillet they're cut from, including filet mignon, tournedos and chβteaubriand. You also 'fillet' a fish to remove the bones.

Filo pastry Paper-thin translucent sheets of pastry commonly used in Greek, Eastern European and Middle Eastern cuisines. It's sold ready-made in rolled layers - fresh from the chiller cabinet, or frozen. The delicate sheets are strengthened by using several layers together. You have to work quickly with filo pastry otherwise it dries out. It's best to keep it in the plastic wrapping or cover it with a damp cloth while you're working with it. The layers are usually brushed with melted butter or oil to help them brown. Filo can be fried or oven baked and cooks very quickly. It can be used to make a wide variety of sweet and savoury dishes. It's perfect for making savoury little parcels such as Greek spanakopita (spinach and cheese triangles), samosas or spring rolls.

It can be used for sweet bakes, tarts and tartlets such as apple strudel or the decadent Greek dish baklava (honey and nut pastry). For a simple canapι, cut shapes from a few layers of filo, deep-fry them and sprinkle with herbs and spices. Try wrapping cuts of meat, fish or chicken in sheets of filo and baking in the oven.

Filter To strain a liquid through a porous paper, fine cloth, etc., to remove small particles, as in making coffee or clarifying fruit juice to make jelly. Water may be filtered through charcoal to remove unpleasant flavours and colours; bacterial filters for water have pores fine enough to remove bacteria.

Filth test Name given to a test originated in the USA for determining the contamination of a food with rodent hairs and insect fragments as an index of the hygienic handling of the food.

Fines herbes A mixture of chopped aromatic fresh herbs used in French cooking, particularly in egg dishes, sauces, salads and soups. The classic combination is chopped chives, chervil, parsley and tarragon. You can buy fines herbes dried.

Fines Herbs–Homemade This is a mixture of chopped aromatic herbs, such as parsley, chervil, tarragon, and chives, in various proportions. The mixture is used to flavor sauces, cream cheese, meat, sautιed vegetables, and omelets. In the past, chopped mushrooms were added, and now some include stalks of celery, fennel, basil, rosemary, thyme, and bay leaf.

Fire point The temperature at which a frying oil will sustain combustion. It ranges between 340 and 360 ‘C for different fats. See also flash point; smoke point.

Firming agents Fresh fruits contain insoluble pectins as a firm gel around the fibrous tissues which keeps the fruit firm. Breakdown of cell structure allows conversion of pectin to pectic acid, with loss of firmness. The addition of calcium salts (chloride or carbonate) forms a calcium pectate el which protects the fruit against softening; these are known as firming agents. Alum is sometimes used to firm pickles.

Fish cakes Chopped or minced fish, bound with egg and flour (or matzo meal) and seasoned with onion, pepper, and sometimes herbs, then deep fried. See also gefillte fish.

Fish cook or poissonier The fish cook—all fish and shellfish items and their sauces

Fish fingers Shaped fish fillets covered with breadcrumbs; approximately 50% fish. Two fish fingers, grilled (55 g) are a rich source of iodine; a source of protein and niacin; contain 5 g of fat, of which one-third is saturated and one-third polyunsaturated; and supply 120 kcal (500 kJ).

Fish ham Japanese product made from a red fish such as tuna or marlin, pickled with salt and nitrite, mixed with whale meat and pork fat and stuffed into a large sausage-type casing.

Fish meal Surplus fish, waste from filleting (fish-house waste), and fish unsuitable for human consumption are dried and powdered. The resultant meal is a valuable source of protein for animal feed, or, after deodorization, as human food since it contains about 70% protein of biological value up to 0.7. That made from white fish is termed white fish meal, distinct from the oily type which is sometimes of very poor quality and is consequently used as fertilizer.

Fish oils These contain long-chain polyunsaturated fatty acids which appear to offer some protection against problems associated with heart disease. The two main ones are EPA (eicosapentaenoic acid; twenty carbon atoms and five double bonds) and DHA (docosahexaenoic acid; twenty-two carbon atoms and six double bonds). Fish oil concentrates containing these fatty acids are sold as pharmaceutical preparations.

Fish sauce A powerful thin brown sauce used in the cooking of numerous countries in Asia. It's made by fermenting small whole fish in brine and drawing off the liquid, which is then bottled. It smells pungent and tastes very salty, although cooking greatly reduces its 'fishiness' and simply adds richness and a layer of flavour to cooked dishes. It's frequently used in the cooking of Thailand, where it's known as nam pla. In the Philippines it's known as patis and shottsuru in Japan. Fish sauce is available in most Asian shops, as well as in supermarkets. If you can't find it, use a light soy sauce.

Fish, fatty or oily Anchovies, herring, mackerel, pilchard, salmon, sardine, trout, tuna, whitebait, containing about 15% fat (varying from 5 to 20% through the year) and containing 10-40 ug vitamin D per 100 g, as distinct from white fish, which contain 1-2% fat and only a trace of vitamin D. See also herring.

Five-spice powder A pungent mixture of five spices commonly used in Chinese cookery; it's a brown powder made of ground star anise, fennel seeds, cloves, cinnamon and Sichuan pepper. It's available from Chinese grocers, and is becoming more widely available in supermarkets too. A good blend should be fragrant and spicy but also slightly sweet.

Flageolet beans Considered the caviar of beans, flageolets are tiny, tender French bush type beans that are very popular in French cooking. They range from creamy white to light green. Flageolets are removed from the pod when tender and just maturing. This bean of French origin is grown in the fertile soil of California. Its versatile flavor compliments lamb, as well as fish and chicken. If you can't find them, substitute navy beans instead.

Flan An open pie with a pastry base containing a sweet or savoury filling in a custard of eggs and cream. Spinach flan or leek and bacon flan are examples. In Spain and Latin America 'flan' is used to refer to the egg custard dessert that we know as crθme caramel.

Flash point With reference to frying oils, the temperature at which the decomposition products can be ignited, but will not support combustion; range between 290 and 330 °C. See also fire point; smoke point.

Flat sours Bacteria such as Bacillus stearothermophilus render canned food sour by fermenting carbohydrates to lactic, formic, and acetic acids, without gas production. This means that the ends of the can are not swelled out but remain flat. Economically they are the most important of the thermophilic spoilage agents; some species can grow slowly at 25 °C and thus spoil products after long storage periods

Flavanones A type of flavonoid found in citrus fruits which provides the health benefits of neutralizing free radicals and possibly reducing the risk of cancer.

Flavin mononucleotide (FMN) A coenzyme in oxidation reactions, chemically the phosphate of vitamin B2 (riboflavin).

Flavin The group of compounds containing the iso-alloxazine ring structure, as in riboflavin (vitamin B2), and hence a general term for riboflavin derivatives.

Flavones A type of flavonoid found in various fruits and vegetables which provides the health benefits of neutralizing free radicals and possibly reducing the risk of cancer.

Flavoproteins Enzymes that contain the vitamin riboflavin, or a derivative such as flavin adenine dinucleotide or riboflavin phosphate, as the prosthetic group. Mainly involved in oxidation reactions in metabolism.

Flavour potentiator A substance that enhances the flavours of other substances without itself imparting any characteristic flavour of its own, e.g. monosodium glutamate and ribotide as well as sugar, salt, and vinegar in small quantities.

Flavour profile A method of judging the flavour of foods by examination of a list of the separate factors into which the flavour can be analysed, the so-called character notes.

Flavours, synthetic Mostly mixtures of esters, e.g. banana oil is ethyl butyrate and amyl acetate; apple oil, ethyl butyrate, ethyl valerianate, ethyl salicylate, amyl butyrate, glycerol, chloroform, and alcohol; pineapple oil is ethyl and amyl butyrates, acetaldehyde, chloroform, glycerol, and alcohol.

Fleur de sel Fleur de sel is a moist salt from France. Available from good delis or some larger supermarkets.

Fleuron Small crescent-shaped piece of puff pastry used as a garnish.

Flip Drink made with beaten egg and milk, with added wine or spirit, and sweetened.

Flitch Side of bacon; half a pig, slit down the back, with the legs and shoulders removed.

Floats Caribbean (Trinidad); fried biscuits made with yeast dough. See also bakes.

Florentine 1. Thin biscuits with nuts and dried fruit coated with chocolate.

2. Garnished with spinach.

Florentine Any French or Italian dish described as 'Florentine' uses spinach as its base. A florentine is also a kind of biscuit made with nuts, honey and dried fruit. When the biscuits are cooked and have cooled they're spread on one side with melted chocolate and left until the chocolate cools and hardens.

Florets Florets are the small, individual flower stems that make up the heads of vegetables such as broccoli and cauliflower.

Floridean starch A polysaccharide (chemically a glucosan) resembling glycogen, obtained from red algae (Florideae spp.).

Flounder There are many varieties of flounder around the world. In the U.S. this category includes the Atlantic fluke, gray sole, Pacific petrale sole, rex sole, and sand dab. All of these are flatfish with both eyes on one side. They can be purchased either whole or as fillets. They are all mild tasting and should be cooked with attention to their delicate structure.

Flour Flour is made from finely ground cereal, such as wheat, barley, oats, rye, rice and maize (corn). In Britain, the word 'flour' usually refers to flour produced from wheat. Wheat flour contains gluten, a protein that forms an elastic network that helps contain the gases that make mixtures (such as doughs and batters) rise as they bake. Different types of flour are needed for different products. Bread flour, or strong flour, for example, has a high protein content and good gluten strength. Plain flour is usually a soft flour and is best for cakes and pastries. Self-raising flour has a standard amount of raising agent (usually a mixture of bicarbonate of soda and cream of tartar) already added to it. Varying degrees of processing in the milling of the grain give wholemeal or wholewheat, brown and white types of flour. Spelt flour is made from an ancestor of modern wheat and, although it contains a small amount of gluten, some people who are intolerant to wheat flour can cope with it.

Flour enrichment The addition of certain vitamins and minerals to flour, to contain not less than: in the UK, vitamin B1, 0.24 mg; niacin, 1.6 mg; iron, 1.65 mg; calcium, 120 mg/100 g; in the USA, vitamin B1, 0.44-0.56 mg; vitamin B2,

0.2-0.33 mg; niacin, 3.6-4.4 mg; iron, 2.9-3.7 mg/100 g; calcium not specified.

Flour strength A property of the flour proteins enabling the dough to retain gas during fermentation to give a 'bold' loaf. 'Strong' flour is higher in protein content, has greater elasticity and resistance to extension, and greater ability to absorb water. A 'weak' flour gives a loaf that lacks volume. See also extensometer, farinograph.

Flour–bread Bread flour is unique in that it contains a high level of protein called gluten. Bread flour contains two proteins, gliadin and glutenin, which co-form gluten under the proper conditio.;s; e.g. water and agitation. Gluten provides the structure and elasticity necessary for a yeast dough. Home bakers who make a great deal of bread will find that bread flour will yield better volume, a tender crust and an evenly distributed, fine grain.

Bread flour is best suited for yeast breads. A longer kneading time is recommended to fully develop the gluten and less flour may be necessary for a smooth, elastic dough. It is not suitable for flaky tender products such as pastries.

Flour–Cake and Pastry Cake and pastry flours are milled from soft wheat. They have lower protein and gluten content than other flours. These products have a fine uniform texture with pastry flour being the courser product of the two.

Pastry flour has less starch than cake flour and is used basically for pastries.

Cake and pastry flour are well suited to products which do not need strong structure. Cakes and pastries, as well as cookies, crackers, and snack foods are made from these flours. Both flours are available in enriched white and whole wheat. Whole wheat varieties of these flours will yield a heavier, more dense product than a comparable enriched white product.

Flour–durum-semonlina The best quality pasta is made from 100% durum wheat. Durum wheat is a high protein, hard wheat which contributes to the characteristics of good pasta. The endosperm of durum is called semolina. It is a granular, hard substance resembling sugar.

Macaroni and spaghetti are made from this. A byproduct of semolina milling is durum flour which is used to make noodles. Both semolina and durum flour are enriched with B-Vitamins and iron.

Semolina and durum flour are sold commercially in specialty food stores. The greatest share of the product is sold to pasta manufacturers.

Flour–Graham This is another term for whole wheat flour. Whole wheat flour is a course-textured flour ground from the entire wheat kernel (bran, germ, and endosperm).

Flour–Hard Wheat Different kinds of wheat flours are selected for those qualities specific to the food product. For example hard wheat flour from hard red winter and hard red spring wheat is usually higher in protein than other wheat flours. Hard wheat flour is more suitable for commercial bread production because it has the qualities to produce a lighter, more porous texture. This is the same reason that hard wheat flour is added to whole wheat and rye flours for bread.

Soft wheat flours, from soft red winter wheat and white winter wheat are sold for family use for biscuit or cake flours. In commercial production it is used for crackers, cakes, cookies, and pastries.

Consumers are seldom aware of the hardness or softness of flour. These are the characteristics of the two types hard wheat falls into separate particles if shaken in the hand while soft wheat flour clumps a bit and tends to hold its shape if pressed together. Hard wheat flour feels somewhat course and granular when rubbed between the fingers. Soft wheat flour feels smooth more like talcum powder.

Flour–Instantized Instantized flour is enriched white, all-purpose flour, which has been specifically ground and sieved. It has a granular texture and uniform particle size. This type of flour blends easily with water.

Flour–Semolina Semolina, the highest protein flour, is the most desirable for making shaped pasta. It is a coarsely ground product from durum wheat which is the hardest wheat variety. While cooking, pasta made from semolina retains its shape and firmness and does not become mushy or sticky.

Flour–Soft Wheat Different kinds of wheat flours are selected for those qualities specific to the food product. For example hard wheat flour from hard red winter and hard red spring wheat is usually higher in protein than other wheat flours. Hard wheat flour is more suitable for commercial bread production because it has the qualities to produce a lighter, more porous texture. This is the same reason that hard wheat flour is added to whole wheat and rye flours for bread.

Soft wheat flours, from soft red winter and white winter wheat are sold for consumer use for biscuit or cake flours. In commercial production it is used for crackers, cakes, cookies, and pastries.

Flour–Unbleached The nutritional value of bleached flour is the same as unbleached flour. Enriched flour of either type contributes carbohydrates, protein, and several other important nutrients. The term "bleaching" is traditional milling industry term that refers to the whitening of flour. Because freshly milled flour may not make consistently high-quality baked products, it is stored for several months for slow natural air oxidation to occur. Oxidation produces a whiter flour and results in products with a finer texture and improved baking quality. Food technologists devised chemical methods to quickly whiten flour and improve baking performance. No trace elements from the bleaching process remain in the final product.

Fluid bed dryer A bed of solid particles is supported on a cushion of hot air jets (fluidized) and the material may be conveyed this way, while being dried. The method achieves intimate mixing without mechanical damage; applied to cereals, tabletting granules, salt, coffee, and dried vegetables.

Flummery Old English pudding made by boiling down the water from soaked oatmeal until it becomes thick and gelatinous. Similar to frumenty. Dutch flummery is made with gelatine or isinglass and egg yolk; Spanish flummery with cream, rice flour, and cinnamon.

Fluoride Fluoride is a natural component of minerals in rocks and soils. Widespread use of fluoride in water supplies and oral health products is credited with the dramatic decline in dental caries among children and adults alike. All water contains fluoride, but it is sometimes necessary to add it to some public supplies to attain the optimal amount for dental health. Fluoride makes tooth enamel stronger and more resistant to decay. It also prevents the growth of harmful bacteria and interferes with converting fermentable carbohydrates to acids in the mouth.

FMN Flavin mononucleotide (chemically riboflavin phosphate), one of the coenzymes derived from vitamin B2.

FMNV Foods of Minimal Nutritional Value. FMNV is defined as: (i) In the case of artificially sweetened foods, a food which provides less than five percent of the Reference Daily Intakes (RDI) for each of eight specified nutrients per serving; and (ii) in the case of all other foods, a food which provides less than five percent of the RDI for each of eight specified nutrients per 100 calories and less than five percent of the RDI for each of the eight specified nutrients per serving. The eight nutrients to be assessed for this purpose are protein, vitamin A, vitamin C, niacin, riboflavin, thiamine, calcium and iron. The Code of Federal Regulations (CFR) Section 210.11 defines FMNV; Appendix B states foods of minimal nutritional value include: soda water, water ices, chewing gum and certain candies.

FNS Food and Nutrition Service. The agency within the USDA that has jurisdiction over federal nutrition and commodity distribution programs.

Foam-mat drying A method of drying food. The liquid concentrate is whipped to a foam with the aid of a foaming agent, spread on a tray and dried in a stream of warm air. It reconstitutes very rapidly with water because of the fine structure of the foam.

Focaccia An Italian olive-oil bread, quite flat and usually round or square. It has an almost cake-like texture and is often flavoured with herbs such as rosemary, sage or basil, perhaps olives or tapenade, and sometimes has a filling of ham or cheese. It's fun to experiment making your own with various toppings and fillings. It's become very popular in the past few years and you should be able to buy various types of focaccia, including a ready-to-bake version, which just needs finishing off in a pre-heated oven for a few minutes. Cut it into generous wedges to serve with olive oil and balsamic vinegar for dipping.

Foie gras Literally French for 'fat liver', this term refers to the rich pβtι made from the liver of ducks and geese that have been force-fed and fattened until their livers become enlarged. The south-west of France is the major foie gras producing area and the method of production isn't practised in Britain. After preparation, the livers are soaked overnight before being marinated in Armagnac, port or Madeira, depending on the chef's recipe.

Foie gras is sold fresh or cooked. For cooked foie gras, the livers are baked in a bain-marie and then chilled. It's a great French delicacy, and very expensive. Foie gras has a rich flavour and the texture is silky smooth. It's usually served in thin slices at the start of a meal with a sweet wine. It has become more widely available to buy in recent years - fresh or mi-cuit (partially preserved) and in cans.

As it's such a luxury it's best eaten simply, just spread on toasted brioche. Small slices can be fried and used to top meat or fish dishes. In recent years, concerns about animal welfare have turned many people, chefs and restaurant-goers alike, against the practice of force-feeding geese and ducks.

Foie gras The literal translation from the French for foie gras is "fat liver." It usually refers to goose liver, which is considered to be the best, but it can be liver from a duck or a goose. Foie gras is a dish made from the livers of fattened geese and ducks that have been force-fed on a special diet in a confined living space, until they are grossly fat and their liver have become enlarged and fatty. The liver is soaked overnight in liquid (water, milk, or port wine). Then the liquid is drained and marinated in Armagnac, Port or Madeira mixed with seasonings. The next step is to cook, usually by baking the livers. The exact preparation can vary by vender or cook. Traditionally it has been served chilled with thin, buttered toast slices and accompanied by sauternes, but now chefs are using foie gras in all kinds of interesting ways in their recipes.

Folacin Folacin acts as a coenzyme (with vitamin B-12 and vitamin C) in the breakdown (metabolism) of proteins and in the synthesis of new proteins. It is necessary for the production of red blood cells and the synthesis of DNA (which controls heredity), as well as tissue growth and cell function.

Folic acid Folic acid, folate, folacin, all form a group of compounds functionally involved in amino acid metabolism and nucleic acid synthesis. Good dietary sources of folate include leafy, dark green vegetables, legumes, citrus fruits and juices, peanuts, whole grains and fortified breakfast cereals. Recent studies show, if all women of childbearing age consumed sufficient folic acid (either through diet or supplements), 50 to 70 percent of birth defects of the brain and spinal cord could be prevented, according to the U.S. Centres for Disease Control and Prevention (CDC.) Folic acid is critical from conception through the first four to six weeks of pregnancy when the neural tube is formed. This means adequate diet or supplement use should begin before pregnancy occurs. Recent research findings also show low blood folate levels can be associated with elevated plasma homocysteine and increased risk of coronary heart disease.

Follow-on formula Follow-on formulas are specially formulated for older infants for use as the liquid part of the weaning diet for infants after the age of four or six months.

Fond The French word for stock - the flavoured liquid base used for making a sauce, stew or braised dish.

Fondant Fondant is a sweet itself and is also used as an icing or filling. It's made from sugar, water and cream of tartar or liquid glucose, which are boiled together until the syrup reaches what is called soft ball stage (when a spoonful of the sugar syrup is dropped into a bowl of cold water it will form a soft ball when rolled between the fingers).

The mixture is kneaded into a smooth dough and then colourings or flavours such as peppermint, lemon or coffee, can be added. It can be rolled into shapes to make sweets or used warm and poured into moulds then coated in melted chocolate. It's often used as an icing or coating for small fruits and is used to ice or decorate cakes.

Fondant can also refer to fondant potatoes - these are potatoes that are sliced and layered in a pan with butter, then sautied over a fairly high heat so they have a crisp outside and a meltingly soft centre.

Fondant Minute sugar crystals in a saturated sugar syrup; used as the creamy filling in chocolates and biscuits and for decorating cakes. Prepared by boiling sugar solution with the addition of glucose syrup or an inverting agent (see invert sugar) and cooling rapidly while stirring.

Fondue A glorious Swiss dish of melted cheese and wine served at the table in a large pot (also called a fondue) set over a burner to keep the cheese warm. Each person spears bite-size pieces of bread with a long-handled fork and dips it into the melted cheese. It's a dish associated with ski chalet cuisine - perfect for eating when you get back tired and weary from the slopes!

Classic dinner party fare during the 1950s and 1960s, it's now enjoying something of a revival. The classic cheeses to use are gruyθre and emmental flavoured with kirsch or white wine - the alcohol keeps the cheese below boiling point so it can be heated without going stringy. It's best to stir the fondue occasionally as you eat so the cheese and wine don't separate. Rubbing garlic around the pot adds a hint of flavour.

Other types of fondue include fondue bourguignon in which cubes of beef are dipped in hot oil at the table until cooked, and then eaten with dips and sauces; and chocolate fondue served with fresh fruit and biscuits for dipping. If you do a lot of entertaining it might be worth investing in a fondue set which includes the pot, stand, burner and forks.

Fontina A very popular semi-soft Italian cows'-milk cheese, fontina is deep golden yellow in colour with a reddish brown rind. It has a firm, slightly springy texture and melts easily, so is great to cook with. It has a delicate flavour and makes a good dessert cheese. When fully matured, it can be grated and used like Parmesan.

Fontina cheese One of the most delicious Italian cheeses. Made of cow's milk and the fat content is from 45% to 50%. Flavor is delicate, somewhat fruity. Frequently melted and excellent with pasta dishes, especially stuffing. When fully cured, it is hard, and used for grating. The process involved in the production of Fontina cheese dates back hundreds and hundreds of years, and it was first officially documented in 1480, when its characteristic form was recorded in a fresco in the castle at Issogne along with other typical products of the valley.

Food Any solid or liquid material consumed by a living organism to supply energy, build and replace tissue, or participate in such reactions. Defined by the FAO/WHO Codex Alimentarius Commission as a substance, whether processed, semi-processed, or raw, which is intended for human consumption and includes drink, chewing gum, and any substance that has been used in the manufacture, preparation, or treatment of food but does not include cosmetics, tobacco, or substances used only as drugs.

Food additive Substances added to food to alter its taste, texture, appearance, keeping qualities, or other properties. Additives have been employed since Roman times; some 3800 are now used, including flavourings (about 3500), colouring agents, emulsifiers, stabilizers, thickening agents, preservatives, antioxidants, flavour enhancers, artificial sweeteners, anticaking agents, and bleaching agents.

Food allergy An immune system response by which the body creates antibodies as a reaction to certain food. Studies show that true food allergies are present in only 1-2% of adults.

Food and Drug Administration (FDA) The Food and Drug Administration is part of the Public Health Service of the U.S. Department of Health and Human Services. It is the regulatory agency responsible for ensuring the safety and wholesomeness of all foods sold in interstate commerce except meat, poultry and eggs (which are under the jurisdiction of the U.S. Department of Agriculture). FDA develops standards for the composition, quality, nutrition, safety and labeling of foods including food and colour additives. It conducts research to improve detection and prevention of contamination. It collects and interprets data on nutrition, food additives and pesticide residues. The agency also inspects food plants, imported food products and feed mills that make feeds containing medications or nutritional supplements that are destined for human consumption. And it regulates radiation emitting products such as microwave ovens. FDA also enforces pesticide tolerances established by the Environmental Protection Agency for all domestically produced and imported foods, except for foods under USDA jurisdiction.

Food and nutritional security Add to the definition of food security the concept that, beyond access to consumption, the organism must possess adequate physiological conditions for the utilization of the food through good digestion, absorption and metabolism of nutrients.

Food and nutritional surveillanca Consists of the collection and analysis of information concerning the food nutritional situation of individuals and collectives, with the purpose of creating measures to prevent or correct existing or potential problems. An essential requisite for the rational justification of food and nutrition programs. See also growth and development, control of coexisting diseases and specific nutritional treatment.

Food bank A large, centralized site of food collection and distribution. Food collected by food banks is generally distributed to food pantries, soups kitchens, and other community organizations that provide food to those in need. Some food banks also provide food directly to those in need and offer additional services.

Food bank network An organization of food banks that coordinates the transfer of donated food and grocery products to where they are needed most. Often a food bank network will coordinate transfer of food to areas of need on a nationwide basis.

Food chain hazard Biological, chemical or physical agent, or food property, that can have adverse effects on health.

Food composition Nutritive value of foods or their content of specific substances such as vitamins, minerals and ohter elements.

Food composition tables Tables of the chemical composition, energy, and nutrient yield of foods, based on chemical analysis. Although the analyses are performed with great precision, they are, of necessity, only performed on a few samples of each type of food. There is, however, considerable variation, especially in the content of vitamins and minerals, between different samples of the same food. Therefore, calculation of energy and nutrient intakes based on use of food composition tables, even when intake has been weighed, can only be considered to be accurate to within about +10%, at best.

Food desert An area where food is non-existent, not healthy or too expensive. It is an issue of access and can be defined by distance and/or transportation being obstacles in obtaining adequate amounts of healthy food. Fresh food deserts refer to a community with limited or no access to fresh fruits and vegetables.

Food enrichment Addition of determined nutrients vitamins, minerals and others to foods with ralatively low contents of those nutritive elements.

Food frequency questionnaire A method of dietary assessment in which subjects are asked to recall how frequently certain foods were consumed during a specified period of time.

Food record A method of dietary assessment in which subjects records the foods that they consume.

Food guide pyramid The Food Guide Pyramid is a graphic design used to communicate the recommended daily food choices contained in the Dietary Guidelines for Americans. The information provided was developed and promoted by the U.S. Department of Agriculture and the U.S. Department of Health and Human Services.

Food insecurity Limited or uncertain access to nutritious, safe foods necessary to lead a healthy lifestyle; households that experience food insecurity have reduced quality or variety of meals and may have irregular food intake.

Food intolerance A general term for any adverse reaction to a food or food component that does not involve the body's immune system.

Food irradiation The exposure of food to sufficient radiant energy (gamma rays, x rays and electron beams) to destroy microorganisms and insects. Irradiation is used in food production and processing to promote food safety.

Food pantry A site where which food is distributed to low-income and unemployed households to relieve situations of emergency and distress. Food pantries are often located in community centres or faith-based organizations.

Food poisoning An acute illness arising from eating contaminated food. Vomiting and diarrhoea are the usual symptoms (see gastroenteritis). Salmonella is the bacterium that most commonly causes food poisoning (salmonellosis); patients usually recover within a few days. Similar food-borne infections are caused by Campylobacter (in poultry, beef, and milk) and Listeria. Another kind of food poisoning is due to toxins produced by such bacteria as Staphylococcus and Clostridium (which is responsible for botulism). Outbreaks of severe food poisoning occurred in Japan, the USA, and Scotland (1996) and NE England (1999) after consumption of food contaminated with toxin-producing E. coli 0157, a disease-causing strain of the normally harmless bacterium Escherichia coli: several of those affected died from kidney failure.

Food policy council A group, usually established by a legislative or executive directive, comprised of representatives from diverse food-related sectors that aims to provide advice, recommendations, and information regarding a community's food system. Food Policy Councils exist at the state, county, and local level. The exact powers and responsibilities of Food Policy Councils vary, however many are able to recommend policy or program changes. Many Food Policy Councils focus on ensuring community food security.

Food preservative The treatment of food to prevent its deterioration and to maintain its nutritional value. Breakdown of food tissues is caused by enzymes, either contained within the food or produced by microorganisms—bacteria, yeasts, and fungi—growing in the food. These organisms can also produce substances that can cause food poisoning. Oxidation and dehydration also contribute to spoilage. Food preservation therefore aims to alter the condition of food to stop the activities of microorganisms and any chemical change. One of the oldest methods is drying or dehydration—used for meat, vegetables, cereals, milk products, etc.

Food quality and safety In Sanitary Surveillance, concerns those attributes related to safety and nutritional value of food. See also healthy dietari practices.

Food Quality Protection Act (FQPA) A law (enacted in August 1996) which significantly amended the Federal Insecticide, Fungicide and Rodenticide Act (FIFRA) and the Federal Food, Drug and Cosmetic Act (FFDCA) and thus provided increased protection for infants and children from pesticide risk. The new safety standard resulting from FQPA is a "reasonable certainty of no harm" standard for aggregate exposure using dietary residues and all other reliable exposure information.

Food rescue The collection of perishable foods from wholesale and retail sources and the food industry. For example, collecting excess produce from supermarkets or prepared foods from hotels, caterers and restaurants.

Food safety Food safety is a relative and not absolute matter. Relative food safety can be defined as the practical, certainty that injury or damage will not result from food or ingredient used in reasonable and customary manner and quantity.

Food safety criteria Principles and standards to assure that foods have good nutritional value and present no physical, chemical and biological contaminants harmful to consumers.

Food safety objective A government-defined target considered necessary to protect the health of consumers (this may apply to raw materials, a process or finished products).

Food safety requirement A company-defined target considered necessary to comply with a food safety objective.

Food science The study of the basic chemical, physical, biochemical, and biophysical properties of foods and their constituents, and of changes that these may undergo during handling, preservation, processing, storage, distribution, and preparation for consumption. Hence, the term food scientist.

Food security Access by all people at all times to enough food for an active, healthy life. Food security includes at a minimum: 1) ready availability of nutritionally adequate and safe foods, and 2) an assured ability to acquire acceptable foods in socially acceptable ways.

Food stamp administration Administration of the Food Stamp Program is shared by the federal and state governments. The USDA monitors state administration of the program, and provides bonus awards to states with the lowest and most improved payment error rates, lowest and most improved negative error rates, highest and most improved participation indices, and highest rates of timeliness in case handling.

Food stamp employment and training program Federal funds made available to the states through the Food Stamp Program for the purpose of providing employment and training programs to food stamp households that would otherwise be ineligible for food stamp benefits.

Food stamp household A person or a group of people living together, but not necessarily related, who purchase and prepare food together.

Food stamp nutrition education (FSNE) This program, administered through FNS at the USDA, aims to improve the diet and nutrition-related skills of food stamp recipients and their families.

Food stamp program The largest nutrition program for low-income Americans that provides an allotted monthly benefit on electronic debit cards. Benefits can be redeemed at many grocery stores, some farmers markets and other retail sites, allowing low-income individuals to obtain food through normal channels of trade. The Food Stamp Program is a **USDA** program that provides an entitlement to states. Benefits are 100% federally funded. Administrative costs are shared between the federal and state governments. Food stamp benefits can only be used for food, and cannot be used to buy: any nonfood item (such as pet food, household supplies, grooming items, etc.); alcoholic beverages and tobacco; vitamins and medicines; any food that will be eaten in the store; and hot foods.

Food standard A set of criteria that a food must meet if it is to be suitable for human consumption, such as source, composition, appearance, freshness, permissible additives, and maximum bacterial content.

Food standards committee Permanent advisory body to the Ministry of Agriculture, Fisheries, and Food in the UK.

Food supplementation Additional quota of foods destined towards prevention or correction of nutritional deficiencies. See food support.

Food support Personal or institutional donations of one or more types of food for people suffering from, or at risk of, malnutrition. The same as food supplementation or, in some countries, food assistance.

Food system Refers to the agricultural production, food distribution, and consumption needs of a particular place (neighborhood, city, county, state or region). See also Community Food System.

Food technology The application of scientific knowledge to the preparation, preservation, and storage of food. Food technology can slow or halt the natural degradation processes of certain foodstuffs and thus make foods available out of season (See food preservation). The palatability or nutritional qualities of many raw food materials can be enhanced by selective processing. For example, cereals may be crushed by milling to produce flour, a process which removes or breaks down the indigestible outer husk of the cereal seeds. The flour can be made more palatable by making it into bread or pasta.

In recent years the market has seen new processing and packaging technologies, allowing an increase in production of, and demand for, 'convenience foods': ready-prepared or easily prepared meals, and foods with an increased shelf life. More recently, advances in technology have led to the extensive use of chemical preservatives, although growing consumer awareness has led the food industry to limit the use of such food additives.

Modern food processing technology has also allowed the production of 'new' foods. possible to produce very good meat analogues from mycoprotein (protein obtained from fungi) and vegetable proteins.

Foodborne disease Infectious or toxic disease caused by agents that enter the body through the consumption of food. The causative agents may be present in food as a result of infection of animals from which food is prepared or contamination at source or during manufacture, storage, and preparation.

There are three main categories: 1. diseases caused by micro-organisms (including parasites) that invade and multiply in the body;

2. diseases caused by toxins produced by micro-organisms growing in the gastro-intestinal tract;

3. diseases caused by the ingestion of food contaminated with poisonous chemicals or containing natural toxins or the toxins produced by micro-organisms in the food.

Forcemeat A highly seasoned stuffing made from chopped or minced veal, pork, or sausage meat mixed with onion and a range of herbs (French: farce, stuffing).

Formula diet Composed of simple substances that do not require digestion, are readily absorbed, and leave a minimum residue in the intestine: glucose, amino acids or peptides, mono- and diglycerides rather than starch, proteins, and fats.

Forslean ForsLean is manufatured by a proprietary process and is a standardized extract from the roots of the Coleus forskohlii plant, the only known plant source of forskolin.

ForsLean is a registered trademark of Sabinsa Corporation and is the only Coleus forskohlii preparation supported by US Patent # 5,804,596 defined as "a method of preparing a forskolin composition...and use of forskolin for promoting lean body mass and treating mood disorders".

Fortification The deliberate addition of specific nutrients to foods in order to increase their content, sometimes to a higher level than normal, as a means of providing the population with an increased level of intake. Generally synonymous with enrichment, supplementation, and restoration; in the USA enrichment is used to mean the addition to foods of nutrients that they do not normally contain, while fortification is the restoration of nutrients lost in processing. See also wine, fortified.

Fortified foods Fortified foods have nutrients added to them that were not present originally. For example, milk is fortified with vitamin D, which helps your body absorb calcium and phosphorus found naturally in milk.

Fortune cookie A tasty Chinese-American wafer cookie with a piece of paper inside with a "fortune" written on it. Fortune means "a prediction of destiny or fate." These cookies are usually used in Chinese-American restaurants after the meal is completed, and the cookie must be broken open to get the fortune. Fortune Cookies are not known in the Chinese food culture, and it wasn't until the 1990s that the fortune cookies actually arrived in China. They were advertised as "Genuine American Fortune Cookies."

Fractional test meal A method of examining the secretion of gastric juices; the stomach contents are sampled at intervals via a stomach tube after a test meal of gruel. It is usual to test for total and free acidity, and in addition peptic activity may be measured.

Fragile X syndrome A syndrome resulting from a fragile or broken site on the X chromosome, often characterized by mental retardation, hypotonia and hyperactivity

Fragrant rice An aromatic long-grain rice favoured in Thai and Vietnamese cooking. It's also known as jasmine rice and is quite similar to Indian basmati, but is slightly stickier. Serve it with Thai-style curries or spicy, saucy dishes. For something different try using it to make a sticky rice pudding.

Frangipane Also know as frangipani. A creamy pastry filling flavored with almonds that is usually baked in a sweet pastry crust with fruit or puff pastry pithiviers. The history of frangipane is traced to a 16th-century Italian nobleman named Marquis Muzio Frangipani, who introduced almond perfume-scented gloves that were all the rage. Pastry chefs tried to capture this popular scent in desserts; hence the birth of frangipane. Later, when the perfume was added to an almond cream dessert, the resulting delicacy was also dubbed frangipane. Today it is most often used to refer to an almond-flavored pastry cream.

Frankfort plane A line extending from the most inferior part of the orbital margin to the left tragion (the tragion is the deepest point in the notch superior to the tragus of the auricle); for length and height measurements, when the head is positioned correctly, the subject's line of sight is parallel to the headboard; also called Frankfort horizontal plane

Free from For a food label or advertising to bear a claim that it is free from fat, saturates, cholesterol, sodium, or alcohol it must contain no more than a specified (low) amount. The precise levels at which such claims are permitted differ from one country to another. In the USA the food so described must contain only a trivial or physiologically insignificant amount of the specified nutrient.

Free meal certification A classification within the child nutrition programs indicating that a child is able to receive meals and snacks at no cost to his or her family. Children from families with income at or below 130 percent of the federal poverty level qualify to receive free meals. In the 2005 2006 school year, a family of four with an annual income below $25,155 would qualify to receive free meals. Children can also be certified to receive free meals through categorical eligibility.

Free radical 1. A free radical is a molecule with an odd number of electrons. Free radicals do not have a completed octet and often undergo vigorous redox reactions. Free radicals produced within cells can react with membranes, enzymes, and genetic material, damaging or even killing the cell. Free radicals have been implicated in a number of degenerative conditions, from natural aging to Alzheimer's disease.

2. A highly reactive chemical species that normally exists for a relatively short time. Some free radicals are formed in the body during processes of oxidation and may be useful, e.g., in killing infectious organisms. Free radicals are also capable of doing extensive damage to tissues unless kept in check by antioxidants. The latter can be enzymes or chemicals, many of which are vitamins obtained from the diet (e.g., vitamins C and E).

Freeze concentration Concentration of a liquid by freezing out pure ice, leaving a more concentrated solution; it requires less input of energy, and causes less loss of flavour, than concentration by evaporation. Used especially in the concentration of fruit juices, vinegar, and beer.

Freeze drying Also known as lyophilization. A method of drying in which the material is frozen and subjected to high vacuum. The ice sublimes off as water vapour without melting. Materials dried in this way are damaged little, if at all.

Freeze-dried food is very porous, since it occupies the same volume as the original and so rehydrates rapidly. There is less loss of flavour and texture than with most other methods of drying. Controlled heat may be applied to the process without melting the frozen material; this is accelerated freeze drying.

Freezing The preservation of food by keeping it frozen. The basic principle in all food preservation is to arrest the development of the microorganisms responsible for the decay of the food. Home deep freezers achieve this by keeping food at a temperature of about -18°C (-0.4°F). On thawing, the deterioration process restarts. Most foods are well preserved by freezing, with little loss in nutritional value, but some with a high water content within the cells of the food, such as strawberries and cucumbers, become soggy after freezing as a result of damage to the cell structure by ice formation. Most vegetables are blanched (boiled for 2-4 minutes) before freezing to arrest the action of enzymes. It is the residual enzymic action that determines the recommended storage time.

French dressing Also known as vinaigrette (French for 'little vinegar') this is a fairly thick salad dressing made from a mixture of olive oil, wine vinegar (red, white or balsamic) and salt and pepper to which various flavourings can be added such as herbs, mustard, honey or chilli. The standard ratio is three parts oil to one part vinegar but it's best to experiment until you find a combination you like.

Drizzle it over raw or warm salads, or salad starters such as avocado halves or pan-fried asparagus. There are plenty of ready-made bottled versions to try, but it's very quick and easy to make - just put all the ingredients in a jar and shake well.

French fry/fries In English, "to french," means to cut into lengthwise pieces. French Fries are short for "frenched and fried potatoes." The English call them 'chips', a word which has a similar meaning (a chipped piece of wood). They are known as pommes de terre in French and fritures or frietkoets in Belgium. Belgians enjoyed their fries served in a paper cone with fries and a beer: The list of different names is as varied as the countries that enjoy them. The origin of the French fry has been the target of much animosity between the French and the Belgians. Some people think the French fry (pommes frites) originated in Belgian and then spread to France. Belgian historians claim to have proof that fries were invented in the region of the Meuse in 1680. The French claim they originated in Paris on the Pont Neuf in the mid 19th century. The French fry is part of most international cuisines, but different countries have different names for them.

President Thomas Jefferson (1801-1809), third President of the United States, is credited with introducing America to French fries in the late 1700s. He described them as "Potatoes, fried in the French Manner." He brought over the method of cooking potatoes from France and served them to his guests. It is thought that America's present day craving for French fries may be traced back to the soldiers stationed in Northern France and Belgium during World War I. The soldiers dubbed the hot and crispy fried snack "French Fries," after the French-speaking people who sold them. Today, one out of every three potatoes grown in the United is sliced into French fries. One-quarter of all meals served in American restaurants come with French fries, as they are the most profitable food item in the restaurant industry.

French toast North American breakfast dish; slices of bread dipped in beaten egg, fried, and served with cinnamon and sugar. Known in France as pain perdu ('bread lost' in egg).

Frenching Breaking up the fibres of meat by cutting, usually diagonally or in a criss-cross pattern.

Fresh For food labelling and advertising purposes, the US Food and Drug Administration has defined fresh to mean a food that is raw, has never been frozen or heated, and contains no preservatives. (Irradiation at low levels is permitted.) 'Fresh frozen' and 'frozen fresh' may be used for foods that are quickly frozen while still fresh, and blanching before freezing is permitted.

Fricassee A delicate creamy dish of chicken and vegetables, often served with rice. The chicken is cooked gently in butter, after which a creamy white sauce (usually made with double cream) is added. It's often garnished with small glazed onions and lightly cooked mushrooms. The term fricassie is often applied to anything cooked in a creamy white sauce - mushroom fricassie for example. The dish does have a 1970s feel to it, but is still found on menus of more traditional restaurants. It's a simple dish to cook at home, too.

Frittata An Italian omelette usually made quite thick with a variety of fillings, such potatoes, mushrooms, courgettes, ham, cheese, and so on. Unlike a French omelette, the ingredients are mixed with the eggs rather than being folded inside them. The frittata is cut into wedges and eaten hot or cold. It's similar to a Spanish omelette, or tortilla.

Fritter A fritter is any piece of raw or cooked meat, fish, fruit or vegetable coated in batter and deep-fried until crisp, golden and cooked through.

Fritter batter is usually made from flour, eggs, milk, salt, pepper and a little oil to help them go crisp. If it's a sweet batter for fruit then a little caster sugar is added and often the fritters are dredged in icing sugar before serving.

Frogs' legs The back and legs of the edible frog, Rana esculenta. A 100-g portion is a rich source of protein; a source of vitamins B 1, B 2, and iron; has a trace of fat; supplies 75 kcal (315 kJ).

Fromage blanc Also called fromage frais. In French it literally translates as "white cheese" and that's what it is. It is a simple cheese made with milk and a culture. The technique is identical to making yogurt. The texture of fromage blanc depends on how long, or if, you drain the cheese after the culture incubates in the milk. Some people know it as a runny cheese that has a texture similar to that of yogurt. In

France is sold next to yogurt in French grocery stores, and like yogurt, it is often flavored with fruit.

Fromage bleu Also called bleu cheese. It is the French name for a group of type-type (blue-veined) cheeses made in the Roquefort area in southeastern France. Roquefort-type cheese made in the U.S. is call "blue cheese."

Fromage frais A fresh, low-fat curd cheese (similar to cottage cheese but processed until the texture is smooth and lump-free) made from pasteurised cows' milk. Fromage frais has very little fat but there are ones that have cream added which make them better for cooking. It's delicious eaten on its own or with honey or fresh fruit purte. It can also be used in desserts or savoury dishes. Use it to make savoury sauces or as a topping for jacket potatoes.

Frosting 1 American name for icing on cakes; in the UK icing made from sugar and egg white (known as American icing).

2 A way of decorating the rim of a glass in which a cold drink is to be served; the edge is coated with whipped egg white, dipped into caster sugar, and allowed to dry.

3 For a margarita cocktail the edge of the glass is frosted by dipping it into lemon juice, then salt.

Fructo oliogosaccharides (FSO) A type of prebiotic/probiotic found in Jerusalem artichokes, shallots and onion powder which may improve gastrointestinal health.

Fructose Also known as fruit sugar or laevulose. A six-carbon monosaccharide sugar (hexose) differing from glucose in containing a ketone group (on carbon-2) instead of an aldehyde group (on carbon1). Found as the free sugar in fruits and honey, and as a constituent of the disaccharide sucrose (together with glucose). It is 1.7 times as sweet as sucrose. Commercially it is prepared by the hydrolysis of the polysaccharide inulin from the Jerusalem artichoke. See also invert sugar.

Fruit The fleshy seed-bearing part of plants (including tomato and cucumber, which are usually called vegetables). They contain negligible protein and fat, with carbohydrate varying from 3% in melon to 25% in banana, and supply varying amounts of vitamin C. Yellow-and orange-coloured fruits (e.g. apricot, peach, papaya) are sources of vitamin A (as carotene).

Fruitcakes They are holiday and wedding cakes, which have a very heavy fruit content. They require special handling and baking to obtain successful results.

Frumenty A 14th century porridge (grain pudding) made with grains of wheat, boiled up into a broth added to which were crushed almonds, milk and egg yolks. It was sometimes eaten with honey on Christmas morning but usually as sauce served with mutton or venison. This would often be more like soup and was eaten as a fasting dish in preparation for the Christmas festivities.

Frying Cooking foods with oil at temperatures well above the boiling point of water. Deep frying, in which a food is completely immersed in oil, reaches a temperature around 185 °C. Nutrient losses are less than in roasting, about 10-20% thiamin, 10-15% riboflavin and nicotinic acid from meat; about 20% thiamin from fish.

Fudge An American invention, it was created in the mid 1800s in the Eastern women's colleges of Vassar, and Wellesly. The first printed record of fudge came in 1896 with Opera Fudge (Bordeaux). Fudge became popular at Eastern women's colleges around the turn of The name may have come from when students "fudged" by making the confection when they were supposed to be in bed.

Fume blanc It is the word used in the United States for Sauvignon Blanc. Robert Mondavi as a marketing ploy invented it.

Fumet A strong-flavoured cooking liquor used for flavouring sauces; fumet usually refers to concentrated mushroom and fish stocks. The liquid left over from cooking is boiled down rapidly to a syrupy consistency, to be added to an accompanying sauce. For meat, poultry and game stocks, the word fond is normally used.

Functional abdominal pain Continuous, nearly continuous, or frequently recurrent pain localized in the abdomen but poorly related to gut function.

Functional bowel disorder A functional gastrointestinal disorder with symptoms attributable to the mid or lower gastrointestinal tract.

Functional component Those components in food that provide special health benefits. The abilities of these functional components may reduce cancer risk, aid digestion, decrease risk of tooth decay or improve various other body functions or reduce disease risk.

Functional constipation A group of functional disorders which present as persistent difficult, infrequent, or seemingly incomplete defecation.

Functional diarrhea Daily or frequently recurrent passage of loose (mushy) or watery stools without abdominal pain or intervening constipation.

Functional disorder A functional disorder refers to a "disorder of functioning" where the body's normal activities in terms of the movement of the intestines, the sensitivity of the nerves of the intestines, or the way in which the brain controls some of these functions is impaired. However, there are no structural abnormalities that can be seen by endoscopy, x-ray, or blood tests. Thus it is identified by the characteristics of the symptoms (e.g., Rome Criteria) and infrequently, when needed, limited tests.

Functional foods Foods that may provide health benefits beyond basic nutrition. Examples include tomatoes with lycopene, thought to help prevent the incidence of prostate and cervical cancers; fiber in wheat bran and sulphur compounds in garlic also believed to prevent cancer.

Fungi Subdivision of Thallophyta, plants without differentiation into root, stem, and leaf; they cannot photosynthesize, and all are parasites or saprophytes. Microfungi are moulds, as opposed to larger fungi, which are mushrooms and toadstools. Yeasts are sometimes classed with fungi.

Species of moulds such as Penicillium, Aspergillus, etc., are important causes of food spoilage in the presence of oxygen and relatively high humidity. Those that produce toxins (mycotoxins) are especially problematical. On the other hand species of Penicillium such as P. cambertii and P. roquefortii are desirable and essential in the ripening of certain cheeses.

A number of larger fungi (mushrooms) are cultivated, and other wild species are harvested for their delicate flavour. The mycelium of smaller fungi (including Graphium, Fusarium, and Rhizopus species) are grown commercially on waste carbohydrate as a rich source of protein for food manufacture.

Fungicide A chemical that is mixed with wax and applied to fruits or vegetables to prevent mold and rot from developing.

Fusion Cooking Fusion cooking is a style that incorporates ingredients and/or methods from at least two different ethnic/regional cooking styles. Originally combining western and Oriental culinary art but now includes all ethnic cuisines. Fusion cooking could be considered modern American cooking. Taste is as important as look. For a long time America was the melting pot of cultures. In the past 10 years, it's become the melting pot of cuisines as well. It's about breaking down cultural barriers, trying new things. Fusion is found in a lot of different places. From the finest restaurants, to the local fast food "Wraps."

G

Gaffelbitar 'Semi-preserved' herring in which microbial growth is checked by the addition of salt at a concentration of 10-12%, and sometimes by the addition of benzoic acid as a preservative.

Gag reflex A normal reflex triggered by touching the soft palate or back of the throat that raises the palate, retracts the tongue and contracts the throat muscles; protects the airways from a bolus of food or liquid

Galactose A monosaccharide occurring in both levo (L) and dextro (D) forms as a constituent of plant and animal oligosaccharides (lactose and raffinose) and polysaccharides (agar and pectin). Galactose is the sugar derived from digesting lactose ('milk sugar").

Galangal Galangal is a member of the ginger family. It's widely used in South-east Asian cuisine, particularly Thai cookery; it's an important ingredient in Thai curry pastes. It can be bought as fresh root, dried root or a dried, ground powder. The root looks a bit like a knobbly Jerusalem artichoke. Use the fresh root as you would ginger, peeling and either grating or chopping it finely. It stores well wrapped in cling film in the larder or fridge for about a week. Galangal is also widely used medicinally as an aid to digestion and for respiratory problems.

Galia melon They resemble a small cantaloupe and have a light golden-yellow skin when ripe. Their flesh is lime green and tastes similar to a sweet honeydew melon.

Gallbladder disease There are several different forms of gallbladder disease 1) Gallstones without symptoms. About 20% of women and 8% of men will develop gallstones. In most of these cases, gallstones do not produce symptoms and thus usually do not require treatment. 2) Biliary colic. This condition occurs when a gallstone intermittently blocks the duct that drains the gallbladder (cystic duct). Biliary colic usually causes severe, steady pain that lasts from 15 to 60 minutes to up to 6 hours. 3) Inflammation of the gallbladder (acute cholecystitis). This condition occurs when a gallstone becomes stuck in the cystic duct, causing severe abdominal pain that lasts longer then 6 hours. It is the most common complication of gallstone disease. 4) Chronic cholecystitis. This condition develops when there is long term (chronic) inflammation of the gallbladder. The wall of the gallbladder may be thickened and rigid. 5) Common bile duct stones (choledocholithiasis). This condition occurs when a gallstone passes through the cystic duct into the common bile duct. About 8 to 15% of people who have gallstones also have common bile duct stones. Most people who have common bile duct stones do not have symptoms. However, people who do have symptoms may develop life threatening complications, such as infection and inflammation of the bile duct or pancreas.

Galliano Italian; liqueur flavoured with herbs, roots, berries, and flowers; the basis of the Harvey Wallbanger cocktail.

Gallon A unit of volume. The imperial gallon is 4.546 litres, and the US gallon is 3.7853 litres; therefore 1 imperial gallon = 1.2 US gallons.

Ganache Ganache is a rich chocolate mixture made by combining chopped semisweet chocolate and boiling cream and then stirring until smooth. The proportions of chocolate to cream can vary, and the resulting ganache can be used as a cake glaze or beaten until fluffy and used as a filling or as the base for truffles and other chocolate confections.

Ganglion Usually, a group of nerve cell bodies lying outside of the central nervous system (CNS); also used for one group of nerve cell bodies within the CNS — the basal ganglia.

Garam masala An aromatic mixture of ground spices used as a base for many Indian dishes ('masala' means spice). The proportion of spices changes according to the dish being cooked but the basic ingredients are cumin, coriander, cardamom, black pepper and cinnamon. The mixture can include other spices (such as caraway, nutmeg or bay leaves), depending on whether the dish includes meat, vegetables or fish. It's usually added towards the end of cooking.

Garlic Garlic is a member of leek and onion family. There are many varieties, differing in size, pungency and colour. The bulb or 'head' of garlic is formed of 12 to 16 bulblets, called cloves. The most widely used European variety has a white/grey skin and is grown in southern France. Garlic grows in warm climates around the world, including the UK - the Isle of Wight holds a garlic festival every year where the brave can try garlic ice cream. Green, or fresh, garlic is usually only available from June to August in the UK; the type that's more commonly sold in the UK is dried garlic (fresh garlic just dried in the sun).

Smoked garlic is dried garlic that has been smoked to give it a golden colour and mellow smoky flavour. You can also buy garlic purie and garlic salt or garlic granules for convenience.

Garlic has many culinary uses. The cloves are separated, peeled and then used whole, chopped or crushed. The more finely the garlic is crushed the stronger it will taste in the dish, but slow oven-baking tends to mellow the flavour - hence the famous chicken with 40 cloves of garlic dish isn't as terrifying as it sounds! Raw garlic is essential in pesto sauce and aioli - garlic mayonnaise. Slivers of garlic can be inserted into lamb before roasting or the purie from roasted garlic can be squeezed from the cloves and stirred into mashed potato with some olive oil. For real garlic lovers, the head can be roasted whole and served as a vegetable.

The easiest way to crush garlic is to place a clove on a board and, using the flat side of a small knife, press down firmly until you have squashed it to a pulp. Sprinkle a little salt on the clove to help the knife grip and make a creamy paste. Using a pestle and mortar, again with a sprinkling of salt, is also a good way. Garlic crushers are fine, but some say that crushing the garlic this way gives it a bitter taste. If the garlic is old, be sure to remove the bitter 'germ' in the centre of the clove.

Garnish A decorative edible accompaniment that is added to a finished dish entirely for eye appeal, such as a sprig of mint or parsley. A garnish may be eaten but that is not its purpose.

Garniture French word for garnish. A garniture becomes part of the dish and is eaten with it.

Gastric emptying The action of the stomach contents emptying into the small intestine. Most energy drinks and supplements are absorbed into the body via the intestine. The carbohydrate content of energy drinks affects their gastric emptying rate. Recommended carbohydrate content is 7% (one scoop of Cytomax in a 16-

ounce bottle = 7%), which allows a gastric emptying rate nearly equal to that of waterHs.

Gastric juices Liquids produced in the stomach to help break down food and kill bacteria.

Gastrin Polypeptide hormone secreted by the stomach in response to foods (especially meat) which stimulate gastric and pancreatic secretion.

Gastro-enteritis Inflammation of the mucosal lining of the stomach and/or small or large intestine, normally resulting from infection. See also gastro-intestinal tract.

Gastroenterologist A doctor who specializes in digestive diseases or disorders.

Gastroenterology The field of medicine concerned with the function and disorders of the digestive system.

Gastroesophageal reflux (GER) Regurgitation of the contents of the stomach into the esophagus, where they can be aspirated; often results from a failure of the esophageal sphincter to close; commonly leads to feeding problems in infants and children with neuromuscular disorders; also gastroesophageal reflux disease (GERD)

Gastrointestinal tract The organ along which food travels from the mouth until the undigested remnants emerge as stools. Mixing and some digestion occur in the stomach where the environment is acidic; most digestion and absorption of nutrients occurs in the small intestine; the large intestine, principally the colon, contains very large numbers of micro-organisms capable of fermenting food components that have escaped digestion in the small intestine.GelA complex solid and liquid food system, interconnected to give a network of intermingled particles.

Gastronomy The study and appreciation of good food and good eating, and a culture's culinary customs, style and lore. Any interest or study of culinary pursuits as relates essentially to the kitchen and cookery, and to the higher levels of education, training and achievement of the chef apprentice or professional chef.

Gazpacho A cold uncooked summer tomato soup (a liquid salad). Usually contains tomatoes, bell peppers, onions, celery, cucumbers, and bread moistened with water. Gazpacho should be drunk slightly chilled, but not iced. As its purpose is to quench thirst as well as nutritious, there should no need to supplement it with a drink. The southern Spanish region of Andalusia is known for this dish. A Spanish refrain says, "De gazpacho no hay empacho" which means there's never too much gazpacho. It hits the spot any time of the day or night. In Andalusia, you will probably eat these cold soups as a first course, just as they have been served for about thirty years in the restaurants and private homes of the large cities in Andalusia. It is still customary in village homes to have gazpacho after the first course and before dessert.

Originally a soup from Andalusia in southern Spain. It probably derives from Roman dish gruel of bread and oil. The name gazpacho may come either from the Latin or Mozarab (Hispano-Romans or "would-be Arab") word "caspa," meaning "fragments, residue, or little pieces," referring to the bread crumbs which are such an essential ingredient. None of the forerunners of gazpacho contained tomatoes, considered basic today. That's because tomatoes were unknown in Spain, until after the discovery of the New World. The base for gazpacho was originally bread, garlic, oil, vinegar, and salt. The Roman legions carrying bread, garlic, salt, olive oil and vinegar along the roads of the Empire, with each soldier making his own mixture to taste. An ancient ritual whereby they approach after each other and then "step back" at the moment of eating. The Moorish influence is evident too, especially in some of the variations on the basic theme, such as ajo blanco, made with ground almonds. Gazpacho was originally poor people's food and was eaten in the fields.

According to historians, the popularity of gazpacho out of Andalusia into the rest of Spain is said to be the result of Eugenia de Montijo, originally from Granada and the wife of the French Emperor Napoleon III in the 1850s. Gazpacho was unknown, or little known, in the north of Spain before about 1930.

Gelatin The word gelatin comes to us from the French word geatine meaning "edible jelly" and gelato meaning" to freeze." In Italian, it's gelatina. An odorless, colourless, tasteless thickening agent is the nutritious glutinous protein material obtained from animal tissues by boiling. Most comes from beef bones, cartilage, tendons, and pigskin.

Gelatine A product derived from the bones of animals, and used as a setting agent for sweet or savoury jellies and pudding fillings. Gelatine comes in powder form or in leaves and is tasteless. Powdered gelatine is sprinkled over cold water and left to soak and swell before being stirred into hot liquid to dissolve.

Leaf gelatine is soaked in a little cold liquid for a few minutes to soften it, then the excess liquid is squeezed out before adding hot liquid to dissolve it. Agar-agar is the vegetarian alternative.

Gelato An Italian word meaning "frozen" and is the same as ice cream in the U.S. It is usually made of whole milk and eggs. This gives it richness without flavors becoming masked by the fat from cream. According to historians, gelato has very ancient origins. It is believed that the Arabs brought what came to be known as sorbetto to Sicily; but gelato is said to have been first created by Bernardo Buontalenti for the court of Francesco de' Medici in 1565. The Greeks and the Turks were also known for preparing lemon-based mixtures that resembled sorbetto (sherbets). Sherbets were thought to have a beneficial effect on the nervous and digestive systems, and were usually served between main courses, more precisely after the first few meat and fish dishes, at the sumptuous banquets of the 18th and 19th century. It was only later that richer ingredients such as egg yolks, sugar, milk, and cream began to be used; to make what is now known as gelati alla crema (ice cream). Gelato is classified according to the ingredients used in making them.

Gene A gene is the unit of heredity in living organisms. Genes are encoded in an organism's genome, composed of DNA or RNA, and direct the physical development and behaviour of the organism. Most genes encode proteins, which are biological macromolecules comprising linear chains of amino acids that effect most of the chemical reactions carried out by the cell. Some genes do not encode proteins, but produce non-coding RNA molecules that play key roles in protein biosynthesis and gene regulation. Molecules that result from gene expression, whether RNA or protein, are collectively known as gene products.

Gene expression The process by which the instructions in genes are converted to messenger RNA, which directs protein synthesis.

General Tso's Chicken Fried boneless dark-meat chicken, served with vegetables and whole dried red peppers in a sweet-spicy sauce. It's not authentically Chinese, but it's nevertheless one of the most popular dishes at Chinese restaurants. Alternate spellings include General Cho, General Zo, General Zhou, General Jo, and General Tzo. It is pronounced "Djo," with the tongue hard against teeth. This dish is thought to have been the invention of Taiwanese immigrants to the United States in the 1970s and was named after General Zou Zong-Tang (1812-1885), a general of the Qing (Manchu) Dynasty of China. He was responsible for suppressing Muslim uprisings. His name was used to frighten Muslim children for centuries after his death.

Generalizability The extent to which the results of a study are able to be applied to the general population of people that is comparable to the population studied. The selective, deliberate alteration of genes (genetic material) by man. This term has a very broad meaning including the manipulation and alteration of the genetic material of an organism in such a way as to allow it to produce endogenous proteins with properties different from those of the normal, or to produce entirely different (foreign) proteins altogether. Other words applicable to the same process are gene splicing, gene manipulation, or recombinant DNA technology.

Genetic engineering Genetic engineering, genetic modification (GM) and gene splicing are terms for the process of manipulating genes, usually outside the organism's normal reproductive process.It involves the isolation, manipulation and reintroduction of DNA into cells or model organisms, usually to express a protein. The aim is to introduce new characteristics or attributes physiologically or physically, such as making a crop resistant to a herbicide, introducing a novel trait, or producing a new protein or enzyme. Examples can include the production of human insulin through the use of modified bacteria, the production of erythropoietin in Chinese Hamster Ovary cells, and the production of new types of experimental mice such as the OncoMouse (cancer mouse) for research, through genetic redesign.

Genetic Genetic may refer to:Genetics, in biology, the science of genes, heredity, and the variation of organismsGenetic (linguistics), in linguistics, a relationship between two languages with a common ancestor languageGenetic algorithm, in computer science, a kind of search technique modeled on evolutionary biology.

Genetic stability A measure of the resistance to change, with time, of the sequence of genes within a DNA molecule or of the nucleic acid sequence within a gene.

Glucose Tolerance Test 1. A test to see if a person has diabetes. The test is given in a lab or doctor's office in the morning before the person has eaten. A first sample of blood is taken from the person. Then the person drinks a liquid that has glucose (sugar) in it. After one hour, a second bloodsample is drawn, and, after another hour, a third sample is taken. The object is to see how well the body deals with the glucose in the blood over time.

2. A test of the body's ability to metabolise carbohydrate by administering a standard dose of glucose under controlled conditions and measuring the blood and urine for sugar at regular intervals thereafter. The glucose tolerance test is usually used to assist in the diagnosis of diabetes or other disorders that affect carbohydrate metabolism.

Genoise An almond powder based sponge. It is usually about a 1/4-inch and wrapped around a cake.

Genome The total hereditary material of a cell, containing the entire chromosomal set found in each nucleus of a given species.

GER Also called acid reflux, a condition where the contents of the stomach regurgitates (or backs up) into the esophagus (food pipe), causing discomfort.

GERD (Gastroesophageal reflux disease) A condition characterized by symptoms and/or tissue damage that results from repeated or prolonged exposure of the lining of the esophagus to acidic contents from the stomach.

German chocolate cake German Chocolate Cake is an American creation that contains the key ingredients of sweet baking chocolate, coconut, and pecans..

Gestational diabetes A type of diabetes mellitus that can occur when a woman is pregnant. In the second half of her pregnancy, a woman may have glucose (sugar) in her blood at a higher than normal level. In about 95 percent of cases, blood sugar returns to normal after the pregnancy is over. Women who develop gestational diabetes, however, are at risk for developing type 2 diabetes later in life.

Ghee Ghee is clarified butter with all of the water and solids removed. Ghee will not scorch or burn and can be cooked at higher temperatures than any oil. It allows cooking with butter at a higher temperature before it will burn. It removes the milk solids from the butter and will last in the fridge for a long time! Ghee can be used in place of butter (it has a nutty more intense flavor). It can also be used for stir-frying as the ghee making process removes the protein solids permitting it to be used in high temperature cooking. It does not require refrigeration if you keep moisture out of it; for example, don't dip a wet spoon into the ghee jar. Ghee is used extensively in good Indian Cuisine. Ghee comes from ancient India; I believe the first reference to ghee comes from the Ayurveda text, which dates back a couple thousand years.

Giardiniera In Italian, the word means "garden style." Italian mixed pickled vegetable assortment or condiment that usually includes cauliflower, carrot, sometimes celery or fennel, and hot or sweet peppers. Generally used as a condiment on sandwiches or antipasto plates.

Giberellins Plant growth substances derived from giberellic acid, originally found in the fungus Gibberella fujikori growing on rice. About thirty giberellins are known; they cause stem extension and allow mutant dwarf forms of plants to revert to normal size, induce flower formation, and break bud dormancy. They are used to accelerate the germination of barley for malting.

Ginger A spice that comes from the rhizome (a thick underground stem) of the Zingiber officinale plant. Ginger can be used fresh (often called root ginger or ginger root) or dried and ground to a powder. Ginger adds a touch of heat to both sweet and savoury dishes and is used in cuisines throughout Asia and Europe.

In South-east Asia and the Indian subcontinent, fresh ginger is frequently added to curry pastes and it's often cooked with fish dishes in China. In Europe, dried ginger is more frequently used in baking, as in the classic parkin of northern England. It can also be used in drinks, as in ginger 'tea' and ginger beer, and can be preserved in sweet syrup (known as stem ginger).

Ground ginger should be replaced frequently because, like other dried spices, it quickly loses its pungency when ground. When buying fresh ginger, look for plump rhizomes that are not wrinkled and store in the fridge.

Ginger, ginger root At one time ginger was as common as salt and pepper and was frequently placed on the table. Hawaii, Fiji, and Costa Rica grow most of the world's ginger supply, which is available throughout the year. In January and February look for its pale, golden flesh; in summer and early fall look for young, baby ginger. In late fall or early winter, the harvest can come from as far away as Fiji. Ginger is thought of as a "hand" and the "fingers" are snapped off. It should feel heavy for its size. There are many types of ginger available today, including fresh and dried. As a general rule, fresh and dried ginger should not be substituted for one another in recipes, as their flavor is very different. Ginger is also available in syrup, crystallized, candied, preserved and pickled (as served with sushi).

The Chinese and Indians first cultivated it. It was one of the important spices that led to the opening of the spice trade routes. The name Ginger comes from the Sanskrit word "sinabera" meaning "shaped like a horn" because of its resemblance to an antler. In the 19th century it was popular to keep a shaker of Ginger on the counter in English pubs so the patrons could shake some into their drinks. This practice was the origin of ginger ale.

Glace de viande It is a meat glaze by French definition, but it is actually a very high end bouillon cube made by reducing unsalted meat stock. The stock is boiled down to about 20% of its original volume or until it is thick, viscous, and syrupy. It is so concentrated a little bit goes a long way.

Glace French word meaning: 1. ice or ice cream;

2. Icing or frosting used on a cake;

3. A cut of mean that has been glazed in a hot oven by constantly basting the meat with its own juices.

Glaze To alter the surface of a product for taste or eye appeal by adding a glossy coat. Glazing can be done by basting the food with a syrupy liquid while it is cooking or by putting a sauce on it and placing briefly under the broiler. To glaze a cold food, you can cover it with a shiny coat of aspic or gelatin.

2. Also coating pastries and cakes with an icing.

Gleaning The collection of crops from farmers' fields that have already been mechanically harvested or on fields where it is not economically profitable to harvest.

Glial cell A type of cell that surrounds nerve cells and holds them in place. Glial cells also insulate nerve cells from each other.

Globe artichoke The globe artichoke is related to the thistle. Its leaves are eaten, along with the bottom part of the flower, called the heart (which you can also buy tinned). It makes a delicious starter simply boiled whole and served with melted butter, mayonnaise, hollandaise or vinaigrette for dipping the leaves into. Break off each leaf and draw the soft fleshy base through your teeth.

Once you've removed all the leaves you can pull or slice off the hairy 'choke' and eat the heart and the meaty bottom with the remaining sauce. See also artichoke for information about Jerusalem and Chinese artichokes.

Globus A sensation of something stuck or of a lump or tightness in the throat.

Glucagon A hormone secreted by the a-cells of the pancreas which causes an increase in blood sugar by increasing the breakdown of liver glycogen and stimulating the synthesis of glucose from amino acids.

Glucans Soluble but undigested complex made of glucose units; found particularly in oats, barley, and rye. See also fibre, soluble; non-starch polysaccharides.

Glucosamine sulphate Glucosamine Sulphate is a compound which is helpful in maintaining joint health in degenerative conditions such as arthritis. It is an effective means of providing glucosamine orally, as a building block for the regeneration of cartilage glycosaminoglycans, lost during the progression of osteoarthritis. It is often used in the management of osteoarthritis and rheumatoid arthritis. When given orally, it is selectively taken up by joint tissues to exert beneficial effects. Glucosamine is clinically proven to retard the progression of degenerative changes in the joints.

Glucose A sugar, most commonly in the form of dextroglucose, that occurs naturally, has about half the sweetening power of regular sugar and does not crystallize easily. Glucose comes from grape juice, honey and certain vegetables, among other things.

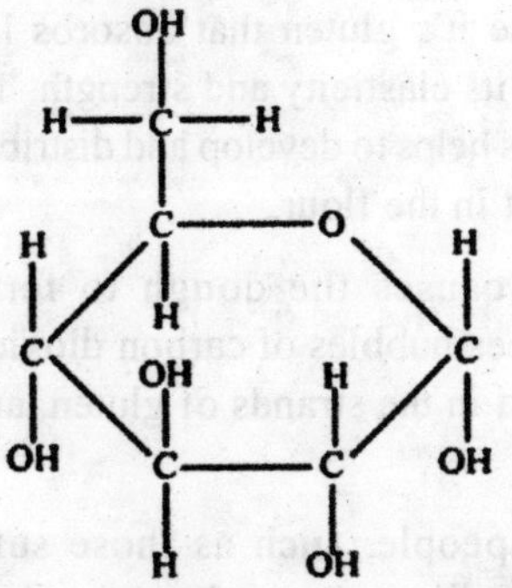

Fig. Structural formula for Glucose

Glucose oxidase Enzyme that oxidizes glucose to gluconic acid, with the formation of hydrogen peroxide. Used for specific quantitative determination of glucose, including urinary glucose excreted in diabetes, and also to remove traces of glucose from foodstuffs (e.g. from dried egg to prevent the Maillard reaction during storage). Originally isolated from the mould Penicillium notatum and called notatin.

Glutamate Glutamate is an amino acid. It is necessary for metabolism and brain function, and is manufactured by the body. Glutamate is found in virtually every protein food we eat. In food, there is "bound" glutamate and "free" glutamate. Glutamate serves to enhance flavors in foods when it is in its free form and not bound to other amino acids in protein. Some foods have greater quantities of glutamate than others. Foods that are rich in glutamate include tomatoes, mushrooms, parmesan cheese, milk and mackerel.

Glutathione 1. A substance found in plant and animal tissues that has many functions in a cell. These include activating certain enzymes and destroying toxic compounds and chemicals that contain oxygen.

2. A small-molecular-weight antioxidant molecule produced naturally in the human body and present in some foods.

Gluten Gluten is a mixture of two proteins present in cereal grains, in particular wheat. It's a key factor in the success in all kinds of baking because it's gluten that absorbs liquid, giving dough its elasticity and strength. The kneading process helps to develop and distribute the gluten present in the flour.

Yeast causes the dough to ferment which produces bubbles of carbon dioxide. These get trapped in the strands of gluten, and the dough rises.

Some people, such as those suffering from coeliac disease, are gluten-intolerant, so they can't eat standard wheat-flour breads. There are gluten-free baked goods available and it's possible to make gluten-free breads and baked goods at home substituting, for example, rice flour for wheat flour.

Wheat gluten is of particular interest to vegans and vegetarians because it's the source of a product called seitan. To make seitan, the gluten is extracted from wheat and then processed to resemble meat. It's more similar to meat in texture than either textured vegetable protein or mycoprotein and is used as a meat substitute in a range of foods.

Gluthathione peroxidases A family of antioxidant molecule produced naturally in the human body and present in some foods.

Glutose A six-carbon sugar (hexose) with a keto group on carbon-3; it is not metabolized and non-fermentable.

Glycaemic index A method for assessing the comparative effects of different carbohydrates on the pattern of changes in the concentration of glucose in the blood following a meal. A dose of 50 g of glucose is assigned a glycaemic index of 100, given by integrating the area under the curve when blood glucose concentration is plotted against time.

Glycerin A syrupy type of alcohol derived from sugar which is used in food flavorings to maintain desired food consistency.

Glycerol A colourless, odorless, syrupy liquid—chemically, an alcohol—that is obtained from fats and oils and used to retain moisture and add sweetness to foods.

Glycogen Glycogen is a polysaccharide that is the principal storage form of glucose (Glc) in animal and human cells. Glycogen is found in the form of granules in the cytosol in many cell types. Hepatocytes (liver cells) have the highest concentration of it - up to 8% of the fresh weight in well fed state, or 100–120 g in an adult. In the muscles, glycogen is found in a much lower concentration (1% of the muscle mass), but the total amount exceeds that in liver. Small amounts of glycogen are found in the kidneys, and even smaller amounts in certain glial cells in the brain and white blood cells. Glycogen plays an important role in the glucose cycle.

Gnocchi A sort of pasta for potato lovers - these are small Italian dumplings usually made from potato, flour (traditionally buckwheat flour) and egg and shaped into small ovals with a ridged pattern on one side. They can also be made from semolina, as Roman cooks do. Gnocchi are often poached and then cooked au gratin (with breadcrumbs and grated cheese) in the oven and served as a hot starter. They are easy to make fresh, but are also widely available in vacuum packs. Serve them in a similar way to pasta with a cheese or tomato-based sauce and freshly grated Parmesan. They can also be added to soups, stews and casseroles.

Goiter Significant enlagement of the thyroid gland, beyond normal limits.

Good Manufacturing Practices (GMP) The Food and Drug Administration's (FDA's) approval mechanism for a process to manufacture a given food or food additive. It is implemented instead of specific regulations (such as those used to dictate processes in simple food manufacturing, as in beef packing), due to the newness of the technology and may later be superceded (due to further advances in the technology).

Gooseberry A small green, grape-sized fruit that is still slightly tart even when ripe. Makes wonderful jams and jellies. The New Zealand gooseberry or Cape gooseberry is a small tart fruit that is enclosed in papery husks.

Gorgonzola An Italian blue cheese made from pasteurised cows' milk. It's pale yellow streaked with greenish-blue veins. It has a distinct smell and can be mild, strong or sharp in flavour depending on its maturity. Gorgonzola is rich and creamy, generally used uncooked. It's often eaten as a dessert cheese but is also good in salads and dips.

Gorgonzola cheese The most popular of the Italian blue cheeses. Made of cow's milk, fat content 45%, and is very soft and tender. Gorgonzola, which has an intricate, complicated method of creation, dates back to the eleventh century. The thick veins are created from the addition of penicillin glaucum, a mold, which is primarily grown in laboratories today. Originally, Gorgonzola was aged in caves, but now it is mass-produced by creating controlled environments. Named after a village in Italy. It is similar to the American blue cheese and the French type. Gorgonzola was made in the Po Valley in Italy in 879 A.D. and Italy became the cheese-making centre of Europe in the 10th Century. According to folk legends dating back to the 10th century: 1. Gorgonzola was invented by an absent-minded dairyman, which let a curd bundle drip all night long. The day after he tried to make up for his mistake by mixing it with the morning curd.

2. Its inception was the result of the herds of cattle that were moved through the village on their way down from the northern Alps. By the time the poor beasts reached the town, they needed badly to be milked. Much of this of milk was then given or traded to local inhabitants. Quite often, curdled milk from the morning milking was mixed with the then cooled milk from the evening.

Gouda cheese Gouda was first made in the vicinity of Gouda, in the Province of South Holland, Netherlands. It can range from semi-soft to firm with a smooth texture. It is made from whole or partly skimmed cow's milk. It is usually shaped like a flattened sphere and it usually has a wax coating (a more mature Gouda has a yellow wax coating and black wax or a brown rind suggests it has been smoked and aged for over a year). Gouda melts quickly when it is shredded and heated.

Goujon Small thin chunky strip of fried food. Originally term was used for fish, but now term is also used for chicken. Chicken cut this way is known as goujon style.

Gourmand A French word for a person who appreciates fine food. Considered to be a step about a gourmet. It is said that basically the word means a "glutton."

Gourmet 1. A gourmet is a person of impeccable taste. A gourmet is not only concerned with the quality of the food and wine he serves, but also with the way the food he chooses harmonizes with each other.

2. Food of the highest quality that is perfectly prepared and presented.

Gout Painful disease caused by accumulation of crystals of uric acid in the synovial fluid of joints; may be due to excessive synthesis and metabolism of purines, which are metabolized to uric acid, or to impaired excretion of uric acid.

Traditionally associated with a rich diet, although there is little evidence for dietary factors in causing the condition. May be exacerbated by alcohol.

Graham crackers Graham crackers are sweetened wheat "biscuits" or "crackers" eaten in the United States. They are flat; about 3 inches square and appear dark golden brown. They are (frequently sweetened with honey). Despite the name, most brands of "graham cracker" today use refined white flour Graham crackers were invented in 1829 by American Presbyterian minister named Sylvester Graham (1795-1851). He was a vegetarian and promoted and preached on temperance and stressed whole-wheat flour and vegetarian diets. He promoted the use of a type of coarsely ground wheat flour, which was high in fiber. The flour became known as "Graham Flour" and the crackers known as "Graham Crackers". Graham thought intense physical desire, regardless of whether you were married or not, would have dire physiological consequences on people. He thought men should remain virgins until age 30 and then should make love only once a month—not at all if they were sickly. To control lust, Graham prescribed a special vegetarian diet, the centerpiece of which was "Graham bread," made from whole-wheat flour. Graham crackers, which Graham invented in 1829, were another manifestation of the same idea.

Grains Grains are the seeds or fruits of various food plants including cereal grasses. The examples of wheat, corn, oats, barley, rye and rice provide a partial list. Grain foods include foods such as bread, cereals, rice and pasta.

Gram A unit of weight in the metric system. There are 28 grams in 1 ounce or 454 grams in 1 pound.

Gram flour A flour made from ground chickpeas. It's pale yellow and powdery and has an earthy flavour best suited to savoury dishes. Gram flour contains no gluten and is widely used in Indian cookery.

Grana Grana is a class of hard grating cheeses from Italy, which were developed in the 13th Century in the Po Valley. One-quarter of Italian milk production goes to making Grana cheese. Most are aged for up to four years, yet they have a smooth texture and "melt in your mouth."

Granadilla An exotic fruit belonging to the passion fruit family, granadillas are twice the size of passion fruit with a smooth, brittle, orange shell and a mild, sweet pulp inside made of a mass of flesh-covered green seeds. Only the seeds are eaten, not the shell. They're available all year round and the refreshing tangy flesh is good eaten straight from the shell, scooped out with a spoon (it tastes a little blander than passion fruit), or used to flavour ice cream, yoghurt, jellies or mousses.

Granita It is an Italian ice. A coarse fruit ice similar to sorbet, without the meringue, which is often flavored with liqueurs. Unlike ice creams or sherbets, granita must be frozen into a pan of plastic or stainless steel with the syrup not higher than 1-1/2" up the sides. It should be stirred from time to time to allow the sides and the top to freeze. Churn before serving, so as to yield a lightly granular texture. Liqueurs may be added if desired. The sugar and/or liqueur will not allow the granita to freeze solid, making it easier to churn before serving. Granita is served in a long-stemmed glass.

Granite These are slushy grainy water ices, usually come in lemon or coffee flavors, are normally found in bars, and are more common in southern Italy.

Granulation tissue Connective tissue that forms on the surface of a healing wound, ulcer, or inflamed tissue surface

Grape Fresh fruit of a large number of varieties of Vitis vinifera. One of the oldest cultivated plants (recorded in ancient Egypt in 4000 BC). Can be grouped as dessert grapes, wine grapes, and varieties that are used for drying to produce raisins, currants, and sultanas (see fruit, dried).Of the many varieties of grape that are grown for wine making, nine are considered 'classic varieties': cabernet sauvignon, chardonnay, chenin blanc, merlot, pinot noir, riesling, sauvignon blanc, smillon, syrah. A 100-g portion is a source of copper; provides 0.5 g of dietary fibre; supplies 60 kcal (245 kJ).

Grape leaves Leaves from grape vines originally planted in the Mediterranean region, but now grown locally. Available in jars, packed in brine, at specialty food stores and some supermarkets. Leaves bought in jars should be soaked briefly in hot water and rinsed well before using. Fresh leaves should be steamed or poached briefly to soften before using.

Grape must The juice pressed from grapes before it has fermented; new wine. Grape must is also used in making traditional balsamic vinegar, which must mature by a long and slow process thought natural fermentation.

Grapeseed oil This is very light oil that cooks at high temperatures. It should have a "grapey" flavor and fragrance. It is excellent for sauting and for fondues.

Grappa An old alcoholic beverage made from the remnants of wine-grape pressings (whatever was leftover, including stems, seeds, and skins). Grappa has been made in Italy since at least the sixteenth century. The first grappa makers were probably frugal farmers seeking a way to use up the leftovers from the winemaking process. Like balsamic vinegar and wine, the price goes up depending on the vineyard, and the aging process. Although grappa is a thoroughly Italian beverage, similar concoctions are produced in other nations, including the United States. In Spain it is aguardiente, the French call it marc, and the Greeks have their raki.

GRAS (Generally Recognized as Safe) GRAS is the regulatory status of food ingredients not evaluated by the FDA prescribed testing procedure. It also includes common food ingredients that were already in use when the 1959 Food Additives Amendment to the Food, Drug and Cosmetic Act was enacted.

Grate To rub hard-textured food against a grater (a tool with small, rough, sharp-edged holes) to reduce to fine particles. Grating works best with firm foods; soft food (such as some cheeses) form clumps.

Gratin A gratin is any dish that's topped with cheese or breadcrumbs mixed with knobs of butter, then heated in the oven or under the grill until brown and crisp. The terms 'au gratin' or 'gratine' refer to any dish prepared in this way. Special round or oval gratin pans and dishes are ovenproof and shallow, which increases a dish's surface area, thereby ensuring a larger crispy portion for each serving!

Gravlax A Swedish dish of salmon cured in a sugar, salt, and dill mixture. It is then sliced thin and served on dark bread with a dill and mustard sauce

Gravy Traditionally, 'gravy' meant simply the naturally concentrated juices that come from meat as it roasts. The juices can also be combined with a liquid such as chicken or beef stock, wine or milk and thickened with flour, cornflour or some other thickening agent to make a thicker, more sauce-like gravy.

Although it frightens a lot of people, making gravy just needs a little practice to get right. Simply add enough flour to the fat and juices in the roasting pan and stir over the heat until the flour has browned and you've scraped any sediment loose. Add up to 570ml (1 pint) of stock and, using a balloon whisk, stir until boiling. Season to taste and simmer for a couple of minutes.

Green goddess dressing A salad dressing that is a mixture of mayonnaise, anchovies, tarragon vinegar, parsley, scallions, garlic, and other spices. It was created at San Francisco's Palace Hotel (now called the Sheraton-Palace) in the 1920s. The Palace Hotel was built in 1875 and was San Francisco's first grant lodging. The hotel chef named the dressing for English actor George Arliss (1868-1846), who stayed there while performing in the play called The Green

Goddess. This play was considered the best play of the 1920-21 Broadway season and it later became on the earliest "talkie" movies in 1930. The actor frequently complemented San Francisco's marvelous weather and proclaimed that it induced a healthy appetite. George Arliss, himself, suggested that the hotel should name a salad or salad dressing after the play.

Green onion A green onion can be classified as a type of scallion. As the name scallion applies to several members of the onion family, including a distinct variety called scallion, immature onions (commonly called green onions), young leeks, and sometimes the tops of young shallots. In each case the vegetable has a white base that has not fully developed into a bulb and green leaves that are long and straight. Both parts are edible.

Gremolata An Italian garnish of raw, finely chopped garlic, parsley and lemon zest. It's usually sprinkled over slow-cooked braised meats, as in the Italian dish osso bucco, but it makes a good garnish for grilled fish or chicken too.

Griddle A flat cast-iron pan traditionally used for breads and scones. More recently griddles tend to have a ridged surface and are used for cooking vegetables, meat and fish. It tends to be thought of as a healthier method of cooking as the fat from the meat drains away down into the grooves.

Grill, grilling Grilling is a high-heat cooking method done directly over live flames (cooking the food in a matter of minutes). Many grilled foods have a wonderful smokey or charred flavor because as the food cooks, fat drips down to the heat source and as it burns on the coals or heat element its fumes and flavors are sent back up to the outside of the food. Usually the food is turned over as it grills, so both sides are directly exposed to the heat source.

Grits The word comes from the Old English grytt meaning "bran," but the Old English greot also meant "something ground." Grits are coarsely ground hominy (corn with the hull and germ removed). Hominy is made from field corn that is soaked in lye water (potash water in the old days) and stirred over the next day or two until the entire shell or bran comes loose and rises to the top. The kernel itself swells to twice its original size. After the remaining kernels have been rinsed several times, they are spread to dry either on cloth or screen dryers. In the Southern United States, it is commonly boiled and served for breakfast or as a dinner side dish. Grits are considered an institution in the South, but rarely found in northern states. Many cookbooks will refer to grits as hominy, because of regional preference for the name.

Grouper Groupers are members of the sea bass family. They are particularly common around coral reefs and rock outcroppings of the inner coastal shelf, which makes them less vulnerable to, trawls or traps. In addition to the southern United States, Mexico, Central and South America, the Mediterranean, and South Africa have important grouper fisheries. They are a white-fleshed and lean fish.

Growth and development The first term refers to the increase in body measurements, such as height and weight. The second is applied to the appearance and improvement of functions, such as language, motor ability, cognitive functions, psychic maturity and others.

Gruyere cheese It is also known as groyer cheese. It is named for the village of Gruyere, in the Canton of Fribourg, Switzerland, which is near the French border. It is a shiny yellow, hard, smooth small-eyed cheese that melts well without separating and is often used for sauces, with grilled meats, poultry, and fish. It is made from cow's whole milk in much the same way as Swiss cheese.

Guacamole An avocado condiment that is made from ripened avocados and lemon or lime juice, diced onion, tomatoes, and cilantro.

Guar gum A substance made from the seeds of the guar plant which acts as a stabilizer in food systems. Is found as a food additive in cheese, including processed cheese, ice cream and dressings.

Guardposts Areas or communities that can be monitored by means of the aplication of a series of nutritional state indicators, providing information which, by analogy, can express the probable situation in similar socio-economic and sanitary contexts.

Guava A native to South America, it is also grown in the U.S. There are many varieties of guavas, and they can range in size from a small egg to a medium apple, all are very sweet. Guavas make excellent jams, preserves, sauces, and sorbets.

Gumbo A delicacy of South Louisiana. It is a thick, robust soup almost always containing a roux, and sometimes thickened with okra or file'. There are thousands of variations, only a few of which are shrimp or seafood gumbo, chicken or duck gumbo, okra and file' gumbo. Generally, gumbos come in two categories, those thickened with okra (thus the name), which comes from an African word for "okra," and those with ground sassafras leaves, known as "file." The earlier gumbos were closer to soups than to the stew often served today. You can make the soup thicker by using more roux or adding more file powder. The ingredients call for oyster liquor, the juice left over from opening oysters, which would have been abundant in an era when many meals began with oysters. Bottled clam juice or fish broth make suitable substitutes. Serve the gumbo over rice.

GYE Guinness Yeast Extract, see yeast extract.

Gyle Alcohol solution formed in the first stage of vinegar production, 6-9% alcohol. Subsequent fermentation with Acetobacter spp. converts the alcohol to acetic acid.

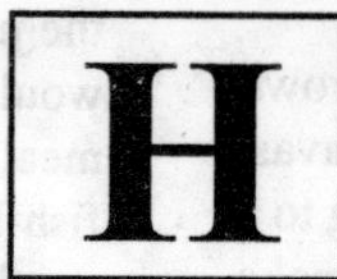

Habanero pepper You might also know this Yucatan-raised, lantern-shaped chile as a Scot bonnet or Bahamian chile. Whatever you call it, with a fire reportedly 60 times that of a Jalapeno, these pods pack a punch. It is the hottest of all chiles in the world. It should be handled only while wearing plastic gloves. Ripe Habaneros, which are dark green, red, or orange-red, have a sweeter flavor and are fruitier than the green, unripe ones.

HACCP (Hazard Analysis and Critical Control Points) The underlying approach under HACCP for preventing foodborne illness and promote quality is to identify the danger spots and try to avoid them. Instead of putting the burden on government to discover that a food safety problem exists, HACCP shifts responsibility onto the industry to ensure that the food it produces is safe. Food producers will have to prevent bacterial contamination from occurring in the first place.

Haddock A white sea-fish similar to cod (and subject to the same problems of overfishing). It has flaky flesh, is available fresh or frozen, whole or as steaks and fillets. It can be cooked just like cod - poached, baked, fried or grilled, and served with or without sauce. Tartare sauce is a classic accompaniment, and haddock is delicious deep-fried for homemade fish and chips. It's also good in fish pie, fishcakes, soup or kedgeree.

You can easily buy haddock smoked, but avoid the dyed stuff (recognisable by its bright yellow hue) because it contains colourings. Buy undyed where possible. An Arbroath smokie is a whole wood-smoked haddock.

Haemin The hydrochloride of haematin, derived from haemoglobin. The crystals are readily recognizable under the mieroscope and are used as a test for blood.

Haemoglobin The red haem-containing protein in red blood cells which is responsible for the transport of oxygen and carbon dioxide in the bloodstream. Because haem contains iron, there is a deficiency of haemoglobin and impaired oxygen transport to tissues in iron deficiency anaemia.

Haemoglobin, glycosylated Haemoglobin linked via lysine to glucose. The reaction occurs non-enzymically, and is increased when blood concentrations of glucose are persistently higher than normal. Measurement of glycosylated haemoglobin is used as an index of the control of diabetes over the preceding 2-3 months. Normally 3-6% of haemoglobin is glycosylated; as much as 20% may be glycosylated in uncontrolled diabetes.

Haemorrhagic disease of the newborn Excessive bleeding due to vitamin K deficiency; in most countries infants are given vitamin K by injection shortly after birth to prevent this rare but serious (potentially fatal) condition.

Haggis Haggis is a Scottish dish made from sheep's offal (windpipe, lungs, heart and liver) of the sheep, which is first boiled and then minced. It is then mixed with beef suet and lightly toasted oatmeal. This mixture is placed inside the sheep's stomach, which is sewn closed. The resulting haggis is traditionally cooked by further boiling (for up to three hours). This is the most traditional of all Scottish dishes, eaten on Burns Night (25th January; the birthday of Scotland's national poet, Robert Burns, 1759-1796) and at Hogmanay (New Year's Eve). Haggis is traditionally served as "haggis, neeps and tatties". The neeps are mashed turnip or swede, with a little milk and allspice added, whereas the tatties are creamed potatoes flavored with a little nutmeg. To add that authentic touch, consume your haggis, neeps and tatties with a dram of good whisky.

Hake The various fish that come under the banner 'hake' are deep-sea members of the cod family and are popular throughout Europe and America. Hake is quite a mild fish, having a more subtle flavour than cod. In France it's known as 'saumon blanc', while in the US it's called ling or whiting (rather confusingly, whiting in Europe is a different, less tasty fish).

One tip - if you're buying your hake frozen, avoid the South American variety, which has a poorer flavour. Hake is easy to prepare, as it has few bones. You'll usually see it for sale fresh or frozen, whole, or as fillets and steaks. It's a reliable fish fried or poached or used in fish soup.

Halibut Halibut is a large flatfish, resembling the turbot in appearance, and is the largest in the flatfish group. They sometimes weigh in at over 500 pounds and six feet in length. The flesh of the halibut is coarser and the flavor is stronger and less refined than the flounder, and especially the sole. Halibut is exclusively a cold-water fish and is found in the North Atlantic and North Pacific oceans. "Hippo of the sea" is how the halibut's Latin family name "hippoglossus" translates.

Halva There are numerous forms of halva, which is basically a 'sweetmeat' or dessert depending on which version you're eating. The Middle Eastern sweet known as halva is made from ground roasted sesame seeds and honey. It's usually made in a slab and is often studded with chopped dried fruit or nuts.

You can buy it in the UK ready-made wrapped in bars. Indian halva is a sweet dessert dish made with semolina, fried in ghee, mixed with spiced syrup and raisins and cooked until light and fluffy. It can also be made with grated vegetables - carrot halva is the most common. The vegetables are cooked with milk or cream and sugar into a thick paste, then flavoured with cardamom or other spices and sometimes nuts.

The name means 'sweetmeat' in numerous languages, so you may see it written as helva, halvah, halwa, halawi and it could take on a slightly different form with a wide variety of spices, nuts, fruits or vegetables being added to it.

Hamburger A grilled, fried, or broiled patty of ground beef that is usually served on a "hamburger bun" and topped with ketchup, onions, and/or other condiments. It is considered a cultural icon in America.

Hangtown Fry This oyster dish includes oysters, eggs, and bacon.

Hard cider Hard cider is a fermented beverage prepared from the juice of apples. The fermentation continues until the sugar is transformed into alcohol.

commercial grade cider - Apple juice or cider is usually more refined than ordinary cider. They remove the yeasts and develop to produce hard cider. They are destroyed by a low temperature method without affecting the vitamin content.

Apple juice is also put through very fine filters. Of course, they usually add preservatives.

fresh or sweet cider - The liquid is fresh cider as long as it remains in its natural state and is not sweetened, preserved, clarified, or otherwise altered. In sweet cider, fermentation is not permitted at all.

Hardtack A hard square biscuit or cracker that is made with flour and water only (unleavened and unsalted bread). Since it's very dry, it can be stored for years without refrigeration. People can live for quite a while on just bread and water. Hardtack is eaten by itself, dipped in coffee, or crumbled into soups. Inexpensive, stable, and easy to transport, hardtack was a staple in military life throughout most of our history. It was also the most convenient food for soldiers, explorers, and pioneers.

Haricot vert The French term for green string beans, Haricot means, "bean," and vert means, "green." They are much thinner than regular green beans and traditionally have a much better flavor. They are also known as French green beans and French beans.

Hartshorn It is also called bakers' ammonia (ammonium carbonate). It is an ammonia compound and not harmful after baking. However, don't eat the raw dough. Your kitchen will stink of ammonia while the cookies bake - but once baked, the cookies will not taste of it. Can be substituted for equal amount of baking powder in any cookies recipe. It is an old-time leavening favoured for cookies, such as German Springerle. It is said to give a "fluffiness" of texture baking powder can't. Its leavening is only activated by heat, not moisture (such as baking powder).

Harvard standard Tables of height and weight for age used as reference Values for the assessment of growth and nutritional status in children, based on data collected in the USA. Now largely replaced by the N.H. (US National Centre for Health Statistics) standards.

Harvey wallbanger A cocktail based on half a measure of Galliano floating on four measures of orange juice and half a measure of vodka.

Hash A dish of chopped pork or beef combined with various chopped up vegetables and seasonings. Hash is often thought of as a dish that you throw into it whatever is left in the kitchen. In the 19th century, cheap restaurants were called "hash houses" and the workers in these restaurants were called "hash slingers."

Haunch A term used in a cut of meat, usually venison. One of the back legs of an animal with four legs that is used for meat (the leg and loin undivided, or, as more commonly called, the hind quarter) - a haunch of veal, venison, or wild boar.

Haute Cuisine Couture It means "Recipe for Comfort" and it relates to the fashion world. It is first and foremost a form of expertise or savoir-faire, involving a craft that has endured for more than one hundred and fifty years. The origins of haute couture date back to Charles Friduric Worth who, in 1858, founded the first true house of haute couture at 7, rue de la Paix, in Paris, creating original models for individual clients. Haute couture involves craftsmanship, the skill of the seamstress and embellisher (feather makers, embroiderers, milliners) who, each season, create the finery of the exceptional.

Haute Cuisine Food that is prepared in an elegant or elaborate manner; the very finest food available. The French word "haute" translates as "high" or "superior." Cuisine translates as "cooking" in general. Literally meaning "high cooking" or high-class cooking, the rich sauces, fine ingredients and exquisite taste of haute cuisine typifies classic French cooking.

Havarti cheese It is a light to pale yellow cheese with tiny holes "eyes" in its smooth body, it melts well when it is shredded. It is similar to Montery Jack cheese.

Hay diet A system of eating based on the concept that carbohydrates and proteins should not be eaten at the same meal, for which there is no scientific basis. It ignores the fact that almost all carbohydrate-rich foods also contain significant amounts of protein. In any case, in the absence of adequate carbohydrate, protein is oxidized as a metabolic fuel (i.e. to provide energy) and therefore not available for tissue building. Also called combining diet or food combining.

Hazard Hazard may mean: Dangers, risks, problems A hazard is a source of potential harm. A hazard has three modes: 1. Dormant (there are no people around; there is no risk)

2. Armed (there is a person or people in the vicinity; there is risk)

3. Active (human reaction time is too slow to combat the effect of the hazard; it is too late to prevent the conseqences of the hazard)

Hazard characterisation The qualitative and/or quantitative evaluation of the nature of the adverse health effects associated with biological, chemical and physical agents which may be present in food. For chemical agents, a close response assessment should be performed. For biological or physical agents, a dose-response assessment should be performed if the data are obtainable.

Hazard identification The identification of biological, chemical and physical agents capable of causing adverse health effects which may be present in a particular food or group of foods.

2. Determining if a chemical or a microbe can cause adverse health effects in humans and what those effects might be.

Hazelnut A type of hard-shelled nut with an oval or round kernel, also known as a filbert. Hazelnuts are high in dietary fibre. Turkey is a major supplier of hazelnuts, along with Spain and Italy, but they do grow wild in the hedgerows around Britain.

Cobnuts, which grow in Britain, are a type of hazelnut. You may be able to buy fresh nuts, particularly native cobnuts, still in their husks, but most are sold dried and processed. Use hazelnuts whole, grated or ground to flavour savoury and sweet dishes.

Finely ground they can be used in place of flour to make a 'torte', or roughly chopped they add crunch to biscuits or meringues. Use them as the basis for a stuffing or simply chop them up with some dried fruits and scatter the mixture on your cereal.

Some recipes might call for 'skinned hazelnuts'. If so, just roast them in the oven for a few minutes; when they've cooled slightly, rub the skins off with your fingers. Hazelnuts have an affinity with chocolate - as in hazelnut and chocolate torte, for example, or hazelnut and chocolate spread.

In Turkey, a sauce to serve with shellfish is made from garlic and hazelnuts. Frangelico is a hazelnut liqueur from northern Italy. Hazelnut oil is delicate in flavour and makes a change from olive oil in a salad dressing.

Headcheese A sausage made from a calf or pig's head and molded in its own jelly and seasoned. In England it is called brawn and in France it goes by the name fromage de tete de porc.

Health As officially defined by the World Health Organization, a state of complete physical, mental, and social well-being, not merely the absence of disease or infirmity.

Health claims Claims that link food—or food components—in the overall diet with a lowered risk of some chronic diseases. Strictly regulated by the Food and Drug Administration, only health claims supported by scientific evidence are allowed on food labels. Since this information is optional, many foods that meet the criteria don't carry any health claim on their label.

Health related quality of life The impact an illness has on quality of life, including the individual's perception of his or her illness.

Healthy dietary practices Uses, habits and costums that define parameters of food consumption according to scientific and technical knowledge concerning good nourishment. See dietary orientation, food composition, and nutritional well-being.

Healthy weight Compared to overweight or obese, a body weight that is less likely to be linked with any weight-related health problems such as type 2 diabetes, heart disease, high blood pressure, high blood cholesterol, or others. A body mass index (BMI) of 18.5 up to 25 refers to a healthy weight, though not all individuals with a BMI in this range may be at a healthy level of body fat; they may have more body fat tissue and less muscle. A BMI of 25 up to 30 refers to overweight and a BMI of 30 or higher refers to obese.

Heart The muscle that pumps blood received from veins into arteries throughout the body. It is positioned in the chest behind the sternum (breastbone; in front of the trachea, esophagus, and aorta; and above the diaphragm muscle that separates the chest and abdominal cavities. The normal heart is about the size of a closed fist, and weighs about 10.5 ounces. It is cone-shaped, with the point of the cone pointing down to the left. Two-thirds of the heart lies in the left side of the chest with the balance in the right chest.

Heart disease Any disorder that affects the heart. Sometimes the term "heart disease" is used narrowly and incorrectly as a synonym for coronary artery disease. Heart disease is synonymous with cardiac disease but not with cardiovascular disease which is any disease of the heart or blood vessels. Among the many types of heart disease, see, for example Angina; Arrhythmia; Congenital heart disease; Coronary artery disease (CAD); Dilated cardiomyopathy; Heart attack (myocardial infarction); Heart failure; Hypertrophic cardiomyopathy; Mitral regurgitation; Mitral valve prolapse; and Pulmonary stenosis.

Heart of palm Heart of palm is the inner, edible portion of the stem of the cabbage (palmetto) palm tree. This palm grows in tropical climates such as Florida (it's the state tree) and Brazil. Hearts of palm are ivory coloured and resemble white asparagus without the tips. They are usually available canned and packed in water. They are rather expensive and have a taste reminiscent of artichoke. Delicious in salads, hearts of palm can also be used in main dishes or fried.

Heartburn A burning sensation in the chest usually caused by reflux (regurgitation) of acid digestive juices from the stomach into the oesophagus. A common form of indigestion, treated by antacids.

Heat of combustion Energy released by complete combustion, as for example, in the bomb calorimeter. Values can be used to predict energy physiologically available from foods only if an allowance is made for material not completely oxidized in the body. For example, the end products of protein oxidation in the body are carbon dioxide, water, and urea; the latter contains non-available energy. See energy conversion factors.

Hedonic regression Hedonic regression, or more generally hedonic demand theory, in economics is a method of estimating demand or prices. It decomposes the item being researched into its constituent characteristics, and obtains estimates of the value of each characteristic. In essence it assumes that there is a separate market for each characteristic. It may be estimated using ordinary least squares (OLS) regression analysis. Often an attribute vector (or dummy variable) is assigned to each characteristic or group of characteristics. Each characteristic within a vector is either included in the regression or not, by multiplying it by either 1 or 0.

Helix A spiral, staircase like structure with a repeating pattern described by two simultaneous operations (rotation and translation). It is one of the natural conformations exhibited by biological polymers.

Hemorrhoids Veins around the anus or lower rectum that are swollen and inflamed.

Herb butter A mixture of butter and mayonnaise blended with parsley, tarragon, dill, watercress, thyme, green pepper, garlic, and other herbs, used as a savoury spread on biscuits or bread.

Herb tea Or tisane, an infusion made from any kind of herb, fruit, or flower. Camomile, lime blossom, and fennel seeds are commonly used. Medicinal or health claims are sometimes made, largely on traditional rather than scientific grounds.

Herbicides Herbicides are a class of crop protection and specialty chemicals used to control weeds on farms and in forests, as well as in non agricultural applications such as golf courses, public tracts of land and residential lawns.

Herbs Soft-stemmed, aromatic plants used fresh or dried to flavour and garnish dishes, and sometimes for medicinal effects. Not clearly distinguished from spices, except that herbs are usually the leaves or the whole of the plant while spices are only part of the plant, commonly the seeds, or sometimes the roots or rhizomes.

Herring A North Atlantic fish that's rich oils. Herring stocks are suffering from the effects of overfishing and ecological changes, so herring is less widely available than it once was. Usually sold whole, herrings can be poached, fried or grilled as well as pickled, marinated, salted and smoked.

The tasty herring is rich in protein and vitamins and omega-3 fatty acids, which are beneficial to health. Available all year round, but best from spring to autumn. Usually sold whole. Ensure freshness by choosing large, firm and slippery fish.

Clean the fish before cooking. It's usual to dispose of the head but the bones are usually soft and edible. Cook by opening fillets out, seasoning with oatmeal and shallow frying in butter. Serve hot or cold.

Herring is perhaps best cooked in white wine or light vinegar - the acid flavours suit the rich flesh. Also good scored, brushed with butter and grilled. The traditional accompaniment is mustard, though horseradish is good too.

Herring roe is also full of flavour. Mackerel or sardines can be used as a substitute in recipes if you can't find herrings.

Heterocyclics Cyclic organic molecules containing one or more hetero atoms (e.g., nitrogen, sulphur, oxygen, etc.).

HHS United States Department of Health and Human Services. The federal agency responsible for administration for health and social service programs at the federal level. HHS also administers the Elderly Nutrition Program and the Nutrition Services Incentive Program.

Hiatal hernia A small opening in the diaphragm that allows the upper part of the stomach to move up into the chest.

Hickory nuts There are 17 varieties of hickory trees, 13 of which are native to the United States, including the pecan nut. The common hickory nut has an extremely hard shell. Hickory nuts have an excellent rich flavor with a buttery quality due to their high fat content. They are a usually sold unshelled. Hickory nuts can be used in a variety of baked goods and in almost any recipe as a substitute for pecans.

High blood pressure Also known as hypertension, high blood pressure is, by definition, a repeatedly elevated blood pressure exceeding 140 over 90 mmHg — a systolic pressure above 140 with a diastolic pressure above 90.

High density lipoproteins (HDL) Plasma lipoproteins containing relatively low concentrations of cholesterol and other lipids; thought to be beneficial because they cycle cholesterol out of tissues.

High fructose corn syrup (HFCS) HFCS are formulations generally containing 42 percent, 55 percent or 90 percent fructose (the remaining carbohydrate being primarily glucose) depending on the product application. HCFS are used in products such as soft drinks or cake mixes.

High in EU legislation (in preparation in 1995) states that for a food label or advertising to bear a claim that it is high in a nutrient it must contain 50% more of the claimed nutrient than a similar product for which no claim is made. Claims may also be made for foods containing more than 12 g of protein, 6 g of dietary fibre or more than 30% of the labelling Reference Amount of a vitamin or mineral /100 g (see Appendix VI). US legislation permits a claim of 'high in' for foods containing more than 20% of the Daily Value for a particular nutrient in a serving.

High Tea High Tea is often a misnomer. Most people refer to afternoon tea as high tea because they think it sounds regal and lofty, when in all actuality, high tea, or "meat tea" is dinner. High tea, in Britain, at any rate, tends to be on the heavier side. American hotels and tea rooms, on the other hand, continue to misunderstand and offer tidbits of fancy pastries and cakes on delicate china when they offer a "high tea." Afternoon tea (because it was usually taken in the late afternoon) is also called "low tea" because it was usually taken in a sitting room or withdrawing room where low tables (like a coffee table) were placed near sofas or chairs generally in a large withdrawing room. There are three basic types of Afternoon, or Low Tea:

Cream Tea - Tea, scones, jam and cream

High-density lipoprotein (HDL) A form of cholesterol that circulates in the blood. Commonly called "good" cholesterol. High HDL lowers the risk of heart disease. An HDL of 60 mg/dl or greater is considered high and is protective against heart disease. An HDL less than 40 mg/dl is considered low and increases the risk for developing heart disease.

High-temperature short-time treatment (HTST) Sterilization by heat from times ranging from a few seconds to minutes; usually applied to flow sterilization, in which the process time is less than about 1 minute; based on the fact that at higher temperatures bacteria are destroyed more rapidly than damage can occur to nutrients and texture.

Hippenmasse A cookie that you fill with chocolate mousse or berries.

Hirschprung's disease A congenital absence of nerves in the smooth muscle wall of the colon that results in buildup of feces, and widening of the bowel (megacolon), symptoms include vomiting, diarrhea, and constipation; surgical repair in early childhood is usually successful

Histamine Histamine is a biogenic amine chemical involved in local immune responses as well as regulating physiological function in the gut and acting as a neurotransmitter. New evidence also indicates that histamine plays a role in chemotaxis of white blood cells.

Histidinaemia Genetic disease due to a defect in the metabolism of the amino acid histidine. If untreated it leads to mental retardation and nervous system abnormalities. Treatment is by feeding a diet very low in histidine.

HIV/AIDS Human immunodeficiency virus (HIV) is the retrovirus that causes acquired immunodeficiency syndrome (AIDS); symptoms of HIV infection can include opportunistic infections, growth problems, diarrhea, developmental regression and immune system dysfunction

HMB HMB is short for beta-hydroxy beta-methylbuyrate. It is a metabolite of L-Leucine, and has been studied for it effects on lean mass and strength.

Hoagie Also known as submarines, heroes, bombers, grinder, torpedoes, and rockets in other parts of the United States. Hoagies are built-to-order sandwiches filled with meat and cheese, as well as lettuce, tomatoes, and onions, topped off with a dash of oregano=vinegar dressing on an Italian roll. A true Italian Hoagie is made with Italian ham, prosciutto salami, and provolone cheese, along with all the works. It was declared the "Official Sandwich of Philadelphia."

Holland Rusks Rusks are known in France as Biscotte and in Germany as Zwieback. A rusk is a slice of yeast bread (thick or thin) that is baked until dry, crisp, and golden brown. In America, rusks are given to babies when teething.

Hollandaise sauce Uses butter and egg yolks as binding. It is served hot with vegetables, fish, and eggs (like egg benedict). It will be a pale lemon colour, opaque, but with a luster not appearing oily. The basic sauce and its variations should have a buttery-smooth texture, almost frothy, and an aroma of good butter. Making this emulsified sauce requires a good deal of practice — it is not for the faint of heart. Biarnaise sauce, which is "related" to hollandaise sauce, is most often served with steak.

Holosides Complexes of sugars that yield only sugars on hydrolysis. As distinct from heterosides which yield other substances as well as sugars on hydrolysis, e.g. tannins, anthocyanins, nucleosides.

Home-delivered meals A program in which volunteers deliver meals to homebound seniors. Home-delivered meals programs are often supported by the Elderly Nutrition Program. Some states also use funds from the Social Services Block Grant to support home-delivered meals programs. These programs are more commonly known as Meals on Wheels.

Homeostasis Homeostasis is the property of an open system, especially living organisms, to regulate its internal environment to maintain a stable, constant condition, by means of multiple dynamic equilibrium adjustments, controlled by interrelated regulation mechanisms. The term was coined in 1932 by Walter Cannon from the Greek homoios (same, like, resembling) and stasis (to stand, posture).

Hominy Hominy is made from dried corn kernels from which the hull and germ have been removed, usually by boiling in lime. The kernels look somewhat like popcorn and have a soft, chewy consistency. It is sold either in canned or dried form.

Hominy grits Cornmeal and hominy grits are made from mature white or yellow corn from which the bran and germ have been removed. Cornmeal is ground corn. For hominy, kernels of hulled corn are either left whole or broken into particles. Hominy grits are grains of hominy broken into small uniform particles. White cornmeal and grits are traditional in the Southern U.S., while yellow corn meal and grits are more likely to be found in the North. Besides colour, there are also differences in flavor in these products.

Homocystinuria A genetic disease affecting the metabolism of the amino acid methionine and its conversion to cysteine, characterized by excretion of homocysteine and its derivatives. May result in mental retardation and early death from atherosclerosis and coronary thrombosis if untreated, as well as fractures of bones and dislocation of the lens of the eye. Treatment (which must be continued throughout life) is either by feeding a diet low in methionine and supplemented with cysteine or, in some cases by administration of high intakes of vitamin B 6 (about 100-500 times the normal requirement).

Homogenization Emulsions usually consist of a suspension of globules of varying size. Homogenization reduces these globules to a smaller and more uniform size. In homogenized milk the smaller globules adsorb more of the protein, which acts as a stabilizer, and the cream does not rise to the top.

Honey A naturally sweet, viscous liquid made from the nectar of flowers, collected by honey bees. Honey comes in numerous varieties with different colours, textures and flavours. The flavour, colour and sweetness is dependent on which type of flower the nectar was collected from.

There's a huge choice available now including Scottish heather honey, acacia honey and chestnut honey, plus a wide range from countries around the globe. Clear or runny honey and set honey have different textures because of the varying amounts and types of natural sugars contained in each of them. Clear honey is often easier to use for cooking because it's easier to pour. Apart from spreading it on your toast, use honey as a sweetener to replace sugar in desserts, drinks and in baking. Stir honey into yoghurt and spoon onto fruit salads or use it as the basis for a sticky marinade for pork or chicken - honey and mustard is a great combination.

Honey also makes a delicious glaze for roast pork, sausages or parsnips. Honey keeps in the larder for up to a year. Clear honey has a tendency to crystallise after time, but just put the jar in a jug of hot water for a minute or so and it will turn clear again.

Hooch, hootch A cheap whiskey. The term, which became widespread during Prohibition. It was derived from the name of a Chinook Indian tribe, the Hoochinoo that made a form of distilled spirits bought by U.S. soldiers who had occupied the Alaskan territory.

Hopping john A southern dish made of black-eyed peas (cowpeas) and rice. It is traditionally served on New Year's Day to ensure good luck for the New Year. The dish was a staple of the African slaves who populated southern plantations (especially those of South Carolina).

Hormone A chemical substance that is secreted into body fluids and transported to another organ, where it produces a specific effect on metabolism.

Horn of plenty A common woodland mushroom, so named because it grows in the shape of a long horn or funnel. It's also known as black trumpet and trompette de la mort. It has a fluted edge and dark gills and is very dark brown, almost black in colour. It looks and tastes like a dark version of the chanterelle mushroom.

Horns of plenty are a bit of a luxury as they only grow wild - and if you do find them in your local farmers' market, or more remarkably, your supermarket, then they'll be very expensive. Nonetheless, they have a delicious rich flavour - good with creamy sauces or in soups or stews, with chicken, polenta or pasta.

For a real treat just fry them in butter and serve them on toast. Gathered from summer through to winter, they're sometimes available dried. Clean them carefully before use to get rid of any grit.

Hors d'oeuvres Means little snack foods, small items of food or light courses, served before or outside of ("hors") the main dishes of a meal (the "oeuvres") which are intended to stimulate the appetite. The terms hors d'oeuvres and appetizers are often used interchangeably, but there is a difference: hors d'oeuvres are the small savory bites, typically finger food, served before a meal, while appetizers appear as the first course served at the table. The name hors d'oeuvres comes from the French and is literally translated as "out of the work," but it's more logical to think of it as meaning "apart from (or before) the meal."

Horseradish A perennial plant originating in eastern and south-eastern Europe, horseradish is cultivated for its tough, twisted root. Horseradish is a member of the mustard family. The root, which is similar in appearance to a parsnip, releases a distinctive aroma when bruised or cut and it has a very hot, peppery flavour that's more powerful than mustard.

Once peeled, the root can be grated and mixed with cream and other ingredients to provide a hot-flavoured sauce to accompany roast beef or fish such as trout. Care must be taken when grating, because the vapours can make the eyes sting.

Horseradish is traditionally made into a sauce to serve with roast beef, venison or well-flavoured fish such as tuna, smoked trout or mackerel. To store, keep fresh horseradish in a paper bag in the fridge for up to one week or cut into smaller pieces and freeze to use as required.

To prepare fresh root, simply peel and then grate as required. Only prepare the amount needed, as once peeled it loses its pungency quite quickly. It's used raw in sauces - cooking destroys its flavour.

Creamed horseradish is a creamy but strongly flavoured combination of horseradish, vinegar and cream. This is the traditional tangy accompaniment to roast beef. It has a slightly runny consistency. Serve with roast beef, steaks or beef stews.

Once opened store creamed horseradish in the fridge for up to one year. Horseradish hot sauce is a mix of horseradish and vegetable oil. It has a very strong flavour and a thicker consistency than creamed horseradish. Serve with venison or well-flavoured fish such as mackerel or tuna. Stir into mashed potatoes for a tangy flavour. Once opened store the sauce in the fridge for up to one year.

Horseshoe Sandwich The sandwich is considered the signature dish or Springfield, Illinois, the home of Abraham Lincoln. This sandwich will make our arteries cringe and your taste buds rejoice. The sandwich starts out with two to three slices of thick toasted bread. On top of that you have two traditional choices: a thick fried ham steak or two large hamburger patties. Then a large amount of freshly made French fries are placed onto the top of it. The secret to this sandwich is the sauce that is poured over the top. Every restaurant and chef seems to have his or her own secret cheese sauce recipe. The name of the sandwich comes from the shape of the ham with the fries representing the horseshoe nails, and the heated steak platter as the anvil. If you order a Pony Shoe Sandwich, it is the same thing, but a smaller or half a Horseshoe portion (usually one slice of toast).

Hot brown sandwich An open-faced turkey sandwich with turkey, bacon, pimientos, and a delicate Mornay sauce. The sandwich is place under the broiler to melt the cheese.

Hot dog Also called frankfurters. A cooked sausage that consists of a combination of beef and pork or all beef, which is cured, smoked, and cooked. Seasonings may include coriander, garlic, ground mustard, nutmeg, salt, sugar, and white pepper. They are fully cooked but are usually served hot. Sizes range from big dinner frankfurters to tiny cocktail size.

Hot fudge sundae It was first served at C.C. Browns in Hollywood by an unknown and long forgotten "soda jerk". This hot and cold sensation is still one of ice cream lover's favourites.

HPA (Hypothalamic-pituitary-adrenal) axis A system within the body that responds to stress by stimulating or inhibiting the release of various hormones, in particular cortisol, into the blood which then stimulates systems essential to self-preservation.

Human Genome Project This project is, in simplest terms, a sequencing of the human genome. Information from the Human Genome Project is making it possible, for example, to identify the exact gene (or genes) that influences a person's susceptibility to a disease, to develop new and better drugs, and to identify thousands of different polymorphisms. The full scope of the Human Genome Project's potential to improve human health is only beginning to be appreciated.

Human milk banks Specialized centres responsible for promoting breastfeeding incentives and for the collection, processing, stocking and quality control of artificially extracted human milk, to later be distributed under a doctor's or nutritinist's prescription.

Humectants Substances such as glycerol, sorbitol, invert sugars, honey which prevent loss of moisture from foods, especially flour confectionery, which would make them unappetizing; they also prevent sugar crystallizing and the growth of ice crystals in frozen foods. They are used in other products too, such as tobacco, inks, glues, etc.

Hummus Hummus is an Arabic and Greek dish made from cooked chickpeas crushed with sesame oil. Sometimes soy sauce is added. One source states it is a combination of garbanzo beans, sesame tahini, lemon, garlic and mild spices. Hummus may be purchased from some health food and grocery stores.

Hunger The uneasy or painful sensation caused by lack of food. The recurrent and involuntary lack of access to sufficient food due to poverty or constrained resources can lead to malnutrition over time.

Hurler syndrome A mucopolysaccharidosis characterized by cerebral degeneration and storage of mucopolysaccharides; symptoms include severe abnormality in the development of skeletal cartilage and bone, characteristic facial features, and severe mental retardation; Hurler syndrome is autosomal recessive, and is usually fatal during childhood

Hurricane This signature cocktail of New Orleans is a potent sweet fruit punch and rum drink that is served in a special hurricane lamp glass that has become one of the most sought-after souvenirs in New Orleans. During celebrations (celebrations seem to be nightly in the New Orleans French Quarter) tourists carry their "to go" Hurricane drink down the streets. Hurricanes are also the cocktail of choice during Mardi Gras, where thousands come to parade and party. The Hurricane was made famous by Pat O'Brien's French Quarter bar. Other restaurants and bars serve this drink but it has become synonymous with Pat O'Brien's, where people line up to get their Hurricane drink.

Hushpuppies A finger-shaped dumpling of cornmeal that is deep-fried (they are traditionally served with fried catfish). Hushpuppies, also known as corn dodgers. They are especially popular throughout the South.

Hybridization of crops The mating of two plants from different species or genetically very different members of the same species to yield hybrids possessing some of the characteristics of each parent. Those (hybrid) offspring tend to be more healthy, productive and uniform than their parents—a phenomenon known as "hybrid vigor."

Hydrogen The most plentiful element in the universe and one present in all organic compounds. Hydrogen is a gas with an atomic number of 1 and the symbol H.

Hydrogenation Hydrogenation is the process of adding hydrogen molecules directly to an unsaturated fatty acid from sources such as vegetable oils to convert it to a semi solid form such as margarine or shortening. Hydrogenation contributes important textural properties to food. The degree of hydrogenation influences the firmness and spreadability of margarines, flakiness of pie crust and the creaminess of puddings. Hydrogenated oils are sometimes used in place of other fats with higher proportions of saturated fatty acids such as butter or lard.

Hydrolysis Not to be confused with electrolysis, the common method of producing hydrogen gas from water. Hydrolysis is a chemical reaction or process in which a molecule is split into two parts by reacting with a molecule of water, which has the chemical formula H2O. One of the parts gets an OH- from the water molecule and the other part gets an H+ from the water. This is distinct from a hydration reaction, in which water molecules are added to a substance, but no cleavage occurs. In organic chemistry, hydrolysis can be considered as the reverse or opposite of condensation, a reaction in which two molecular fragments are joined for each water molecule produced. As hydrolysis may be a reversible reaction, condensation and hydrolysis can take place at the same time, with the position of equilibrium determining the amount of each product. In inorganic chemistry, the word is often applied to solutions of salts and the reactions by which they are converted to new ionic species or to precipitates (oxides, hydroxides, or salts).

Hyperalgesia Lowered threshold to pain.

Hypercholesterolemia Hypercholesterolemia (literally: high blood cholesterol) is the presence of high levels of cholesterol in the blood. It is not a disease but a metabolic derangement that can be secondary to many diseases and can contribute to many forms of disease, most notably cardiovascular disease. It is closely related to the terms "hyperlipidemia" (elevated levels of lipids) and "hyperlipoproteinemia" (elevated levels of lipoproteins).

Hyperglycemia Hyperglycemia or High Blood Sugar is a condition in which an excessive amount of glucose circulates in the blood plasma. The term is from Greek: hyper-, prefix meaning "too much"; -glyc-, root meaning "sweet"; -emia, suffix meaning "of the blood".

Hyperlipidemia Hyperlipidemia, hyperlipoproteinemia or dyslipidemia is the presence of elevated or abnormal levels of lipids and/or lipoproteins in the blood. Lipids (fatty molecules) are transported in a protein capsule, and the density of the lipids and type of protein determines the fate of the particle and its influence on metabolism.

Hypertension High blood pressure, defined as a repeatedly elevated blood pressure exceeding 140 over 90 mmHg. High blood pressure (hypertension) is "the silent killer." Chronic high blood pressure can stealthily cause blood vessel changes in the back of the eye (retina), abnormal thickening of the heart muscle, kidney failure, and brain damage. No specific cause for high blood pressure is found in 95% of patients. High blood pressure is treated with salt restriction, regular aerobic exercise, and medications.

Hypertriglyceridemia In medicine, hypertriglyceridemia (or "Hypertriglyceridaemia") denotes high (hyper-) blood levels (-emia) of triglycerides, the most abundant fatty molecule in most organisms. It has been associated with atherosclerosis, even in the absence of hypercholesterolemia (high cholesterol levels). It can also lead to pancreatitis in excessive concentrations. Very high triglyceride levels may also interfere with blood tests; hyponatremia may be reported spuriously (pseudohyponatremia).

Hypervigilance Increased vigilance. An intensified state of paying attention to or focusing on specific things. May severely limit a person's ability to focus on specific tasks or engage in reflective thinking when their focus is on scanning for threatening stimuli. A person with a functional GI disorder or incontinence may be hypervigilant when their focus is on scanning for bodily sensations or indications that signal symptom onset.

Hypoglycemia A deficiency of sugar in the blood caused by too much insulin or too little glucose.

Hypothermia Low body temperature (normal is around 37°C). Occurs among elderly people far more readily than in younger adults, often with fatal results. Also used in connection with deliberate reduction of body temperature to 28 °C to permit heart and brain surgery.

Hypothyroidism Underactivity of the thyroid gland, leading to reduced secretion of thyroid hormones and a reduction in basal metabolic rate. Commonly associated with goitre due to iodine deficiency. In hypothyroid adults there is a characteristic moon-faced appearance, lethargy, and mental apathy. In infants, hypothyroidism can lead to severe mental retardation, cretinism. See also thyrotoxicosis.

Hypotonia Diminished muscle tone.

Hyssop A strong-flavoured aromatic herb from the Mediterranean region, similar to rosemary or lavender. During the Middle Ages it was popular as a flavouring for soups and stuffings, but now its main use is in the distillation of liqueurs, such as Chartreuse.

It's less common now so quite hard to come by, but the young leaves can be used in cooking - chopped and scattered on salads, sprinkled on meat or oily fish dishes or used to flavour soups, stews and fruit dishes. It's said to help aid digestion of fatty or rich food and hyssop tea is said to be good for chesty coughs. Bees are attracted to its beautiful blue flowers and it makes excellent honey.

I

Iatrogenic A condition caused by medical intervention or drug treatment; iatrogenic nutrient deficiency is due to drug-nutrient interactions.

Ice cream It is a frozen dessert made from cream, or a mixture of cream, milk, sugar, and usually eggs. It can also be made from combination of milk products (usually cream combined with fresh, condensed or dry milk), a sweetening agent (sugar, honey, corn syrup or an artificial sweetener) and flavorings such as pieces of chocolate, nuts, fruit, etc. Ice cream contains air, the more the air the lighter it will be.

Ice milk It is made in much the same way as ice cream, except that it contains less milk fat and milk solids. The result is a lowered calorie count and it has a lighter, less creamy texture.

Ices This dessert are fruit juices or purees of fruit that are blended with sugar syrup and frozen.

Icing A term often interchangeable with "frosting" and preferred in America to describe the sugar-and-water mixture used to decorate and cover cakes. It may also contain other ingredients and flavorings. The word is akin to "ice" for the icing becomes firm or glazed after being applied.

IDACE An association of National Dietetic Foods Industry associations within the European Union.

IDFA Infant and Dietetic Foods Association, based in the UK.

Idiocy Physical, motor and mental retardation brought about by grave iodine deficiency during the fetal period and the first months of life.

IFM The International Association of Infant Food Manufacturers represents manufacturers of foods for infants and young children.

IGBM The Interagency Group on Breast-feeding Monitoring, an ad hoc organization based in London.

Ile flottante Literally 'floating island', this is one of the great desserts of classic French cuisine. It's a very light meringue floating on a sea of custard sauce. The meringue is made from egg whites, sugar, vanilla extract and usually cream of tartar, and cooked in a bain-marie. There are lots of versions that stem from this classic, with various additions of caramel, jam, fruit or fruit purie.

Ileostomy A surgically created opening of the abdominal wall to the ileum, allowing the diversion of fecal waste.

Ileum The lower third of the small intestine, adjoining the colon.

Illness A subjective state of feeling unwell that may include impairment of normal physiological and social function.

Imaging Tests that produce pictures of areas inside the body.

Imam bayildi A Turkish dish of stuffed aubergines. The name roughly translates as 'the imam (priest) fainted'. According to legend, a certain imam was so moved by the fragrant smell of the dish that he fainted from sheer joy!

The stuffing is made with a mixture of aubergine pulp, onions and tomato, which is piled into the halved aubergine, roasted and basted occasionally with oil until meltingly soft. The key is to cook the dish enough so the ingredients remain distinct but are not reduced to mush.

Immune system The cells and tissues which are responsible for recognizing and attacking foreign microbes and substances in the body.

Immunoglobulins Large proteins from which antibodies are formed, and which are then capable of combining with foreign substances (antigens).

In vitro In vitro (Latin: (with)in the glass) refers to the technique of performing a given experiment in a test tube, or, generally, in a controlled environment outside a living organism. In vitro fertilization is a well-known example of this. Many experiments in cellular biology are conducted outside organisms or cells, thus, the conditions and, therefore, results may not correspond to those inside. Consequently, experimental results are often annotated with in vitro or its opposite in vivo as it applies.

In vivo In vivo (Latin: (with)in the living) means that which takes place inside an organism. In science, in vivo refers to experimentation done in or on the living tissue of a whole, living organism as opposed to a partial or dead one. Animal testing and clinical trials are forms of in vivo research.

Incidence Describes the occurrence of a disease or disorder in a population. It is a rate, showing how many new cases of a disease occurred in a population (typically a susceptible population called the "at-risk population") during a specified interval of time (usually expressed as number of new cases per unit time per fixed number of people; e.g., number of new cases per 1,000 persons in one year).

Income eligibility Individuals and households qualify for the federal nutrition programs by providing information about the household's income. Based upon the household income, a child may be certified to receive free or reduced-price school meals. In general, in order to be eligible for the Food Stamp Program, household income cannot exceed 130% of the federal poverty level. Children from households with an income below 135% of poverty can receive Free Meal Certification. Children from households with an income between 135% and 180% of poverty can receive Reduced Price Meal Certification.

Indian Taco Originally known as Navajo Tacos, but since Indian tribes other than the Navajo Nation have also adopted these as their own, they obtained the universal name of Indian Taco. Indian Tacos are a combination of beans or ground beef, chopped lettuce, sliced tomato, shredded cheddar cheese, and an optional green chile sitting atop plate-sized rounds of crispy Navajo or Indian Fry Bread. The Navajo Taco was voted the State Dish of Arizona in a 1995 poll conducted by the Arizona Republic newspaper. No plates or silverware are needed, as you just fill the fry bread with your desired fillings, roll it up, and then eat this delicious food. Eating Indian Tacos is considered very macho and requires some dedicated chewing.

Induction period The lag period during which a fat or oil shows stability to oxidation because of its content of antioxidants, natural or added, which are oxidized preferentially. After this there is a sudden and large consumption of oxygen and the fat becomes rancid.

Infant formula A breast-milk substitute, formulated industrially in accordance with national legislation or applicable Codex Alimentarius standards, that satisfies the normal nutritional requirements of infants up to between four and six months of age, and adapted to their physiological characteristics.

Inflammation Redness, swelling, pain, and/or a feeling of heat in an area of the body. This is a protective reaction to injury, disease, or irritation of the tissues.

Inflammatory bowel disease (IBD) A term that includes ulcerative colitis and Crohn's disease, marked by chronic inflammation and ulceration of the lining of the large intestine and/or the small intestine

Infuse To extract the flavour from herbs, spices, tea or coffee either by pouring on boiling water and allowing the water to take on the flavours before drinking hot, or by bringing the mixture to the boil and allowing it to cool.

Infusion An infusion is the flavor that's extracted from any ingredient such as tea leaves, herbs, or fruit by steeping them in a liquid such as water, oil, or vinegar.

Insalata The Italian word for "salad."

Insecticide Insecticides are a class of crop protection and specialty chemicals used to control insects on farms and forests, as well as non agricultural applications such as residential lawncare, golf courses and public tracts of land.

Inserted genes Genes introduced into the DNA of a recombinant organism which are not present at the same position in the DNA of the organism before genetic modification.

Insoluble fiber A type of dietary fiber found in wheat bran, cauliflower, cabbage and other vegetables and fruits which helps move foods through the digestive system and thereby may decrease the risks of cancers of the colon and rectum. Insoluble fiber may also help reduce the risk of breast cancer.

Institutional review board (IRB) In the U.S. a group of scientists, doctors, clergy, and consumers at each health care facility that participates in a clinical trial. IRBs are designed to protect study participants. They review and must approve the action plan for every clinical trial. They check to see that the trial is well designed, does not involve undue risks, and includes safeguards for patients.

Insufficient height Delay in growth in stature, when compared with the normal parameters for sex and age.

Insulin Insulin (from Latin insula, "island", as it is produced in the Islets of Langerhans in the pancreas) is a polypeptide hormone that regulates carbohydrate metabolism. Apart from being the primary effector in carbohydrate homeostasis, it has effects on fat metabolism and it can change the liver's ability to release fat stores. Insulin's concentration has extremely widespread effects throughout the body.

Integrated pest management (IPM) Integrated pest management is the coordinated use of pest and environmental information along with available pest control methods, including cultural, biological, genetic and chemical methods, to prevent unacceptable levels of pest damage using the most economical means, and with the least possible hazard to people, property and the environment.

Intentional food additives Those added to foods on purpose, such as the chemicals used to ensure longer shelf life or food colourings.

Interleukin Interleukins are a group of cytokines (secreted signaling molecules) that were first seen to be expressed by white blood cells (leukocytes, hence the -leukin) as a means of communication (inter-). The name is something of a relic though; it has since been found that interleukins are produced by a wide variety of bodily cells. The function of the immune system depends in a large part on interleukins, and rare deficiencies of a number of them have been described, all featuring autoimmune diseases or immune deficiency.

Internal validity Internal validity is a form of experimental validity 1.. An experiment is said to possess internal validity if it properly demonstrates a causal relation between two variables (2,3). An experiment can demonstrate a causal relation by satisfying three criteria: That the "cause" precedes the "effect" in time (temporal precedence), that the "cause" and the "effect" are related (covariation), and that there are no plausible alternative explanations for the observed covariation (nonspuriousness).

International code of marketing of breast-milk substitutes Also WHO CODE. Its aim is to contribute to safe and adequate nutrition for infants through the protection and promotion of breastfeeding and by ensuring the proper use of breast-milk substitutes, when needed, through adequate information and appropriate marketing and distribution.

Interstitial cystitis A long-lasting condition also known as painful bladder syndrome or frequency-urgency-dysuria syndrome. The wall of the bladder becomes inflamed or irritated, which affects the amount of urine the bladder can hold and causes scarring, stiffening, and bleeding in the bladder.

Intervention Anything meant to change the course of events for someone (e.g., drug, surgery, test, treatment, counseling, etc.)

Intervention trials Trials in which one or more factors that may affect health are altered, with the aim of demonstrating beneficial effects compared with a control group not receiving the intervention.

Intracellular In cell biology, molecular biology and related fields, the word intracellular means "inside the cell". It is used in contrast to extracellular (outside the cell). The cell membrane (and, in plants, the cell wall) is the barrier between the two, and chemical composition of intra- and extracellular milieu can be radically different. In most organisms, for example, a Na+/K+ ATPase maintains a high potassium level inside cells while keeping sodium low, leading to chemical excitability.

Intestinal permeability The barrier properties of the lining of the intestines, which prevent harmful substances from passing through into the body.

Intestinal pseudo-obstruction A motility disorder with symptoms like those of a bowel blockage, but with no physical evidence of blockage or obstruction. Symptoms may include cramps, stomach pain, nausea, vomiting, bloating, fewer bowel movements than usual, and loose stools.

Intestinal Relating to or occuring in the intestines.

Intestines Also known as the gut or bowels, is the long, tube-like organ in the human body that completes digestion or the breaking down of food. They consist of the small intestine and the large intestine.

Investigational In U.S. clinical trials, refers to a drug (including a new drug, dose, combination, or route of administration) or procedure that has undergone basic laboratory testing and received approval from the Food and Drug Administration (FDA) to be tested in human subjects. A drug or procedure may be approved by the FDA for use in one disease or condition, but be considered investigational in other diseases or conditions. Also called experimental.

Iodide A salt of the mineral iodine. iodine An essential mineral, a trace element; the reference intake is about 140 µg per day. Iodine is required for synthesis of the thyroid hormones, which are iodo-tyrosine derivatives. A prolonged deficiency of iodine in the diet leads to goitre.

Iodine is plentifully supplied by sea foods and by vegetables grown in soil containing iodide. In areas where the soil is deficient in iodide, locally grown vegetables are also iodide deficient, and hence goitre occurs in defined geographical regions, especially inland upland areas over limestone soil. Where deficiency is a problem, salt may be iodized to increase iodide intake.

Iodine Making thyroid hormones that control metabolism. Lobster, shrimp, bread, milk and iodized salt.

Ion An atom or group of atoms that has lost or gained one or more electrons, and thus has an electric charge. Positively charged ions are known as cations, because they migrate towards the cathode (negative pole) in solution, while negatively charged ions migrate towards the positive pole (anode) and hence are known as anions.

Irish coffee A coffee drink made from strong black coffee, sugar and Irish whiskey, topped with fresh whipped cream and sometimes garnished with a coffee bean. It's served in a warmed Irish coffee glass - a tall glass with a handle.

Iron An essential mineral. Iron is necessary for the transport of oxygen (via hemoglobin in red blood cells) and for oxidation by cells (via cytochrome). Deficiency of iron is a common cause of anemia. Food sources of iron include meat, poultry, eggs, vegetables and cereals (especially those fortified with iron). According to the National Academy of Sciences, the Recommended Dietary Allowances of iron are 15 milligrams per day for women and 10 milligrams per day for men. Iron overload can damage the heart, liver, gonads and other organs. Iron overload is a particular risk in people who may have certain genetic conditions (hemochromatosis) sometimes without knowing it and also in people receiving recurrent blood transfusions. Iron supplements meant for adults (such as pregnant women) are a major cause of poisoning in children.

Iron deficiency Organic state of micronutrient deficit that occurs when dietary onsumption of bioavailable iron is low, when blood losses are high or when requirement is increased due to infection or fever or, worse yet, when two or more of these conditions exist simultaneously, diminishing the body's stores of iron and resulting in the appearance of anemia.

Iron Making hemoglobin in blood and myoglobin in muscle, which supply oxygen to cells.

Irritable bowel syndrome A functional bowel disorder in which abdominal discomfort or pain is associated with defecation or a change in bowel habit, and with features of disordered defecation.

Ischemia In medicine, ischemia (Greek ισχαιμία, isch- is restriction, hema or haema is blood) is a restriction in blood supply, generally due to factors in the blood vessels, with resultant damage or dysfunction of tissue. It may also be spelled ischaemia or ischζmia.

ISDI The International Special Dietary Foods Industry is an international federation of industry associations that represents manufacturers of foods for special dietary purposes, including those intended for infants and young children. Its function is to represent the industry by developing common industry positions, to establish and maintain standards for special dietary foods, to act as industry spokesperson to UN agencies, and to communicate with consumer organizations. Members include regional, national and international special interest dietary associations as well as manufacturer's associations.

Isoflavones Daidzein, Genistein A type of phytoestrogen found in soybeans and soy based foods which may reduce menopause symptoms.

Isomerose Trade name of high-fructose corn syrup: 70-72% solids, 42% fructose, 55% glucose, 3% polysaccharides. See fructose syrups.

Isotonic Solutions with the same osmotic pressure (concentration of solids); often refers to a solution with the same osmotic pressure as body fluids. Hypertonic and hypotonic refer to solutions that are more and less concentrated.

J

Jalapeno pepper Named after Jalapa, the capital of Veracruz, Mexico, these smooth, dark green (scarlet red when ripe) have a rounded tip and are about 2 inches long and 3/4 to 1 inch in diameter. Although not as hot as other chile peppers, most people love the flavor this pepper has. Heat range is 3-6, depending on the variety. Besides their flavor, jalapenos are quite popular because they're so easily seeded (the seeds and veins are extremely hot). They're available fresh and canned and are used in a variety of sauces, sometimes stuffed with cheese, fish or meat, and in a multitude of dishes. In their dried form they are known as chipotles. Pickled, it is called cscabeche.

Jam A conserve of fruit boiled to a pulp with sugar; sets to a pectin jelly on cooling. (Known in the USA as jelly.) Standard jam, with certain exceptions, contains a minimum of 35 g of fruit per 100 g; extra jam, with certain exceptions, contains 45 g.

Jambalaya Jambalaya is a rich dish, which varies widely from cook to cook, but usually contains rice. It is said that Louisiana chefs "sweep up the kitchen" and toss just about everything into the pot for this rice dish that is highly seasoned and flavored with any combination of beef, pork, fowl, smoked sausage, ham, or seafood, as well as celery, green peppers and often tomatoes. Jambalaya, is the dish most obviously associated with the brief period of Spanish domination in New Orleans. Celestine Eustis, writing at the turn of the twentieth century, refers to it as a "Spanish Creole dish." It is now considered the hallmark of Cajun cuisine.

Jambon It is the French word for "ham" which consists of the hind leg of the pig, separated from the carcass at about the second joint of the vertebrae.

Jambonneau A French cut of the pork carcass that consists of a portion of the foreleg or a knuckle from the foreleg or hind leg that is cured and pickled or salted.

Jejunostomy (J-tube) A method of enteral feeding in which a tube is surgically placed in the small intestine.

Jejunum The portion of small intestine between the duodenum and the ileum

Jelly bean Historians seem to think that jelly beans were introduced between 1896 and 1905. It is believed the jelly centre is a descendent of a Mid-Eastern confection known as Turkish Delight that dates back to Biblical times. The shell coating is an offspring of a process called panning, first invented in 17th century France to make Jordan Almonds. The panning process, while done primarily by machine today, has remained essentially the same for the last 300 years. It wasn't until the 1930's that jelly beans became a part of Easter traditions. Jelly beans quickly earned a place among the many glass jars of "penny candy" in general stores where they were sold by weight and taken home in paper bags. It wasn't until the 1930's, however, that jelly beans became a part of Easter traditions.

Jerk A term used for an island style of barbecue that includes marinating the meat in a green pesto-like mixture of herbs, spices, and very hot peppers.

Jerk seasoning A spicy Jamaican seasoning used to marinate fish, pork, chicken, and beef. The mix includes a blend of chiles, allspice, thyme, and lime juice or rum. Some jerk mixtures (jerk rub) are thick and are rubbed over meats before cooking. Other blends have more liquid added so that they can be used for marinating and basting. The slaves used this method to preserve their meat.

Jerusalem artichoke It resembles the globe artichoke in flavor but is actually a member of the sunflower family. See artichoke.

Jicama It is also known as the Mexican potato. Jicama is a very firm, bulbous root vegetable that is brown on the outside with pearly white meat. It can be enjoyed either raw of cooked. It is slightly sweet to taste and it is very crunchy (it will remain so even after cooking). Great in salads and for using in dips.

Johnny cake Also called Jonny Cake. Johnny Cakes are the New England equivalent of the tortilla. The simplest recipes call for nothing but corn meal, boiling water, and a little salt. The batter should be fairly thin so that when fried on a hot griddle, the batter spreads out no more than a quarter of an inch thick. The origin of the name is something of a mystery and probably has nothing to do the name John. They also were called Journey Cakes because they could be carried on long trips in the traveler's saddlebags and baked along the way. There is some thought that they were originally called Shawnee Cake and the colonist slurred the words into Johnny Cake. Modern historians have also found that the word joniken, an American Indian word meaning corn cake could possible be the origin of the name. The settlers of New England learned how to make Johnny Cakes from the local Putexet Indians, who showed the starving Pilgrims how to grind and use corn for eating.

Jo-Jo Potatoes Potatoes cut into thick wedges then seasoned (sometimes breaded) and deep-fried. Often served with broasted chicken.

Julienne To cut food into thin sticks which are also called matchsticks. Food is cut with a knife or mandoline into even slices, then into strips. French chef Jean Julien is said to have introduced the "julienne" method or preparing vegetables.

Juniper berries The darkish berries of the juniper tree provide one of the main flavourings for gin. These spicy, aromatic berries are also used, fresh or dried, crushed or whole, to flavour casseroles, marinades and stuffings. They are a good complement to pork - especially pork pβtιs - as well as rabbit, beef and duck. They can also be used in sweet dishes such as fruitcake.

Jus This French word is roughly the equivalent of 'juice', but it has more specific meanings in cookery, referring either to the juices that occur during the cooking process (in particular when roasting meat) or the juice squeezed from raw vegetables or fruit.

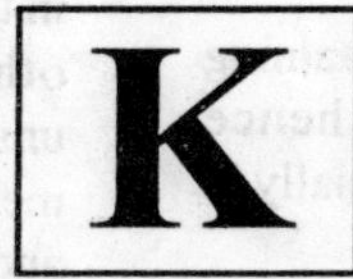

Kabinett German and Austrian wine classification, used for highquality wines. In earlier years monastic wine producers used to set aside their best wine in a special cupboard or small room (the kabinett).

Kale Scottish name for any type of cabbage; in England it means specifically open-headed varieties of cabbage with curly leaves, also known as curly kale or borecole. Distinct from sea kale or Swiss chard.

Kalia Polish; chicken broth flavoured with juice from pickled cucumbers and garnished with diced chicken, celery root, parsley root, and carrots.

Karo syrup Trade name for a dextromaltose preparation made from maize starch, used as carbohydrate modifier in milk preparations for infant feeding. Consists of a mixture of dextrin, maltose, glucose, and sucrose.

Kataifi Greek; pastry in thin strands; the dough is squeezed through a perforated disc onto a hot metal plate, on which it is dried in long strands. Also the name for rolls made from these pastry strands, filled with chopped nuts and sugar, baked and served drenched with syrup.

Katemfe The Sierra Leone name for an intensely sweet African fruit, Thaumatococcus daniellii; also known as the miraculous fruit of Sudan (not the same as miracle berry). The active principle is a protein named thaumatin.

Kebab A kebab is essentially small chunks of meat threaded onto a skewer and grilled or cooked over coals. Kebabs can be served on their own with dips or sauces, with rice, or removed from the skewer and used to stuff an open pitta bread.

Kebabs are part of the culinary tradition of the Caucasus, the Middle East, the Indian subcontinent and other parts of Asia, as well as numerous other cuisines. Vegetables can be used instead of or as well as meat. Kebabs are particularly good for barbecuing because you can satisfy all kinds of tastes on a single skewer from veggie kebabs to chicken, lamb, beef or fruit.

A kofta kebab is made using flavoured, minced meat that is formed in a long sausage shape around the skewer. A doner kebab is thin slices of marinated lamb packed tightly onto a revolving vertical spit to form a solid mass from which slices of meat are cut off the outside as it browns and used to fill an open pitta bread along with salad and hot sauce.

Kedgeree Traditional British breakfast dish, originally from India and probably a corruption of the Hindustani name 'khichri', a favourite Indian dish. The British version is different from the Indian version and is made with rice, cooked and flaked smoked haddock, hard-boiled eggs, garam masala and turmeric, which gives the dish its characteristic sunshine yellow colour.

Kelp Large brown seaweeds of the genus Laminaria. Occasionally used as food or food ingredient but mostly the ash is used as a source of alkali and iodine. Sometimes claimed as a health food with unspecified properties.

Kephalins Or cephalins; phospholipids containing ethanolamine, hence phosphatidylethanolamines. Found especially in brain and nerve tissue.

Kepler extract of malt Trade name for one of the earliest of the malt extracts, intended as a dietary supplement and to aid the digestion, since it was rich in diastase compared with ordinary malt extracts.

Keratin The insoluble protein of hair, horn, hoofs, feathers, and nails. Not hydrolysed by digestive enzymes, and therefore nutritionally useless. Used as fertilizer, since it is slowly broken down by soil bacteria. Steamed feather meal is used to some extent as a supplement for ruminants.

Keshy yena Caribbean; baked Edam or Gouda cheese with a variety of fillings. The name derives from the Spanish queso relleno, stuffed cheese.

Ketchup Often called catsup in the US, this thick, slightly sweet and spicy sauce is a traditional American accompaniment for French fries, hamburgers and many other foods. It's usually made from tomatoes, vinegar, sugar and spices, but other flavours such as mushroom ketchup or various fruit ketchups are available.

It's sold in glass or plastic squeezy bottles and, as well as being used as a condiment, can be an ingredient in its own right - in homemade barbecue sauce, for example.

Ketone bodies Acetoacetate, [í-hydroxybutyrate and acetone; acetoacetate and acetone are chemically ketones; although íhydroxybutyrate is not, it is included in the term ketone bodies because of its metabolic relationship with acetoacetate.

In the fasting state (from about 4 hours after a meal), fatty acids are mobilized from adipose tissue as a metabolic fuel. Most tissues have only a limited capacity for fatty acid oxidation; however, the liver can oxidize more than is required for its own metabolic needs. Acetoacetate and í-hydroxybutyrate are formed from fatty acids in the liver, and are transported in the bloodstream for use as metabolic fuels by other tissues. Acetoacetate is chemically unstable and breaks down to acetone, which is metabolically useless, and is excreted in the urine and on the breath.

Ketones Chemical compounds containing a carbonyl group (C=O), with two alkyl groups attached to the same carbon; the simplest ketone is acetone (dimethylketone, $(CH_3)_2$ -C=O).

Ketonic rancidity Certain moulds of the genera Penicillium and Aspergillus species attack fats containing short-chain fatty acids and produce ketones with a characteristic odour and taste, so-called ketonic rancidity. Fats such as butter, coconut, and palm kernel are most susceptible.

Key lime A tart, golf-ball size, and yellow-green citrus fruit that is native to Southern Florida. The juice is yellow and very tart, more so than standard limes. They grow in Florida, the Keys and other tropical places in the Caribbean. Key lime is used in making Key Lime Pie. The key lime tree, which is native to Malaysia, probably first arrived in the Florida Keys in the 1500s with the Spanish. Key limes look like confused lemons, as they are smaller than a golf ball with yellow-green skin that is sometimes splotched with brown. They are also know as Mexican or West Indian limes. When a hurricane in 1926 wiped out the key lime plantations in South Florida, growers replanted with Persian limes, which are easier to pick and to transport. Today the key lime is almost a phantom and any remaining trees are only found in back yards and their fruit never leave the Florida Keys. Key limes are also grown for commercial use in the Miami area.

Kidney One of a pair of organs located in the right and left side of the abdomen which clear "poisons" from the blood, regulate acid concentration and maintain water balance in the body by excreting urine. The kidneys are part of the urinary tract. The urine then passes through connecting tubes called "ureters" into the bladder. The bladder stores the urine until it is released during urination.

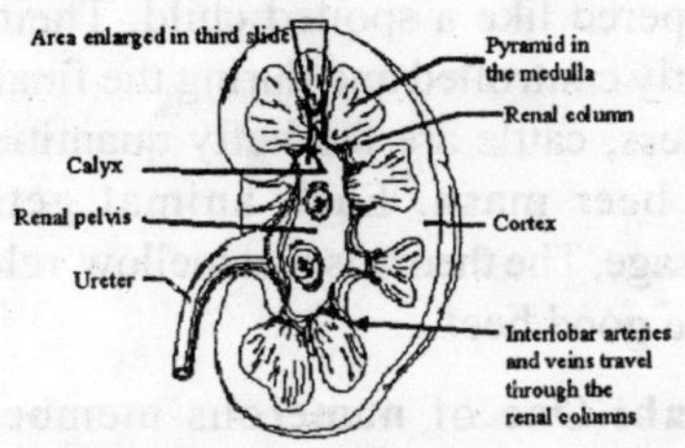

Fig. Regions and Structure of Kideny

Kids cafe A program operated by America's Second Harvest that aims to provide free and prepared food and nutrition education to hungry children. Through the Kids Caft program, food banks and food rescue organizations coordinate with community service organizations that serve children. Some Kids Cafes utilize CACFP to provide food.

Kinilaw Cuisine Kinilaw cuisine is a true Philippine cuisine wiuh influences as far back as pre-colonial times with trans-Pacific trade and exchanges of culture. Later in the 16th century, a strong link with Europe and South America through Spanish colonists had the most tremendous impact on today's Philippine cuisine. This marriage of culinary heritages must be described and considered as a real "fusion cuisine." Regardless of the origin, over the centuries dishes have been transformed, added and changed in so many ways to what has become today's Philippine cuisine. Anything alive and anything fresh can be used for Kinilaw cuisine (crustaceans, fish, meat, vegetables, fruit, flowers, insects, fowl, and snakes; food as rare and unusual as balatan (sea cucumber), lima lima (spider conch), kohol (river snail), abatud (larva of coconut beetle), butbut (sea anemone), guso (seaweed) goat, dog, carabao, venison, wild boar, heart, liver, tripe, animal skin, puso ng saging (banana core) and uncountable other ingredients).

Kipper To kipper means to cure, usually fish, by cleaning, salting and drying or smoking. It also means a male salmon during or shortly after spawning. When a herring is kippered it is first butterflies, cured in brine, and then cold smoked. It has a Smokey, salty flavor and is usually given an artificial golden colour. When a salmon is kippered in the U.S. it is a chunk, steak or fillet of salmon soaked in brine, hot smoked and dyed red. In Europe a split salmon is soaked in brine and cold smoked.

Kippered herring Also called kippers. These are herrings that have been split down the middle and cold-smoked in a solution of brine.

Kirsch From the German 'kirsch' meaning cherry, this is a clear liqueur distilled from cherries and their almond-flavoured stones, often used in sponge cakes, for macerating and to flavour dishes containing fruit. It's often added to fondue and is used in the dish cherries Jubilee - poached cherries flambıed with kirscl..

Kitchen bouquet It is the brand name of a concentrated browning and seasoning sauce. Small amounts of it can be added to gravy to enrich its flavor and enhance its colour. It can also be used to enhance the colour of microwave foods, which don't normally brown. There are other brands on the market, which accomplish the same thing.

Kiwifruit or kiwi fruit The kiwifruit (Actinidia Deliciosa) belongs to the berry family of fruits. It's about the size of a large egg, and is covered by a brown, fuzzy skin. The fruit's rough exterior gives no hint of the beauty within. The inside of a kiwi is bright green, with a yellow centre, dotted by small, black seeds. It is a native of China where it was called Yang Tao. It was introduced into New Zealand in 1906 and has been commercially cultivated there ever since. New Zealanders called the vines Chinese gooseberries, for the original fruit was small, prickly, with a distinctive but unrefined taste. It took more than 40 years to develop the fruit of today. To aid marketing, the name was changed to kiwifruit (this established the fruit as an exotic fruit internationally). This name not only identifies New Zealand but also describes the appearance of a New Zealand native, the tiny Kiwi bird.

Knead The process of working dough by mixing, stretching, and pulling. Kneading is most often used in bread dough, and is a necessary step in order to develop the gluten. To knead, gather your dough into a ball. Using the heel of your hands, press down on the dough. Pull up the part of the dough that was flattened by your hands and fold it back over on itself. Keep repeating the process, turning the dough periodically.

Knee height The distance from the top of the patella to the bottom of the foot; sometimes used as an estimator of stature

Knish The knish is a pastry of Jewish origin consisting of a piece of dough that encloses a filling of seasoned mashed potatoes. Basically they are a mashed potato pie. When sold by the street corner vendors in New York City, they are fried and square shaped. The baked ones are usually round shaped, and are usually made at home and some knish bakeries. Eastern European Jews developed the knish. During the early 1900s, when hundreds of thousands of Eastern European Jews Emigrated to America and settled in New York City, they brought with them their family recipes for knishes. Knishes were made at home until Yonah Schimmel, a rabbi from Romania, began to sell them at Coney Island in New York City, and also from a pushcart on the Lower East Side. In 1910, he opened his original knish bakery located on East Houston Street.

Kobe beef Kobe beef is considered the most exclusive beef in the world. Technically speaking, there's no such thing as Kobe beef, it is merely the shipping point for beef from elsewhere in Japan. What is called "Kobe beef" comes from the ancient province of Tajima, now named Hyogo Prefecture, of which Kobe is the capital. Real beef connoisseurs, however, still refer to it as Tajima beef. This beef comes from an ancient stock of cattle called "kuroge wagyu" (black haired Japanese cattle). Today they are raised on only 262 small farms, most of which pasture fewer than five cows, and the largest of which run only 10 to 15 animals. Each animal is pampered like a spoiled child. Their diets are strictly controlled and during the final fattening process, cattle are fed hefty quantities of sake and beer mash. Each animal gets a daily massage. The theory is that mellow, relaxed cows make good beef.

Kohlrabi One of numerous members of the brassica family, a pale green or purple, bulb-shaped vegetable that tastes a bit like a mild turnip. It's grown more for its bulb-like stem than for its greens leaves, although these can be eaten too if they're attached when you buy it. Kohlrabi can be substituted for turnip in any recipe, and is good steamed or boiled, sliced and stir-fried and added to stews or soups.

Kosher food The word kosher means "fit or proper." It refers to food that is proper for the Jewish people to consume as set out in the laws of Kashrut (the kosher dietary laws) in the Old Testament. It is against the law for Jewish people to eat blood of mats that have been cooked with milk or with anything derived from milk.

Kosher salt A pure, refined rock salt used for pickling because it does not contain magnesium carbonate (because it does not cloud brine solutions). Also used to kosher items. Also known as coarse salt or pickling salt.

Kosher The selection and preparation of foods in accordance with traditional Jewish ritual and dietary laws. Foods that are not kosher are traife.

The only kosher flesh foods are from animals that chew the cud and have cloven hoofs, such as cattle, sheep, goats, and deer; the hindquarters must not be eaten. The only fish permitted are those with fins and scales; birds of prey and scavengers are not kosher. Moreover, the animals must be slaughtered according to ritual before the meat can be considered kosher. From Hebrew kosher, right (Deut. 14: 3-21). kosher for Passover See Passover.

Koulibiac Also spelled 'coulibiac', this is a Russian pie filled with fish, vegetables, rice and hard-boiled eggs. European cooks have adapted and varied the recipe in many ways, making it with brioche dough or puff pastry and filling it with various additions such as chicken and mushrooms, onions, parsley and shallots. Salmon koulibiac is especially popular. It's a handy dish for entertaining because it can be made in advance and left in the fridge covered in cling film until you're ready to warm it in the oven.

Kringle Kringles are hand-rolled circular, butter-layered Danish pastry that enclose a fruit or nut layer, and topped with sugar icing.

Kugel It is a baked pudding, in the style of the British puddings, as opposed to a light dessert such as rice or chocolate pudding. Koogel actually means "ball" or "cannonball" in German. It came to have this name because of the small round pot in which such puddings used to be cooked. This round, covered pot would be placed in the larger pot of cholent, a slow-cooking stew of chunks of meat, marrow bones, beans, barley, potatoes and the like.

Classic ones are made with noodles or grains (sometimes even leftover bread). They often have a sweet ingredient such as raisins or apples, but some are savory. Today, they are even made with a variety of vegetables in a style reminiscent of quiche or casseroles. What is characteristic of all of them, though, is that they are made without water, using fats and/or eggs to bind the ingredients, and they still are capable of being either slow-cooked or of being kept warm on a warming plate.

Kumquat A small citrus fruit originating in central China but now cultivated in the Far East, Australia and America. Kumquats - sometimes called Chinese oranges - can be eaten whole, including the skin, or used for pickling and preserves. They're as sharp in taste as lemons. Choose small, shiny fruits. Wash and eat them whole, poach them in sugar syrup and serve with ice cream, or use in a fruit salad. They're particularly good in stuffings for poultry.

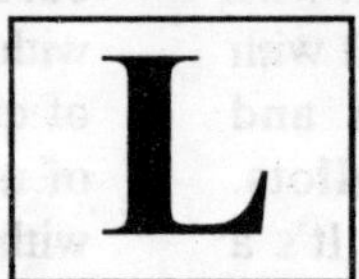

Laboratory study Research done in a laboratory. These studies may use test tubes or animals to find out if a drug, procedure, or treatment is likely to be useful. Laboratory studies take place before any testing is done in humans.

Laboratory test A medical procedure that involves testing a sample of blood, urine, or other substance from the body. Tests can help determine a diagnosis, plan treatment, check to see if treatment is working, or monitor the disease over time.

Lactase The enzyme that hydrolyses lactose to glucose and galactose; normally present in the brush border of the intestinal mucosal cells; deficiency of lactase is alactasia, leading to lactose intolerance.

Lactation The process of synthesizing and secreting milk from the breasts.

Lactic acid, buffered A mixture of lactic acid and sodium lactate used in sugar confectionery to provide an acid taste without inversion of the sugar, which occurs at lower pH.

Lactobacillus A type of prebiotic/probiotic found in yogurt and some other dairy products which may improve gastrointestinal health.

Lactoferrin Iron-protein complex in human milk (only a trace in cow's milk), only partly saturated with iron; has a rτle inhibiting the growth of E. coli and other potentially pathogenic organisms.

Lactometer Floating device used to measure the specific gravity of milk.

Lac-tone Trade name; protein-rich baby food (26% protein) made in India from peanut flour, skim milk powder, wheat flour, and barley flour, with added vitamins and calcium.

Lactose A sugar naturally occurring in milk, also known as "milk sugar," that is the least sweet of all natural sugars and used in baby formulas and candies.

Fig. Lactose

Lactose intolerance Lactose intolerance is an inherited inability to properly digest dairy products, due to a deficiency in the amount of the enzyme, ί galactosidase in the small intestine. This enzyme is necessary for the hydrolysis of lactose (a disaccharide) into its constituent monosaccharides, glucose and galactose. Symptoms of lactose intolerance, including abdominal cramps, flatulence and frothy diarrhea, can increase with age.

Lactose intolerance Lactose intolerance is an inherited inability to properly digest dairy products, due to a deficiency in the amount of the enzyme, β-galactosidase in the small intestine. This enzyme is necessary for the hydrolysis of lactose (a disaccharide) into its constituent monosaccharides, glucose and galactose. Symptoms of lactose intolerance, including abdominal cramps, flatulence and frothy diarrhea, can increase with age.

Lactospore LACTOSPORE is a lactic acid bacillus preparation manufactured and distributed by the SABINSA CORPORATION. The following link reviews the background, nutritional and therapeutic aspects and current status of the use of lactic acid bacillus preparations, and presents arguments for the superiority of LACTOSPORE over other such products in the market, known as "probiotics", used in microbiotherapy.

Lactulose A disaccharide of galactose and fructose which does not occur naturally but is formed in heated or stored milk by isomerization of lactose. About half as sweet as sucrose. Not hydrolysed by human digestive enzymes but fermented by intestinal bacteria to form lactic and pyruvic acids. Thought to promote the growth of Lactobacillus bifidus and so added to some infant formulae; in large amounts it is laxative. Because of the bacterial fermentation, it is also used to acidify the colon and hence prevent the absorption of ammonia in patients with liver failure. See also lactitol.

Ladies' fingers An alternative name (because of its appearance) for okra, an ingredient that's widely used in Indian, Middle Eastern, Caribbean and southern US cookery where it's an essential ingredient in gumbo.

A long green pod with a slightly fuzzy skin, it's full of edible creamy seeds. Okra exudes a glutinous juice in cooking which thickens stews and braised dishes. It's not as popular in the UK as elsewhere but is usually available in supermarkets and grocers. Choose stems that snap cleanly and don't bend.

Okra can be eaten raw in salads or cooked with curries or vegetable stews - add a handful of chopped okra to a ratatouille.

Lagniappe Used primarily in southern Louisiana and southeast Texas, the word lagniappe refers to an "unexpected something extra." It could be an additional doughnut (as in "baker's dozen"), a free "one for the road" drink, and an unanticipated tip for someone who provides a special service or possibly a complimentary dessert for a regular customer. Creole term for something extra.

Lamb (French: agneau; German: Lammfleisch.) Meat from sheep (Ovis aries) younger than 12-14 months. A 150-g portion is a rich source of protein, niacin, iron, zinc, copper, and vitamin B 12; a good source of vitamins B 1, B 2, and B 6; different cuts contain up to 30 g of fat of which half is saturated; supplies 400-600 kcal (1700-2500 kJ).

Lamb's lettuce Or corn salad, a hardy annual plant, Valerianella locusta or V. olitoria used in salads in winter and early spring. A 50-g portion is a rich source of vitamins A (as carotene) and C; supplies 5 kcal (20 kJ).

Lamington or lemmington The word lamington means layers of beaten gold. An Australian dessert of little cubes or squares of sponge cake, dipped in chocolate, then rolled in coconut. In Victoria (State of Australia) they often add a layer of raspberry or plum jam. They are served with tea in the afternoon. Lamington's are so popular in Australia that the cakes are a favourite means of raising money for school groups, church's, and scouts and girl guides. These money making adventure are called Lamington Drives.

Langoustine The French name for the Dublin Bay prawn (which isn't actually a prawn at all, but a small lobster, Nephrops norvegicus). It's also known as Norway lobster and is sometimes called scampi. (Scampi has also become a widely used name referring to tail pieces of prawn that are dipped in batter and deep-fried.).

Langoustines are available fresh or frozen, in and out of their shells. If bought fresh, cook them by boiling or grilling. You're more likely to find fresh ones in good fishmongers and although they're pricey, they're delicious.

Language access The ability of LEP individuals to receive the benefits and services of government programs. To comply with recent federal guidance, administrators of food and nutrition programs can make benefit programs accessible by employing bilingual staff, making available interpreter services, and translating and printing applications and notices in a variety of languages.

Laparoscopy The insertion of a thin, lighted tube (called a laparoscope) through the abdominal wall to inspect the inside of the abdomen and remove tissue samples.

Larch gum A polysaccharide of galactose and arabinose (ratio of 1: 6), found in the aqueous extract of the Western larch tree (Larix occidentalis); a potential substitute for gum arabic, since it is readily dispersed in water.

Lard compounds Blends of animal fats, such as oleostearin or premier jus, with vegetable oils, to produce products similar to lard in consistency and texture. See also lard substitutes.

Lard Lard is the layer of fat located along the back and underneath the skin of the hog. Hog-butchers prepare it during the slaughtering process and preserve it in salt. In Italy it is used mainly (either minced or in whole pieces) to prepare various kinds of sauces and soups, to cook vegetables and legumes, or to lard beef or poultry. In order to remove any excess of salt, lard should be blanched by placing it in cold water, bringing it to a boil and then letting it cool entirely under cold running water.

Lardons Lardons are small, chunky cubes of bacon (smoked or unsmoked) used to flavour dishes such as quiches. They can also be fried and scattered in salads. They're often sweated with onions as a base for soups or stews. They give a good salty depth of flavour to robust dishes such as coq au vin.

They're sold vacuum-packed in most supermarkets, but if you can't find them then thick rashers of bacon cut into dice will do. They will keep in the fridge for about three days.

Large intestine The long, tube-like organ that is connected to the small intestine at one end and the anus at the other. The large intestine has four parts cecum, colon, rectum, and anal canal. Partly digested food moves through the cecum into the colon, where water and some nutrients and electrolytes are removed. The remaining material, solid waste called stool, moves through the colon, is stored in the rectum, and leaves the body through the anal canal and anus.

Lasagna, lasagne 1. Pasta in flat, very wide strips that is almost always used in baked dishes.

2. A dish made by baking such pasta with layers of sauce and fillings such as cheese or meat. Like many things, the origins of pasta and how lasagna was first made are lost in the mists of prehistory. We can only assume that pasta was "invented" by the peoples living in the Mediterranean area some time after our ancestors had learned to cultivate cereals and to grind them into flour. However, the origins of "macaroni" in Italy go back as far as the time of the Ancient Romans who gave the credit to the 'Gods'. Some historians say that "maccheroni" is derived from the Sicilian word "maccarruni" meaning "made into a dough by force." Other historians think the word "lasagne" came from the Greek "lasanon," a chamber pot. The Romans adopted the word for any cooking pot; lasagne is the pasta dish cooked in the lasanum.

Lasagne Rectangular sheets of Italian pasta, about the size of a standard envelope. The baked dish that incorporates them is also called lasagne and is usually prepared with alternate layers of Bolognese sauce, lasagne sheets and bіchamel sauce, topped with grated Parmesan cheese and baked in the oven until browned.

Lasagne can be made with many different fillings, such as roasted vegetables, spinach, aubergine, fish or chicken. A simple tomato sauce could be used in place of bichamel or different cheeses can be grated on top.

There are various types of lasagne sheets to choose from - the simplest is made from durum wheat semolina and water. Lasagne all'uovo is made with eggs and is slightly ridged. Lasagne verde is made with spinach and is dark green in colour. Lasagne sheets are available fresh, semi-fresh or dried and some need to be pre-cooked in boiling water for a few minutes before baking, so it's best to follow the packet instructions to get it right.

Lassi A traditional Indian drink that used to be made from buttermilk poured into earthenware crocks, with salt added to help combat dehydration in the hot climate. It's now made from thin yoghurt, often sweetened with sugar or rosewater or sometimes spiced with cumin. To make your own, dilute plain yogurt, with water or milk, add salt or sugar to taste, then blend vigorously with crushed ice.

Lavender To learn about Lavender, check out Linda Stradley's web page on Lavender.

Laver Edible seaweed. Laver bread is made from the seaweed Porphyra spp., by boiling in salted water and mincing to a gelatinous mass. It is made into a cake with oatmeal or fried. Locally known in S. Wales as bara lawr.

Laxative Or aperient, a substance that helps the expulsion of food residues from the body. If 'strongly' laxative it is termed purgative or cathartic. Dietary fibre and cellulose function because they retain water and add bulk to the contents of the intestine; Epsom salts (magnesium sulphate) also retain water; castor oil and drugs such as aloes, senna, cascara, and phenolphthalein irritate the intestinal mucosa.

Lead A mineral of no nutritional interest, since it is not known to have any function in the body. It is toxic and its effects are cumulative. May be present in food from traces naturally present in the soil; as contamination of vegetables grown near main roads, which absorb volatile lead compounds from car exhaust fumes; from shellfish that have absorbed it from seawater; from lead glazes on cooking vessels; and in drinking water where lead pipes are used. Traces are excreted in the urine.

Leaf Lard is made from the residue of kidney and back fat after the preparation of neutral lard by heating with water above 100 °C in an autoclave. Prime Steam Lard is fat from any part of the carcass, rendered in the autoclave.

Leathers, fruit (Mango leathers, tomato leathers, etc.). Fruit purıes dried in air in thin layers, 4-5 mm thick, then built up into thicker preparations.

Lebkuchen German, Swiss; gingerbread, often baked in carved moulds, traditionally eaten at Christmas.

Lecithin A by product of the refining for soybean oil and is also found in eggs, red meats, spinach and nuts. Historically, lecithin has been used commercially in food processing as an emulsifier, instantizing agent and lubricating agent. Lecithin is a source of choline when digested; and is a critical component of the lipoproteins which transport fat and cholesterol molecules in the blood stream. Lecithin (choline) promotes synthesis of high density lipoproteins (i.e., HDLP also know as "good" cholesterol) by the liver, when it is consumed by humans.

Lectins Proteins from legumes and other sources which bind to the carbohydrates found at cell surfaces. They therefore cause red blood cells to agglutinate in vitro, hence the old names haemagglutinins and phytoagglutinins.

Raw or undercooked beans of some varieties of Phaseolus vulgaris (red kidney beans) cause vomiting and diarrhoea within 2 hours of consumption due to the high level of lectins, but they are rapidly inactivated by boiling.

Leg In popular usage, the leg extends from the top of the thigh down to the foot. However, in medical terminology, the leg refers to the portion of the lower extremity from the knee to the ankle.

Legumes Members of the family Leguminosae eaten by man and domestic animals. Consumed as dry mature seeds (grain legumes or pulses) or as immature green seeds in the pod. On boiling, the dried seeds double in weight, so a 100-g cooked portion is approximately 50 g as a dried product.

Legumes include the groundnut Arachis hypogaea, and soya bean, Glycine max, grown for their oil and protein, the yam bean Pachyrrhizus erosus, and African yam bean Sphenostylis stenocarpa, grown for their edible tubers as well as seeds.

Lemon Very sharp, acidic citrus fruit with a shiny yellow skin and sour but zingy flavour. Lemons are rich in vitamin C but with a low sugar content. They're available all year round and used in both sweet and savoury dishes.

The aromatic zest or outer rind and juice can be used in marinades, to flavour drinks such as lemonade, in marmalade, chutneys, pickles and a wide variety of desserts, such as mousses, syllabubs, soufflıs, cakes, pies and tarts - lemon meringue pie and tarte au citron, for instance.

Lemon is a good accompaniment to fish and can also be used in place of vinegar as a salad dressing. The zest is often incorporated into stuffings for meat and Moroccan preserved lemons can be used to flavour stews.

Lemons can be bought waxed or unwaxed. Choose unwaxed lemons if you're using the zest or adding slices to drinks or using as a garnish. Waxed are fine if you're just using the juice. If you can't buy unwaxed then a good scrub with a vegetable brush will remove most traces of wax. Use a potato peeler or a zester to remove the rind, taking care not to remove any of the white pith with the zest, because it's very bitter.

Lemon balm As its name suggests, this leafy, green herb has a lemony flavour and fragrance. It works well with fish, poultry and vegetables as well as in salads, stuffings and drinks. It's a member of the mint family and makes a very refreshing infusion or tea. Only buy it fresh, however, because it loses virtually all of its flavour when dried.

Lemon curd Cooked mixture of sugar, butter, eggs, and lemons. Legally (UK regulations) must contain 4% fat, 0.33% citric acid, 1% dried egg or equivalent, 0.125% oil of lemon or 0.25% oil of orange, and not less than 65% soluble solids.

Lemon Drop Martini In large west coast cities, especially San Francisco, the Lemon Drop Martini is the popular drink, a lemon drink that is truly reminiscent of the childhood candy. It is sometimes known as adult lemonade. This addictive drink is a mixture of fresh lemon juice, vodka, sweet vermouth or Triple Sec, sugar, and served ice cold in a sugar-rimmed martini glass. This drink came into vogue during the 1970s and was developed at a now defunct bar called Henry Africa's in San Francisco, a well known singles" bar. Since it was basically a singles bar that catered to single men and women, they developed and pushed "girl drinks." They are drinks that are potent, but sweet enough to cover the taste of alcohol. It is felt that it was named after the candy, lemon drops, of the same name.

Lemongrass It is also known as citronella. Lemongrass is native to Malaysia and grown throughout Southeast Asia and California. It is a stiff tropical grass that resembles a large fibrous green onion (the stalks are too tough to eat buy when simmered in liquid, they impart a distinctive fragrance and taste). It is an essential herb in southeast Asian cooking. It adds a lemony flavor to dishes.

Lentil These are tiny bean-like seeds. They are one of the first plants used for foods. The Egyptians and Greeks cooked these small legumes and so did the Romans. Pliny, the Roman naturalist, recommended them as a food that produced mildness and moderation of temper.

LEP Limited English Proficient. Individuals who do not speak English as their primary language and who have a limited ability to read, speak, write or understand English are described as

LEP. Executive Order 13166 says that LEP individuals should have meaningful access to federally conducted and federally funded programs and activities.

Leukotrienes Chemical mediators of the inflammatory response, released by various white blood cells and by mast cells.

Liaison The process of thickening a sauce, soup, or stew. This is a mixture of cream and egg yolks that is used to thicken soups and sauces. Egg yolks must be tempered with hot liquid before adding to the liquid in order to prevent curdling. This process is also referred to as a "binder."

Licorice Its botanical name is Glycyrrhiza, from the Greek meaning "sweet root." The taste of the licorice root is so distinctive that its sweetness is detectable in water even when diluted to 1 part licorice to 20,000 parts water. Licorice has a long and honourable history in the service of mankind. The earliest usage of Licorice was back in the first syllables of recorded time. Licorice freaks throughout history have included Pharaohs and Prophets. Men discovered generous supplies in KingTut's tomb, while Egyptian hieroglyphics record the use of Licorice in a popular beverage in the days when the Bible was still being written! Alexander the Great, the Scythian armies, Roman Emperor Caesar, and even India's great prophet, Brahma, are on record endorsing the beneficial properties contained in Licorice. Warriors used it for its ability to quench thirst while on the march, while others (including Brahma and venerable Chinese Buddhist sages), recognized Licorice's valuable healing properties. Natural licorice can be effective medicine. For over 3000 years, licorice root has been used as a remedy for peptic ulcers, sore throats and coughs in eastern and western medicine. Licorice root has been used since the third century BC to help dissipate coughs.

Liederkrantz cheese It is a semi-soft aromatic cow's milk cheese created by New York cheese maker, Emil Frey, in 1882. This cheese is most commonly enjoyed with beer, dark bread, and onions. Borden Foods purchased the trademark and is its sole producer.

Life expectancy Life expectancy is heavily dependent on the criteria used to select the group. In countries with high infant mortality rates, the life expectancy at birth is highly sensitive to the rate of death in the first few years of life. In these cases, another measure such as life expectancy at age 5 (e5) can be used to exclude the effects of infant mortality to reveal the effects of other causes of death. Typically, life expectancy at birth is specified. If the data on infant mortality rates are suspect for some reason, such as the underreporting of births or of infant deaths, then life expectancy at age 1 (e1) or age 2 (e2) might also be used.

Light (or lite) As applied to foods usually indicates:

1. a lower content of fat compared with the standard product (e.g. breadspreads, sausages);

2. Sodium chloride substitutes lower in sodium (see salt, light);

3. Low-alcohol beer or wine. US legislation restricts the term 'light' to modified foods that contain one-third less energy or half the fat of a reference unmodified food, or to indicate that the sodium content of a low-fat, low-calorie food has been reduced by half. See also fat-free; free from; low in; reduced.

Lignans A type of phytoestrogen found in flax, rye and various vegetables which may provide the health benefits of lowering LDL cholesterol, total cholesterol and triglycerides thereby protecting against heart disease and some cancers.

Lillet French light vermouth made from red or white Bordeaux wines in which fruit peel and herbs are steeped; aged in oak casks.

Lima beans Lima beans come in two varieties; the Fordhook and the baby lima. The Fordhook is meatier and fatter than the baby limas with has a bolder flavor. Fresh limas can be found sometimes in June, July, and August. They should be shelled just before using.

Limbic system A network of brain regions involved in the regulation of the function of internal organs, emotions, and the maintenance of homeostasis.

Limburger cheese Limburger is a semi soft, surface-ripened cheese with a characteristic strong flavor and aroma. It was first made in the Province of Luttich, Belgium and is named for the town of Limburger, where originally much of it was marketed.

Lime This small, green citrus fruit is used mainly for its juice. It can be added to savoury dishes, as in Asian cuisine, curries in particular. It has a stronger, more sour taste than lemon. Lime juice and zest can be used in marinades and salsas or just squeezed over finished dishes. It's used in ceviche to effectively 'cook' the raw fish.

It's used in cocktails such as the mojito (fresh mint and whole limes crushed together with sugar syrup, angostura bitters, rum, ice and soda), rum punch and margarita. Key lime pie is a famous dessert from Florida where a special variety of limes called Key limes are used to make it - though standard limes are fine if you want to try our recipe below!

Lime leaves Sometimes called kaffir lime leaves, these are the leaves of a wild lime tree which have an unusual figure-of-eight shape - double leaves joined tip to end. They have a spicy, lemon flavour and give a distinctive citrus scent to soups and curries in Thai and Indonesian cooking. They're used in Asian cooking in a similar way that bay leaf is used in Western cooking - pretty much thrown in to all kinds of dishes! They're becoming more widely available, fresh and dried, but substitute lemongrass if you can't find them.

Limoncello Limoncello is the generic name for an Italian citrus-based lemon liqueur that is served well chilled in the summer months. An absolute natural product acquired by the infusion of lemon skins in pure alcohol. It has become Italy's second most popular drink after Campari. It is wonderful as a palate cleanser or as an after dinner drinks. Keep your bottles of Limoncello in the freezer until ready to serve. The ingredients are simple and few, and making a batch doesn't require much work, but you'll need some time. In most recipes, Limoncello must steep for (80) eighty days. It has long been a staple in the lemon-producing region along the Italian Amalfi Coast in Capri and Sorrento. The Amalfi Coast is known for its citrus groves and narrow winding roads. Authentic Limoncello is made from Sorrento lemons, which come from the Amalfi Coast. Families in Italy have passed down recipes for this for generations, as every Italian family has their own Limoncello recipe.

Linguine A flattened spaghetti-like pasta. It's best served with a medium-thick sauce which will cling to the thin strands well. Cream-based sauces go well with linguine and it's often served with seafood. Allow about 75g/2½oz of pasta a person. Use spaghetti if you can't find linguine, although it's available from most supermarkets either fresh or dried.

Lipid Lipids are a class of hydrocarbon-containing organic compounds essential for the structure and function of living cells. Lipids are characterized by being water-insoluble and soluble in nonpolar organic solvents. Although the term lipid is often used as a synonym for fat, the latter is in fact a subgroup of lipids called triglycerides.

Lipid peroxidation A process in which unsaturated fat-soluble substances (lipids) are oxidised to form radicals and therefore capable of causing extensive tissue damage. The polyunsaturated fatty acid components of lipids are particularly prone to oxidation in this way. The process can occur in foods before they are eaten or can take place in the body.

Lipoproteins Particles composed of specialised proteins and lipids (triglycerides, phospholipids and ccholesterol) which enable lipids (which are water insoluble) to be carried in blood plasma.

Lipid pneumonia A condition marked by inflammatory and fibrotic changes in the lungs due to the inhalation of oil

Lipolytic rancidity Spoilage of foods as a result of hydrolysis of fats to free fatty acids on storage (by the action of lipase, either bacterial lipase or the enzyme naturally present in the food). Since the enzyme is inactivated by heat, this type of rancidity occurs oniy in uncooked foods.

Liquefied herring Herring reduced to liquid state by enzyme action at slightly acid pH; used as protein concentrate for animal feed.

Liqueurs Distilled, flavoured, and sweetened alcoholic liquors. For example, curaŋao (30% (weight/volume, w/v) alcohol, 30% sugar); cherry brandy (19% alcohoı, 33% sugar); advocaat (13% alcohol, 30% sugar, 0.75% nitrogen).

Liquid diet Diet consisting of foods that can be served as liquids or strained purees, prescribed in acute inflammation of the gastrointestinal tract and for patients unable to consume normal foods, especially after surgery.

Liquorice Used in confectionery and to flavour medicines; liquorice root and extract are obtained from the plant Glycyrrhiza glabra; stick liquorice is the crude evaporated extract of the root. The plant has been grown in the Pontefract district of Yorkshire since the sixteenth century; hence the name Pontefract cakes for the sugar confection of liquorice. See also glycyrrhizin.

Listeria Listeria monocytogenes is a Gram positive bacterium, found in at least 37 mammalian species, as well as 17 species of birds and possibly some fish and shellfish. The bacteria can be isolated from soil, and is resistant to heat, freezing and drying.

Listeria has been associated with foods such as raw milk, soft ripened cheeses, ice cream, raw vegetables, raw and cooked poultry, raw meat and raw and smoked fish. Unlike other pathogenic bacteria, such as salmonella, listeria can survive and grow at temperatures as low as 5°C (41°F).

Acute infection with listeria may result in flu like symptoms including persistent fever, followed by septicemia, meningitis, encephalitis, and intrauterine or cervical infections in pregnant women. Possible gastrointestinal symptoms include nausea, vomiting and diarrhea, alone or couple with other symptoms (mentioned above).

Liver Usually from calf, pig, ox, lamb, chicken, duck, or goose; a 150-g portion (fried or stewed) is an exceptionally rich source of iron and vitamins A, D, B 2, B 6, and B 12; a rich source of protein, zinc, copper, selenium, niacin, and vitamin B 1; also, unusually for meat, a good source of vitamin C; contains 10 g of fat of which one-third is saturated; supplies 300-380 kcal. The vitamin A content of liver is high enough for it to pose a possible hazard to unborn children, and pregnant women have been advised not to eat liver. See vitamin A toxicity. Fish liver is a particularly rich source of vitamins A and D, and fish liver oils (especially cod and halibut) are used as sources of these vitamins as nutritional supplements.

Lobster A large seawater crustacean. Lobster is considered the king of the crustacean family and has a jointed body and limbs covered with a hard shell. The American or Northern lobster is caught from Newfoundland to the Carolinas, but lobster is the essence of the Main seacoast. Lobster and Maine are all but synonymous. For centuries, lobsters were so abundant that they were usually considered food for the poor. According to regional legend, John D. Rockefeller Sr. rescued the lobster in 1910. The legend is that a bowl of lobster stew, meant for the servants' table, was accidentally sent upstairs (where it was rapturously received). From then on, it was given a permanent place on his menu. Back in New York, what was good enough for John D. was good enough for the rest of society.

Lobster Newberg A rich lobster dish in an elegant sauce. It is usually served over buttered toast points.

Lobster Thermidor Select pieces of lobster sautıed with shallots and mushrooms, and then deglazed with white and place back in the shell. Lobster

Thermidor was introduced on January 24, 1894, at Chez Marie, a well-known Paris restaurant. On that evening Victorien Sardou's play "Thermidor" had its first performance at the theatre called Comedie-Francais. Marie decided to launch his new dish by giving it the name of the play "Thermidor." The play was called "Thermidor" after one of the months of the French republican calendar.

Locoweed Astralagus and Oxytropus spp., common in arid areas of the western USA. Toxic to cattle, causing locoism: neurological damage, abortion, and birth defects. Apparently caused by an alkaloid, swainsonine, which is also found in mouldy hay.

Lofenalac Trade name for food low in phenylalanine for treatment of phenylketonuria.

Loganberry A hybrid between a blackberry and raspberry, the loganberry is a large soft dark-red berry, a little bigger than a raspberry. It has a less subtle flavour than a raspberry and can be quite tart, so needs plenty of sugar when used in desserts. Use it as you would other summer berries - eaten fresh with sugar or cream, in desserts, jams and coulis. In savoury cooking it goes particularly well with game dishes.

Loin A loin is a cut of meat that comes from the back of the animal. It's sold as a roasting joint, with or without bones, as well as chops and steaks which are good for grilling and barbecues. You'll occasionally find the word loin describing some fish, such as tuna loin or monkfish loin.

London broil London broil is actually a dish and a cut of meat. For the dish, large pieces of flank steak (from the lower hindquarters) or top round (from the inner portion of the hind leg) are cut into pieces, marinated, grilled, or broiled, and then sliced across the grain. In the market, you'll find many thick cuts of meat — including top round and sirloin tip — labeled "London broil."

Longitudinal A study in which an individual or a group of individuals is observed over a period of time

Lovage Also known as sea parsley, the leaves and stem of the lovage plant add an intense celery-like flavour to soups, stews and stocks or pork and poultry dishes. It can also be used to enhance potato dishes.

Low calorie sweetener Low calorie sweeteners are non nutritive sweeteners, also referred to as intense sweeteners. Low calorie sweeteners can replace nutritive sweeteners in most foods at a caloric savings of approximately 16 calories per teaspoon. Thus, caloric reduction may be achieved when low calorie sweetened foods and beverages are substituted for their full calorie counterparts. Examples of low calorie sweeteners in use in the U.S. food supply are saccharin, aspartame and acesulfame K.

Low-density lipoproteins (LDL) Plasma lipoproteins containing high concentrations of lipids (which are low in density compared to that of water), including cholesterol. Increased concentrations are a risk factor for coronary heart disease.

Lumen Lumen can mean:Lumen (unit), the SI unit of luminous fluxLumen (anatomy), the cavity or channel within a tubular structureThylakoid lumen, the inner membrane space of the chloroplast141 Lumen, an asteroid discovered by the French astronomer Paul Henry in 1875Lumen (band), an American post-rock band.

Lox Lox is the term used for salmon that has been cured in pure salt for about two months and then is soaked to get rid of the excess salt. Lox is not smoked.

Lugar Pilot Program A pilot program that operated in thirteen states to streamline reimbursement and paperwork for the Summer Food Service Program (SFSP). The program was expanded to nineteen states in the Child Nutrition and WIC Reauthorization Act of 2004, and is now known as the Simplified Summer Food Service Program.

Lutefisk Also called lyefish. It is dried cod that has been soaked in a lye solution for several days to rehydrate it. It is then boiled or baked and served with butter, salt, and pepper. The finished lutefisk usually is the consistency of jello. In the United States, Norwegian-Americans traditionally serve it for Thanksgiving and Christmas. In many homes, lutefisk takes the place of the Christmas turkey. Today the fish is celebrated in ethnic and religious celebrations and is linked with hardship and courage.

Lutein Lutein is one of over 600 known naturally occurring carotenoids. Found in green leafy vegetables such as spinach and kale, lutein is employed by organisms as an antioxidant and for blue light absorption. Lutein is covalently bound to one or more fatty acids present in some fruits and flowers, notably marigolds (Tagetes). Saponification of lutein esters yields lutein in approximately a 2:1 weight-to-weight conversion.

Lychee A fruit that originated in China and is now grown in the Far East and the West Indies. It's about the size of a small plum and has a thin, hard, rough shell that comes off easily. The white, juicy flesh has a similar texture to grapes but is more chewy, with a delicate scent. There is a large dark brown stone in the centre.

In Europe, fresh lychees are available from November to January, but they're most often sold tinned, preserved in sugar syrup.

Lyc-O-Mato An all-natural extract of red, ripe tomatoes. Lyc-O-Mato is valued as a dietary supplement and functional food ingredient because it provides a full complement of tomato carotenoids and other nutrients to benefit good health. The synergy of the natural tomato lycopene, phytoene, phytofluene, beta-carotene, phytosterols, and vitamin E results in enhanced activity and this means greater health benefits for you.

Lycopene Lycopene is a carotenoid related to the better known beta carotene. Lycopene gives tomatoes and some other fruits and vegetables their distinctive red colour. Nutritionally, it functions as an antioxidant. Research shows lycopene is best absorbed by the body when consumed as tomatoes that have been heat processed using a small amount of oil. This includes products such as tomato sauce and tomato paste. Also, see functional foods.

Lymphocyte A type of white blood cell. Lymphocytes have a number of roles in the immune system, including the production of antibodies and other substances that fight infection and diseases.

Lyonnaise A la lyonnaise describes various dishes, usually sautied, characterised by the use of chopped onions cooked in butter until golden and often finished off with vinegar and sprinkled with chopped parsley. Lyonnaise sauce is a classic French sauce made with onions and white wine, then strained and served with meat or poultry.

Lysine An essential, basic amino acid obtained from many proteins by hydrolysis.

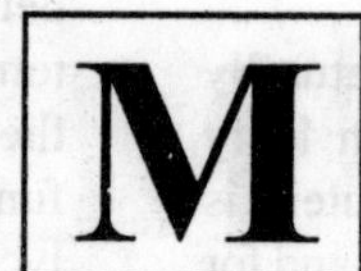

Macadamia A relatively expensive nut that 's native to Australia but is now grown commercially in Hawaii and California, particularly for the American market where they're widely used in cookies, ice cream and cakes.

The shell is incredibly hard to crack, but inside is a creamy, almost buttery, white nut with a flavour that tastes somewhere between hazelnut and coconut. In Asia macadamia nuts are used in curries and stews.

Macadamia nut The macadamia tree is a native of Queensland, Australia. It has an extremely hard shell, a buttery texture, and a high fat content. It is now grown extensively in Hawaii. It is also a staple in Indonesia where it is known as Keriri, Buah or candle nut.

Macaroon A small round cookie that has a crisp crust and a soft interior. It may be made from almonds, though coconut is common in the U.S. They may also be flavored with coffee, chocolate, or spices. Amaretti, from Italy, are also a type of macaroon. They originated in an Italian Monastery around 1792. The Carmelite nuns to pay for their housing when they needed asylum during the French Revolution baked these cookies. The Carmelite nuns followed the principle: "Almonds are good for girls who do not eat meat." During the Revolution, two nuns who hid in the town called Nancy, made and sold macaroons. They became known as the "Macaroon Sisters."

Mace This is the lacy outer layer (or 'aril') that covers the nutmeg, a nut-like seed of the nutmeg tree. Mace is sold either in blades or ground. It adds a mild nutmeg flavour to soups and sauces as well as sausages, pβtis and fish dishes.

Macerate Similar to marinating, this means to soak raw, dried or preserved fruit or vegetables in liquid (usually alcohol, liqueur, wine, brandy or sugar syrup) to soften or take away bitterness, and to allow the ingredients to absorb the flavours of the liquid.

You can serve macerated fruits as they are with some cream or ice cream, or use them to make fritters or compotes.

Dried fruits for winter compotes are often macerated. Ensure you completely cover fruits that discolour with the liquid and don't leave soft fruits too long or they'll turn to mush.

Mache Means "corn salad." It is a salad green (not actually corn), having small, white to pale bluish flowers and edible young leaves. Mache leaves are tender, velvety green with either a mild or sweet, nutty flavor. It is also sometimes called field salad, field lettuce, feldsalat, lamb's tongue, and lamb's lettuce. It is considered a gourmet green and usually is expensive and hard to find. This plant grows wild in Europe and is used as a forage crop for sheep and is a pest in wheat and cornfields. However, skilled chefs, who love these early spring greens, desire it. Mache is very perishable, so use immediately. Cook it like spinach, or use it in fruit and vegetable dishes. Makes a nice salad by itself when dressed with a peanut oil based dressing or light vinaigrette.

Mackerel A firm-fleshed, oil-rich fish with a torpedo-like shape and beautiful silvery-blue skin. It's delicious and nutritious - packed with omega-3 fatty acids.

Fresh mackerel is usually sold whole with or without the head on. It can be grilled, fried, barbecued or poached and is perfect for stuffing and oven-baking. It also suits being pickled, marinated, salted and smoked.

Smoked mackerel is very inexpensive and is delicious torn into salads or whizzed in a blender with some crθme fraξche or ricotta cheese, lemon juice and pepper to make smoked mackerel pβtι. Mackerel served with gooseberry sauce is a traditional English dish.

Macrobiotic diet A system of eating associated with Zen Buddhism; consists of several stages finally reaching Diet 7 which is restricted to cereals. Cases of severe malnutrition have been reported on this 'diet'. It involves the Chinese concept of yin (female) and yang (male) whereby foods, and even different vitamins (indeed, everything in life) are predominantly one or the other and must be balanced.

Madeira Madeira is a fortified wine that comes from the island of the same name. Different grape varieties are used to make the four types (Sercial, Verdelho, Bual and Malmsey), which range from dry to sweet. It can be served chilled and drunk as an aperitif, but is also used extensively in cooking in the same way as you would dry sherry.

Madeleines Buttery French sponge cakes traditionally baked in scallop-shaped Madeleine moulds. They're made with sugar, flour, melted butter and eggs, often flavoured with lemon or almonds. The English version is often baked in dariole moulds and topped with jam, desiccated coconut or icing sugar.

Magnesium A mineral involved in many processes in the body including nerve signaling, the building of healthy bones, and normal muscle contraction . About 350 enzymes are known to depend on magnesium.

Mahi Mahi This is a type of dolphin fish, not to be confused with the dolphin that is a mammal. The Hawaiians named it mahi mahi to avoid this misunderstanding. It is a moderately fatty fish with firm, flavorful flesh and it is usually available as steaks or fillets. It tastes best when grilled or broiled.

Mai Tai It is a potent cocktail that combines light and dark rums with different frit juices of choice served over ice. The Mai Tai is considered the unofficial and favourite drink of the State of Hawaii. It seems that every bartender in the Hawaiian Islands has his own secret recipe and that every tourist seems to sample as many as possible. It was created in San Francisco, California in 1944 by restaurateur, Victor J. Bergeron, the original owner of Trader Vic's Restaurant. Supposedly he created it for a couple of Tahitian friends, Harn and Carrie Guild. On tasting the drink, Carrie reportedly exclaimed, "Mai Tai Roa Ae" meaning in Tahitian, "Out of this world The Best." In 1953, Bergeron introduced the Mai Tai at the Royal Hawaiian, Moana, and Surfrider Hotels in the Hawaiian Islands. Victor Bergeron is reported to have said, "There's been a lot of conversation over the beginning of the Mai Tai, and I want to set the record straight. I originated the Mai Tai. Many other have claimed credit. All this aggravates my ulcer completely. Anyone who says I didn't create this drink is a dirty stinker."

Maldon sea salt An exceptional sea salt that comes from the Maldon area of Essex. Sea salt is produced as the sea washes over rocks and then recedes with the tide, leaving pools of water.

The sun evaporates the water and leaves the salt in the form of crystals that can be used in cooking or preserving, as whole crystals or ground.

It's an absolutely pure salt that tastes of the sea and its sparkling white crystalline flakes are delicious used in all kinds of savoury cooking. Fill your salt mill or crush the flakes between your fingers and scatter over hot chips, jacket potatoes or other foods to give a pretty finish and a delicious salty bite. It has a pronounced and distinctive 'salty' taste so use less than you would with ordinary salt.

Malnutrition A failure to achieve proper nutrient requirements, which can impair physical and/or mental health. It may result from consuming too little food c.: a shortage or imbalance of key nutrients (e.g., micronutrient deficiencies or excess consumption of refined sugar and fat). (American Dietetic Association)

Malt Mixture of starch breakdown products containing mainly maltose (malt sugar), prepared from barley or wheat.

The grain is allowed to sprout, when the enzyme diastase (amylase) develops and hydrolyses the starch to maltose. The mixture is then extracted with hot water, and this malt extract contains a solution of starch breakdown products together with diastase. Malt extract may remain as the concentrated solution or evaporated to dryness.

Manchego One of Spain's best-known cheeses, made from ewes' milk. It originated in La Mancha but is now made all over the UK. It's sold fresh or slightly aged in olive oil, and has a deep yellow rind and creamy white interior. It's firm to the touch with a buttery nutty taste that's slightly sour. It's a good grating cheese that melts well.

Manganese Essential for reproductive function, physical growth, normal formation of bones and cartilage and normal brain function. Whole grains and cereals, fruits, vegetables and tea.

Mango Mango trees are evergreens that will grow to 60 feet tall. Most of the mangos sold in the United States are imported from Mexico, Haiti, the Caribbean, and South America. Today there are over 1,000 different varieties of mangos throughout the world. Mango cultivation has now spread to many parts of the tropical and sub-tropical world, where they grow best. The mango originated in Southeast Asia where it has been grown for 4,000 years. Because the mango seed can't be dispersed naturally by wind or water due to it's large size and weight, it is believed that people who moved from one region to another transported the fruit to new areas. The spread of Buddhism assisted in the distribution of mangoes in Southeastern Asia. Mangoes were carried to Africa during the 16th century and later found their way aboard Portuguese ships to Brazil in the 1700's. Later, in 1742, mangoes were found growing in the West Indies. In 1860, mangoes were successfully introduced to Florida along the East Coast, where only a few varieties were grown.

Mangosteen A tropical fruit from South-east Asia, the mangosteen is the size of a small peach with a leathery skin which, when peeled away, reveals five sweetly scented white segments which have a very delicate taste and melt in the mouth. Eat as it is or add a few to a tropical fruit salad.

Maple sugaring The term "maple sugaring" is part of the history of maple. In many areas of the region where the most maple products are made, the expression "sugaring" has survived since the earliest times, when sugar was the product made instead of maple syrup, which is the most popular variety of maple produced by the sugar makers of today. In the early days, sugar was more easily kept in the primitive containers available, and more safely stored for later use. Journals of the explorers and settlers from as early as 1609 indicate that the native North American Indians were the first sugar makers. "Indian sugar" and "Indian molasses" are terms that were used by the settlers. In later February or early March, at the time of the "Maple Moon," Indian families made sugaring camps in areas where maple trees were plentiful. Gashes were cut in the sugar maples and sap was caught in hollowed out logs or birch bark containers were cut and folded at the corners so as to avoid breaking and consequent leakage. Indian women and children did most of the work. Sugaring was a time of celebration for Indian families. After the cold winter, the Maple Dance brought on warmer weather.

The early settlers who came to Northeastern North America made maple sugar in much the same way as the Indians. Most sugaring was done in outdoor camps, set up in groves of maple trees. Thomas Jefferson, the third president of the U.S., was enthusiastic about maple sugar and established a grove of maples at his Monticello home (one of those maples remains standing on a hill at the plantation today). Abolitionist friends of Jefferson thought the cultivation of sugar maple might bring West Indian slavery to an end. Maple sugar was known as "sugar not made by slaves."

Maple syrup It is the first finished product made from boiled map of the maple tree. This is the form most widely used in recipes. A maple tree is usually 30 years old or more and at least 10 inches in diameter before it is tapped. Depending on its size, a tree may have from one to four taps, each of which yields an average of 10 gallons of sap each season. Before the French even colonized the New World; maple sap was already being collected by the American Indians who used it as a sweet beverage. Although they knew how to tap the trees and collect maple sap, their primitive earthenware, however, were not allowing them to boil the sap quite enough to produce maple syrup. Some historians believe that the American Indians taught the process of sugar making to Europeans; others, rather believe that this discovery can be attribute to a certain doctor named Michel Sarrazin, a military surgeon, who arrived to the Canadian country in 1685. Although nothing proves that he might be the father of sugar making; the fact remains that the maple syrup production spread through the French colony. Maple syrup was considered a precious elixir used as medicine to strengthen the chest. It is now considered a delicacy in the U.S., but in colonial days it was used extensively as an ordinary sweetener. The Indians taught the first white settlers how to tap Maple trees in the spring, and then evaporate the sweet sap until it became maple syrup.

Maquechoux This is a dish that the Cajun people of Louisiana got from the Native American tribes that populated southwest Louisiana. It's a wonderful vegetable dish featuring fresh corn. The recipe is varied the by adding chicken, or even crawfish tails.

Marengo A chicken or veal dish made with cognac or white wine, tomatoes, eggs, crayfish, garlic, olive oil and bread. Chicken Marengo is said to have been created by Napoleon's chef Dunand, who was ordered to create a meal for Napoleon while he was on the battlefield in the Italian town of Marengo in 1800. Napoleon apparently enjoyed it so much that he asked for it to be served after every battle.

Margarine Margarine was invented in the 1860s by a French chemist as a cheap replacement for butter. Nowadays it's bought as a product in its own right, frequently in the belief that it's a healthier option than butter. All margarine contains as much fat as butter, but some are lower in cholesterol and saturated fats.

However, the health benefits of many of these types of spreads has been called into question in recent years because most of them are made with hydrogenated (chemically hardened) vegetable oils and this process is believed to convert the polyunsaturated fat into trans-fats which have a negative effect on cholesterol and are now thought to be linked with heart disease even more than saturated fat.

Aside from this, margarine is a highly processed food made by combining water and vegetable oils and usually containing emulsifiers, preservatives, additives, artificial colourings and flavourings and salt.

There are many types available using different fats and with differing flavours and uses. Some are purely vegetable-based, containing no animal products at all, and are labelled dairy-free or vegan. Others contain a mixture of animal and vegetable fats. Some are designed for spreading, and others are hard and designed for baking so always read the packaging before cooking with margarine.

Margarita The basic or classic Margarita is made using fresh lime juice, orange liqueur, and tequila served in a salt-rimmed glass. Whether plain, salted, straight up, on the rocks, or frozen, Margaritas are made in an array of flavors and colours. Several Mexican bars and bartenders have staked a claim to its origin. 1. The strongest claim comes from Ciudad Juarez, Mexico in 1942. Francisco "Pancho" Morales (1919-1997) is credited with inventing the drink while working in Tommy's Bar. A woman came in and asked for a "magnolia" a drink he had not heard of. Pretending to know what she wanted, he whipped up a cocktail of tequila, cointreau, and lime juice.

2. Margarita Sames claimed to have invented the drink in 1948 at a poolside Christmas party at her Acapulco vacation house. The game at the party was to make a new drink concoction and have the party guests test and rate the result. The result was a success with her guests and quickly spread throughout the southwest United States.

3. Another claim is from Carlos Herrera, owner of the Rancho La Gloria, located between Rosarito Beach and Tijuana. In the latter 1930s, Herrera would fix various tequila drinks for a showgirl named Marjorie King. She liked one particular drink so much that he named it Margarita, the Spanish name for Marjorie.

4. The final story is from a bartender in Virginia City, Nevada who named the drink after his girlfriend, Margarita Mendez, who hit someone over the heat with a whiskey bottle and died in the crossfire that pursued.

Marinate To steep fish, meat or vegetables in a highly seasoned and flavoured liquid (the marinade) usually containing oil, wine or lemon juice, herbs and spices, in order to tenderise and add flavour.

Marinating can transform bland, cheap or tough cuts of meat. It can be cooked or uncooked and can take as little as half an hour or as long as a couple of days depending on the recipe. After the food is marinated you can add the strained liquid to an accompanying sauce, but always cook it thoroughly before serving.

Marjoram Dried leaves of a number of aromatic plants of different species, used as seasoning for poultry, meats, and cheese dishes. The most widely accepted marjoram herbs are the perennial bush Origanum majorana and the annual sweet marjoram Majorana hortensis. Spanish wild marjoram is Thymus mastichina.

Marlin This is the big catch for big-game sport fishermen and catching it's a huge challenge! Found in the waters off Hawaii, Florida, Venezuela and Australia, marlin is available in other parts of the world sold as steaks. These are best cooked under the grill, on a barbecue or as kebabs. The firm flesh can be used interchangeably for tuna in most recipes.

Marmalade Marmalade is a jellylike preserve that contains pieces of citrus fruit and rind. The word is first recorded in English in the early sixteenth century. The word is borrowed from Portuguese marmalada 'quince jam', from marmelo 'a quince'. The original marmalades were made from quince and the Portuguese word "marmelada" means "quince jam." The world's first known book of recipes, called "Of Culinary Matters," written by the Roman gastronome Marcus Gavius Apicius in the first century, includes recipes for fruit preserves. Marmalade is thought to have been created in 1561 by the physician to Mary, Queen of Scots, when he mixed orange and crushed sugar to keep her seasickness at bay. It has also been suggested that the world "marmalade" derives from the words "Marie es malade" (Mary is sick). In the late 18th century in Scotland, James Keiller bought a considerable quantity of oranges off a ship that had come to Dundee from Spain. The oranges were cheap, the reason being, as he soon discovered, that they were very bitter because they were Seville oranges. Unable to sell them he took them home to his wife. She experimenented in her kitchen and came up with what we know as marmalade.

Marmite 1. Marmite is a British product that is a concentrated yeast paste. It can be used on toast, sandwiches, or as an added ingredient in stews and casseroles. It is 100% vegetarian and it contains virtually no fat or sugar. Marmite has a distinctive savory taste, unlike anything else. It remains a popular food in Britain.

2. A French cast iron or earthenware soup pot with a lid.

Marsala Marsala is a wine imported from Sicily. It is Italy's most famous fortified wine that ranges from dry to sweet. Dry Marsala makes a tasty aperitif. Sweet Marsala is used as a dessert wine and also to flavor. It is also a popular cooking wine.

Marshmallows Marshmallow is a confection made from the root of the marsh mallow plant. When we think of traditional holiday meals, sweet potatoes with marshmallows always come to mind. The plant name is really old, first found in an Old English medical book written around 1000 A.D., when it was spelled merscmealwe. As a candy, marshmallows date back at least to the late nineteenth century. Originally the marsh mallow plant was mixed with eggs and sugar and then beaten to foam. Today they are generally made of gelatin, water, sugar, egg whites, corn syrup, vanilla extract, and artificial sweeteners. In the 1920s, marshmallows were introduced as a topper for sweet potatoes. While sweet potatoes and marshmallows were not originally created for the holiday meal, it has become a tradition.

Martini The Martini consists of gin and a varying amount of dry white vermouth, depending on personal taste, and is served in the traditional glass with a V-shaped profile. It can be garnished with an olive, a twist, or a cocktail onion. The Martini has become Americans most popular hard-liquor drink and an American icon. The cocktail has been represented in film, literature, and pop culture as the cocktail of choice for the cool, the suave, and the connected. In the 1920s, the Martini really became popular during the Prohibition era. Prohibition ruined the restaurant business in cities and it changed the way Americans drank. Across the country general liquor consumption was down, but city dwellers drank more per capita, and the trend was towards a mass binge on hard liquor. An illegal truckload of gin carried higher profit margins than beer or wine and because it was easier to counterfeit than whiskey. Just as there are many recipes for Martinis, there are also several stories or legends on how it originated: 1. In 1862, a gold miner came into the bar of the Occidental Hotel in San Francisco, threw a gold nugget on the table and asked the legendary bartender, "Professor" Jerry Thomas to shake up something special for him. This recipe that Jerry Thomas made was later produced in an 1887 reprint of Thomas' Bartending Book (it did not appear in his first edition of the book). A mock court held in San Francisco, called the Court of Historical Review, ruled that the Martini was invented in San Francisco, but not before a Martini was drank by the presiding judge.

2. In 1870, a gold miner stopped at Julio Richelieu's saloon in Martinez, California, and put a fistful of gold nuggets and an empty bottle on the bar, and asked for Champagne, a beverage not available. The bartender told the miner he had something much better than Champagne and served him a drink, which he said, was a "Martinez Special." To this day, Martinez, California claims to be the birthplace of the Martini. A court in Martinez, California overturned Court of Historical Review's decision that the Martini was invented in San

Francisco, and the in 1992, the citizens of the town erected a brass plaque in downtown Martinez proclaiming their town as the birthplace of the Martini.

3. An Italian bartender, Martini di Taggia, at New York's Knickerbocker Hotel claims t have invented the drink in 1912. It is said that he was the first to mix a Martini with dry, not sweet, vermouth.

4. Also bartender, William F. Mulhall, wrote of mixing both sweet and dry Martinis at New York's Hoffman House around the same time.

5. The English also claim the name derived from the Swiss Martini & Henry rifle used by the British army between 1871 and 1891.

6. The Italians also like to take credit for the origin being from the Martini & Rossi Vermouths. The Oxford English Dictionary states that the earliest use of the word was in 1894 and states that the word comes from Martini & Rossi Vermouth citing an advertisement for Heublein's Club Cocktails.

Marzipan A thick paste (also known as almond paste) made from ground almonds, sugar and whole egg or egg whites and used in making cakes and pastries. It's used as a topping for simnel cake or as a base for the icing on a Christmas or wedding cake.

It can be made with egg yolk for a richer colour or coloured with food colouring and flavoured, then used to make petits fours. It can be also be moulded into the shape of fruits, vegetables, and so on, to make little sweets.

Ready-made marzipan is sold in plastic-wrapped blocks in the baking section of most supermarkets.

Mascarpone A thick, creamy, soft Italian cheese with a high fat content (40 per cent). It can be used in savoury and sweet dishes. It's good for stirring through savoury sauces to thicken and add a distinct rich flavour. Serve it with fresh fruit, use it in cheesecakes, as a cake filling, or as a topping for desserts.

Mascarpone is an essential ingredient in the Italian coffee trifle tiramisu. It can be flavoured with various ingredients such as lemon or lime juice and zest, crushed nuts or dried fruits to add taste and texture.

Mast cell degranulation The release from within the cell of granules, or small sacs, containing chemicals that can digest microorganisms and activate other cells to fight infection.

Mast cells Tissue cells which when connected to immunoglobulin E antibodies release histamine or other substances causing allergic symptoms.

Mayonnaise A thick, creamy, cold sauce or dressing made by beating oil and egg yolks, usually with some wine vinegar, salt, pepper and mustard. Used to dress salads or combined with seafood, poultry, eggs or vegetables to make cold starters or main dishes.

Mayonnaise forms the basis of all kinds of other sauces and dressings such as tartare sauce, aioli (garlic mayonnaise), Thousand Island dressing and rumoulade. Although it's available ready-made in jars, tubs and tubes the flavour doesn't compare with homemade and once you have the knack it's simple. It's easier to make if you have a blender as the key is to blend the oil in drop by drop to prevent the mayonnaise from curdling, which can be an exhausting job with a hand whisk!

Because eggs can contain salmonella, it's important to ensure that you use pasteurised egg in dishes in which eggs will be uncooked or only lightly cooked. Pasteurised egg can be bought in liquid or powder form. Commercially produced mayonnaise is almost always made with pasteurised egg, but if you're unsure, check with the retailer or manufacturer.

Meal pattern Meals served under the child nutrition programs must fulfill certain nutrition standards established by the USDA. The meal pattern outlines the specific types (fluid milk, dairy, fruit/vegetable, bread/bread alternative, and meat/meat alternative) and serving size of food that fulfill these guidelines. The meal pattern varies based upon type of meal (breakfast, lunch/supper or snack) and age of the child being served. For example, in the CACFP, the breakfast meal pattern for children aged 6 12 is 1 fluid milk serving, 1 fruit or vegetable serving, and 1 bread/bread alternative.

Meat Generally refers to the muscle tissue of animal or bird, other parts being termed offal. 150-g portions of meat of all types (different cuts and different species including game and poultry), excluding bone, are rich sources of protein and niacin; most are rich sources of vitamin B 2 and iron; sources or good sources of vitamin B 1.

Venison, horse meat, goose, and game birds are exceptionally rich in iron; pork is exceptionally rich in vitamin B 1. The fat content and proportions of fatty acids differ considerably between individual carcasses, species, and cuts of meat.

Seealso beef, lamb, veal, pork, rabbit, hare, goat, horse, venison, duck, chicken, goose, partridge, turkey, pheasant, grouse, quail, pigeon; and heart, kidney, liver, oxtail, sweetbread, tongue, tripe.

Meat, curing Pickling with the aid of sodium chloride (salt), sodium nitrate (saltpetre), and some sodium nitrite, which permits the growth of only salt-tolerant bacteria and inhibits the growth of Clostridium botulinum. The nitrite is the effective preserving agent and the nitrate is converted into nitrite during the process. The red colour of cured meat is due to the formation of nitrosomyoglobin from the myoglobin of muscle.

Mediators Substances within the body, such as hormones, that can transmit messages to nerve or muscle tissue to stimulate a response.

Medicinal paraffin Liquid paraffin, a mineral oil of no nutritive value since it is not affected by digestive enzymes and passes through the intestine unchanged. Used as a mild laxative because of its lubricant properties.

Medium chain triglycerides known as the "fatless fat", these fat molecules are easily mobilized in the bloodstream to provide long-lasting energy, rather than being stored as fat. They also help limit the conversion of excess carbohydrates into fat. One of the "Lean Lipid" ingredients in Muscle Milk.

Megacolon abnormal widening of the colon that may be inborn or may result from chronic constipation or obstipation

Megrim This is a flatfish from the brill and turbot family. It can be cooked like sole or plaice, but doesn't match them for flavour or texture. It's inexpensive, but giving it flavour is up to you. Good for using in fishcakes and stock rather than taking centre stage.

Melba The name given to various dishes dedicated to Dame Nellie Melba, the famous 19th-century Australian opera singer. The best known is Peach Melba, created by the famous chef Escoffier when he was chef at the Savoy in London to celebrate her visit to London. The original was an elaborate dish of a swan of ice with peaches on top of a bed of ice cream and topped with spun sugar. Today, the dessert consists of peach halves on a bed of vanilla ice cream topped with raspberry puree.

Melba toast is thinly sliced bread that has been toasted twice to dry it to a crisp. You can make it at home but there are lots of good ready-made ones available at supermarkets. Serve them with soft-textured foods that are good for dipping or spreading such as herb butter, pβtι or soup.

Mental retardation Significantly subaverage intellectual functioning, accompanied by deficits in adaptive functioning and manifested before age 18 years; subaverage intellectual functioning is defined as an IQ score of 70 or below (e.g., on the WISC-R, Stanford-Binet, K-ABC or other individually-administered psychometric test)

Menu Commonly used to mean the list of foods and dishes served by a restaurant, but correctly a set meal (with options) or dish of the day, as opposed to ΰ la carte.

Meringue Meringue refers to a mixture of whipped egg whites and sugar and the light sweet confections made from this mixture when it's oven-baked. Recipes might call for a specific type of meringue. The three main types are ordinary meringue (the simplest, sometimes called meringue Suisse, which is just egg whites and sugar whisked until stiff); Italian meringue, which is made with a hot sugar syrup; and cooked meringue, which is made by whisking the egg whites with icing sugar in a bowl set over simmering water. Meringue is used as a topping on pies and tarts as in lemon meringue pie or Baked Alaska - a thin sponge base topped with ice cream then covered in meringue and baked. Or it can be piped into shapes or spooned into nest shapes then baked in a low oven to make meringues. These then form the component of various dishes such as Eton mess - crushed meringues mixed with raspberries or strawberries and cream, or pavlova - a large meringue nest topped with whipped cream and fresh fruit.

Meringue can be crisp and dry throughout or crisp outside and marshmallowy inside depending on the ratio of sugar to egg whites and the temperature at which the meringue is baked. They keep for a good few weeks in an airtight container. The Food Standards Agency recommends that pasteurised egg should be used in any dish in which the egg won't be completely cooked. Pasteurised egg is available in frozen, liquid or powder form and eggs pasteurised in their shells are also available.

Mesclun This is the name given to a mixture of salad greens. The term comes from the Provenηal word for 'mixture' and refers to a mix of young field greens such as wild and cultivated chicory, lamb's lettuce and dandelion leaves, but may also include rocket, chervil, purslane and oak leaf lettuce. The idea is to create a good balance of strong- and mild-flavoured greens.

Meta-analyses A method of summarizing previous research by reviewing and combining results from multiple studies.

Metabolism The entire set of enzyme catalyzed transformations of organic nutrient molecules (to sustain life) in living cells. Conversion of food and water into nutrients that can be used by the body's cells, and the use of those nutrients by those cells (to sustain life, grow, etc.).

Methionine An essential amino acid; furnishes (to organism) both labile methyl groups and sulphur necessary for normal metabolism.

Fig. Methionine

Methyl cellulose A number of gummy substances, produced through reaction between cellulose and methyls. It is found in fruit butters and jellies and serves to keep these products from separating.

Micellar Casein Technically referred to as Total Milk Protein but marketed as Micellar Casein. Fresh skim milk is ultra filtered, in much the same process used to make whey protein, to produce a pure un-undenatured milk protein. The resulting material contains 80% casein and 20% whey. This probably the least processed of all milk proteins. Often used in formulations where a time release effect is required.

Micronutrients Nutrients required by the body in extremely small quantities milligrams or micrograms such as iodine, vitamin A, zinc and iron.

Micronutrient deficiency Organic state of lack of nutritive elements, such as vitamin A, iron, iodine and zinc, requised by the body in very small quantities measurable in mg/day.

Microorganisms Simple unicellular and structurally similar representatives of the plant and animal kingdoms. With few exceptions, the unicellular organisms are invisible to the naked eye and generally have dimensions of between a fraction of a micron and 200 micron.

Microwave cooking Rapid heating by passing high frequency waves from a magnetron (in the UK 2450 or 896 MHz (million cycles/second)) through the food or liquid to be heated. Water absorbs the microwaves very well, so food with a high water content cooks more rapidly; fat absorbs the energy more slowly, so foods consisting of mixtures of fat and water cook unevenly. The cooking time is short and microwaves do not cause browning, so the food may not develop flavours associated with longer cooking times. Metal containers reflect the microwaves and cannot be used.

Milk Thistle Milk Thistle (Silybum marianum), is a member of the family Asteraceae and is a tall herb with prickly leaves and a milky sap that is native to the Mediterranean region of Europe. Milk thistle is among the most ancient of all known herbal medicines, having been used as a remedy for centuries.

Millefeuille Literally 'thousand leaves' this is a light and airy pastry dessert made of thin layers of puff pastry, whipped cream and jam or some other filling such as fresh fruit. Millefeuilles are usually small rectangular pastries but can also be made as large gateaux.

Milli As a prefix for units of measurement, one thousandth part (i.e. 10-3); symbol m. See Appendix I.

Milligram (Mg) Abbreviation for milligram, a unit of weight in the metric system. There are 1,000 milligrams in one gram.

Milling The term usually refers to the conversion of cereal grain into its derivative, e.g. wheat into flour, brown rice to white rice.

Flour milling involves two types of rollers: 1. break rolls are corrugated and exert shear pressure and forces which break up the wheat grain and permit sieving into fractions containing varying proportions of germ, bran, and endosperm;

2. reducing rolls are smooth and subdivide the endosperm to fine particles. See also flour, extraction rate.

Mincemeat A spicy preserve comprising a mixture of dried fruit, apple, suet and candied fruit and spices steeped in rum or brandy. It has been part of British cookery for centuries and did originally contain meat, though now the only meat present is in the suet. It's the traditional filling for individual mince pies, served warm at Christmas, but can also be used to fill tarts, pastries or even pasta.

There are some excellent ready-made versions available (including ones made with vegetarian suet) but nothing beats homemade, and it's very simple to make.

Mineral water Drinking water that comes from a protected underground water source and contains at least 250 parts per million of total dissolved solids, such as calcium.

Minestrone A thick Italian soup containing a mixture of vegetables, beans and pasta or rice. The name derives from the Italian word 'minestra' meaning thick soup. Made in the Italian way there should be just enough stock to float the mixture of vegetables and pasta.

Mint sauce A thin savoury sauce made from chopped mint, vinegar and sugar, traditionally served in England as an accompaniment to roast lamb.

Mirepoix A mixture of diced vegetables - usually onion, leek, carrot and celery - and sometimes bacon and herbs. It's sautied in butter and is the basis of many sauces, soups and stews. It's often used as a foundation for braising meat, poultry or fish as well. Mirepoix is the classic French mix, but nearly all cuisines have their own. Italians for instance have 'soffritto', which is usually onions, carrots and celery sautied in olive oil rather than butter.

Mirin Mirin is a sweetened sake or rice wine with a light syrupy texture, used in Japanese cooking. It gives a mild sweetness to sauces and dishes and is particularly good with grilled food because the alcohol burns off, leaving just the sweet taste. Sherry could be used as an alternative, but mirin is becoming more widely available.

Miso Miso is used as condiment, miso paste is a paste made by adding a culture to soybeans and water, and sometimes grains such as barley. It is rich in B vitamins and is typically used in soups or stews, and in sauces and marinades.

Mitochondria Specialized subcellular structures located within body cells that contain oxidative enzymes needed by the cell to metabolize foodstuffs into energy sources. Organic Being composed of, or containing matter of plant or animal origin.

Molasses A thick, dark, heavy syrup that is a by-product of sugar refining. It's far less sweet than syrup or honey and the darker the molasses, the less sugar it contains. Molasses has a slightly bitter flavour that's favoured in traditional North American recipes such as Boston baked beans and it also goes into the making of rich fruit cakes, gingerbread and treacle toffee.

Molybdenum As a component of three different enzymes, it's involved in the metabolism of nucleic acids (DNA and RNA) iron and food converts food into energy. Helps breakdown toxic build ups of sulfites in the body. May help prevent cavities.

Monk's beard No fashionable menu is complete without monk's beard, or barbarata de fratea. Known in the UK as 'goat's beard' or 'Johnny go to bed at noon', these little green shoots are grown in Tuscany, where they're only in season for five weeks of the year.

Monounsaturated fat Fats that are in foods are combinations of monounsaturated, polyunsaturated, and saturated fatty acids. Monounsaturated fat is found in canola oil, olives and olive oil, nuts, seeds, and avocados. Eating food that has more monounsaturated fat instead of saturated fat may help lower cholesterol and reduce heart disease risk. However, it has the same number of calories as other types of fat, and may still contribute to weight gain if eaten in excess.

Mooli A long white Japanese vegetable of the radish family, also known as daikon. It's crunchy, with a mild peppery flavour, similar to watercress. Unlike other radishes it's as good cooked as it is raw. In Chinese and Japanese cookery it's used for vegetable carving as well as cooking. Mooli is sometimes available in larger supermarkets, but you're more likely to find it in Asian or Caribbean food shops.

Morbid obesity This is a state of adiposity or overweight, in which body weight is 100 percent above the ideal and a body mass index of 45 or greater.

Morbidity A disease or the incidence of disease within a population. Morbidity also refers to adverse effects caused by a treatment.

Morel Morels are wild mushrooms found all over the British Isles. With a creamy white stem and conical cap they grow in dry, sandy areas so it's important to wash them well to get rid of any grit. They're often used dried (but never raw) and are excellent in all mushroom dishes and as additions to stews and casseroles. They're particularly good with chicken and are considered among the best mushrooms, along with ceps and chanterelles.

Mornay sauce A bechamel sauce enriched with egg yolks and flavoured with grated gruyere cheese. It's used to coat dishes to be glazed under the grill or browned in the oven, including poached eggs, fish, shellfish and vegetables.

Mortadella A large, cooked Italian salami originating from Bologna. It's made with finely minced pork, garlic, salt and pepper stuffed into a natural casing and is sometimes studded with pistachios or green olives.

Motility Spontaneous movement. A term used to describe the motor activity of smooth muscles in the gastrointestinal (GI) tract

Moussaka A classic aubergine casserole associated with Greece. It's made using minced lamb, slices of aubergine, potatoes and onions, covered with a creamy white sauce and oven-baked until golden. There are many variations, including vegetarian moussaka.

Mousse A mousse is a light fluffy mixture, either sweet or savoury; it can be served hot or cold. There are no hard and fast rules, but sweet mousses are often flavoured with chocolate or fruit puree and many contain whipped cream.

Savoury mousses usually contain purıed or blended fish or meats such as salmon, shellfish, chicken or ham. Sweet mousses tend to be made with beaten egg whites while savoury mousses use gelatine.

Some mousses just need setting in the fridge while other recipes might call for them to be baked in the oven. Use pasteurised eggs if making a mousse in which the egg is not thoroughly cooked.

Mozzarella An Italian fresh or unripened cheese traditionally made from water buffalo's milk (Mozzarella di Bufala) around the Naples area.

Mozzarella is now also made predominantly from cows' milk and is made all over Italy as well as in other countries, including the UK (where some producers are making mozzarella from water buffalo milk). It's a firm but creamy cheese that tastes like fresh milk with a slightly sour edge to it. It melts well and has a unique stretchiness, making it the classic pizza topping cheese.

It's too soft to grate but cut thin slices and layer them in pasta bakes or put a slice on top of pieces of meat or chicken before grilling them. Italy's classic salad - insalata Caprese - is made with slices of mozzarella and ripe tomatoes drizzled with extra virgin olive oil and scattered with torn basil leaves and a little salt.

Mozzarella is sold in rounds about the size of a small fist. Because it has no rind it's packed in plastic bags, surrounded by water to keep it fresh. You're more likely to find buffalo mozzarella from good delis or cheese shops and also look out for small mozzarella balls called 'bocconcini' which are sold in tubs.

MRP A product designed to replace or add to meals. A meal replacement will provide quality protein, carbohydrate, vitamins and minerals.

MSG (Monosodium glutamate) MSG is the sodium salt of glutamic acid. Glutamic acid, or glutamate, is one of the most common amino acids found in nature. In the early part of the century, MSG was extracted from seaweed and other plant sources. Today, MSG is produced in many countries around the world through a fermentation process of molasses from sugar cane or sugar beets, as well as starch and corn sugar.

Mulligatawny A classic Anglo-Indian dish. Mulligatawny is a spicy soup based on chicken or mutton/lamb stock. According to Madhur Jaffrey, the original mulligatawny soup can be traced back to the early days of the East India Company in Madras, and was more like a curry. The word is based on the Tamil name for 'pepper water', 'milligu-thannir', also called 'rasam'.

Recipes for mulligatawny soup abound; some use apples or other fruits, some use nuts, some even use oatmeal, along with meat and vegetables. The common denominator is spiciness and 'curry' flavours from curry powder or a mixture of dried spices.

Multi-benefit outreach Outreach initiatives aimed at connecting low-income families to the range of income support programs and services. Multi-benefit outreach efforts can help low-income families learn about the variety of support programs available while decreasing stigma and simplifying the outreach and enrollment process. Multi-benefit outreach campaigns often provide information about programs such as: EITC, food stamps and other nutrition programs, free and low-cost health insurance, child care assistance, and energy assistance.

Muscular dystrophy A general term for a number of hereditary, progressive degenerative disorders affecting skeletal muscles, and often other organ systems; types of muscular dystrophy include Duchenne and Becker muscular dystrophy, spinal muscular atrophy and myotonic dystrophy

Mustard A condiment made from the seeds of the mustard plant, of which there are three varieties black mustard (spicy and piquant), brown mustard (less piquant), and white or yellow mustard (much less piquant but more pungent).

The familiar hot taste of mustard is released when the crushed seeds are mixed with a liquid. The crushed seeds are usually steeped in water, wine, vinegar and must (the unfermented juice of grapes) before being mashed to a paste with various flavourings.

Different blends of mustard include English, American and French varieties. Available in jars, tubes and cans, they keep indefinitely. English mustards are stronger in flavour than most, and are based on a blend of brown and white seeds, flour and turmeric for colour.

The hot, pungent flavour is excellent with cold meats, steak, roast beef, gammon or sizzling sausages. The uses of mustard are so various that it's worth keeping a few different types in the cupboard. French mustards such as the creamy, slightly hot Dijon; Meaux, which is made from mixed mustard seeds; and the thick, dark brown Bordeaux, best known as French mustard, together with English mustard, are widely used as condiments but can be used to add piquancy to sauces, dressings or marinades. Simply stirring a spoonful of mustard into mayonnaise or crθme fraçche transforms it into a tasty sauce to accompany almost anything!

Myasthenia gravis A neuromuscular disorder, with onset primarily in adulthood, characterized by fluctuating muscle weakness, especially in the face and throat

Mycotoxins Toxins produced by fungi. More than 350 different mycotoxins are known to man. Almost all mycotoxins possess the capacity to harmfully alter the immune systems of animals. Consumption by humans and animals of certain mycotoxins (e.g., via eating infected corn, nuts, peanuts cottonseed products, etc.) can result in liver toxicity, gastrointestinal lesions, cancer and muscle necrosis.

Myelomeningocele A congenital defect that results in a hernia (containing the spinal cord, the meninges and cerebral spinal fluid) along the spinal column, also called spina bifida

Myenteric plexus Unmyelinated fibers and cell bodies in the muscular coat of the esophagus, stomach, and intestines

Myocardial Infarction Also called a heart attack; results from permanent damage to an area of the heart muscle. This happens when the blood supply to the area is interrupted because of narrowed or blocked blood vessels.

Myotonic dystrophy An inherited (autosomal dominant) neuromuscular disorder that occurs in adults, characterized by progressive muscle weakness and wasting and myotonia; onset is usually in the third decade

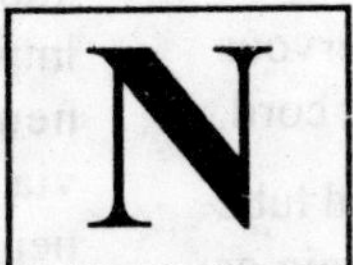

Nam pla This is a thin brown fish sauce that's fundamental to Thai food. It's made by fermenting small whole fish (usually anchovies) in brine and drawing off the liquid, which is then bottled. It smells quite fishy and tastes very salty so use it sparingly as a flavouring and as a condiment (although cooking greatly reduces its fishiness and simply adds a richness and depth of flavour to dishes).

It's a staple in Asian cooking with slightly differing versions in each country. Nam pla is widely available in Asian markets and supermarkets but if you can't find it, substitute a light soy sauce.

Nashi Also called an Asian pear, this fruit has a flavour somewhere between an apple and a pear, combining the shape and crispness of an apple with the grainy texture and flavour of a pear. It's excellent in fruit salads or served with a cheeseboard. In cooking, use it as you would with any other apple or pear recipe.

Nasograstro tube (NG-tube) A method of enteral feeding in which a tube is placed through a nasal passageway into the stomach.

Nasturtium Edible flowers are great for adding colour and peppery flavour to dishes. The nasturtium is an annual flowering plant whose edible leaves and orange, red and yellow petals have a flavour that's similar to watercress. Sprinkle them in salads or use as a garnish for any savoury dish to add colour and bite. The flower buds and seeds, picked when soft and pickled in vinegar, can be used as a substitute for capers. You're most likely to find nasturtiums at specialist food shops or farmers' markets.

Natural toxins A naturally occurring substance (e.g., produced in some cases by disease causing microorganisms) which is poisonous to certain other living organisms.

Natural water Bottled drinking water not derived from a municipal water supply; it can be mineral, spring, well or artesian-well water.

Navarin A classic French stew of lamb or mutton with potatoes and other root vegetables, often carrot or turnip. It's traditionally cooked using cuts of young spring lamb and new vegetables. Fresh peas and beans are sometimes added at the end of cooking. The stew is skimmed of any fat on its surface and is left to cook for a few minutes more until the vegetables are just tender.

Neotame A versatile, new no-calorie sweetener composed of two elements of protein, the amino acids L-aspartic acid and L-phenylalanine, combined with two organic functional groups,'a methyl ester group and a neohexyl group. It is approximately 7,000 to 13,000 times sweeter than sugar and as such captures the "essence of sweetness." with only a very small amount required for use. The chemical composition of neotame makes it stable for use in baking. The FDA has recently approved Neotame for use in a variety of food products and as a tabletop sweetener.

Net carbohydrates A term developed by manufacturers to describe the carbohydrates that have a significant impact on blood sugar levels.

Neural Having to do with nerves or the nervous system, including the brain and the spinal cord.

Neural tube defect In simple terms, a neural tube defect (NTD) is a malformation of the brain or spinal cord (neurological system) during embryonic development. Infants born with spina bifida, where the spinal cord is exposed, can grow to adulthood but usually suffer from paralysis or other disabilities. Babies born with anencephaly, where most or all of the brain is missing, usually die shortly after birth. These NTDs make up about 5 percent of all U.S. birth defects each year. According to the CDC, the use of sufficient folic acid is enough to eliminate the risk of NTDs.

Neuroepithelial Having to do with tissue made up of sensory cells, such as tissue found in the ear, nose, and tongue.

Neurogenic bladder Loss of normal bladder function because of nervous system impairments (e.g., spinal cord injury, myelomeningocele); bladder may be underactive (unable to empty well) or overactive and spastic (emptying by uncontrolled reflexes)

Neurogenic bowel Loss of normal bowel function because of nervous system impairments (e.g., spinal cord injury, myelomeningocele); bowel may be overactive, leading to rectal distention or underactive, leading to constipation, and incontenence

Neuron Neurons (also neurones or nerve cells or nerve fibers) are a major class of cells (parenchyma) in the nervous system. In vertebrates, neurons are found in the brain, the spinal cord and in the nerves and ganglia of the peripheral nervous system. Their main role is to process and transmit information. Morphologically, a prototypical neuron is composed of a cell body, a dendritic tree and an axon. In the classical view of the neuron, the cell body and dendritic tree receive inputs from other neurons, and axon transmits output signals. Neurons have excitable membranes, which allow them to generate and propagate electrical impulses. Neurons make connections with other neurons and transmit information to them via synaptic transmission. Different types of neurons have different shapes, possess specific electrical properties adopted for their function and use different neurotransmitters.

Neuronoal intestinal dysplasia (NID) A variety of conditions in which nerve cells (ganglion) are present in the colon but may be abnormal in their position, number, maturity, or appearance.

Neuropeptide A member of a class of protein-like molecules made in the brain. Neuropeptides consist of short chains of amino acids, with some functioning as neurotransmitters and some functioning as hormones.

NHANES National Health and Nutrition Examination Survey; a series of periodic surveys that collect height, weight and other information on the US population; data from NHANES was used to construct the 1977 NCHS growth charts and the 2000 CDC Growth Chart United States

Nibbed almonds These are specially prepared skinned almonds cut into pieces about 2mm square. They're mostly used for decoration. Brown them for a minute in a hot oven to add colour and to bring out their true nutty flavour.

Niceritol A derivative of the vitamin, niacin (chemically penta-erythritol tetranicotinate) used in large doses (several grams) to reduce plasma cholesterol levels.

Nickel An ultra-trace mineral; known to be essential for experimental animals, although its function is not known. There is no information on requirements. Metallic nickel is used as a catalyst in the hydrogenation of fats.

NIDDK or National Institute of Diabetes and Digestive and Kidney Diseases One of the 27 NIH Institutes and Centres, the NIDDK conducts and supports basic and applied research and provides leadership for a national program in diabetes, endocrinology, and metabolic diseases; digestive diseases and nutrition; and kidney, urologic, and hematologic diseases.

NIH or National Institutes of Health The focal point of biomedical research in the United States. NIH conducts research in its own laboratories; supports the research of non-Federal scientists in universities, medical schools, hospitals, and research institutions throughout the country and abroad; helps in the training of research investigators; and fosters communication of medical information.

Nitrite Nitrite is a safe food additive that has been used for centuries to preserve meats, fish and poultry. It also contributes to the characteristic flavor, colour and texture of processed meats such as hot dogs. Because nitrite safeguards cured meats against the most deadly foodborne bacterium of all, Clostridium (C.) botulinum, its use is supported by the public health community. The human body generates much greater nitrite levels than are added to food. Nitrates consumed in foods such as carrots and green vegetables are converted to nitrite during digestion. Nitrite in the body is instrumental in promoting blood clotting, healing wounds and burns, and boosting immune function to kill tumor cells.

Nitrogen A nonmetallic element that constitutes nearly four fifths of the air by volume, occurring as a colourless, odorless, almost inert diatomic gas in various minerals and in all proteins. It is used in a wide variety of important manufacturers, including ammonia, nitric acid, TNT and fertilizers.

Nitrogen conversion factor Factor by which total nitrogen content of a material (the factor measured chemically) is multiplied to determine the protein; depends on the amino acid composition of the protein of the food. For wheat and most cereals it is 5.8; rice, 5.95; soya, 5.7; most legumes and nuts, 5.3; milk, 6.38; other foods, 6.25. Errors arise if part of the nitrogen is present as non-protein nitrogen. In mixtures of proteins, as in dishes and diets, the factor of 6.25 is used. 'Crude protein' is defined as N x 6.25.

Nitrosamines Compounds bearing the nitroso group on the N of amines. Found in trace amounts in mushrooms, fermented fish meal and smoked fish, and in pickled foods, where they are formed by reaction between nitrite and secondary amines. They cause cancer in experimental animals, but it is not known whether the small amounts in foods affect human beings, especially since they have also been found in human gastric juice, possibly formed by reaction between amines and nitrites or nitrates from the diet.

No till farming A methodology of crop production in which the farmer avoids mechanical cultivation (i.e., only one pass over the field). The plant residue remaining on the field's surface helps to control weeds and reduce soil erosion, but it also provides sites for insects to shelter and reproduce, leading to a need for increased insect control.

Noisettes This term has several meanings it's the French word for hazelnut, so 'pommes noisettes', for example, are hazelnut-sized balls of potato, cut with a melon baller, lightly fried and browned in butter. These are generally used as a garnish. 'Noisette' also means nut-brown, as in beurre noisette, butter heated until it turns to a brown nut colour. Noisettes are also small neat round steaks cut from a rolled and tied boneless rack of lamb or mutton. They're very tender and can be fried in butter and served with a variety of garnishes. The name is also given to small round cuts of beef or veal.

Nonblinded Describes a clinical trial or other experiment in which the researchers know what treatments are being given to each study subject or experimental group. If human subjects are involved, they know what treatments they are receiving.

Noodles A type of pasta made with flour and water and sometimes eggs, cut into thin strips. The strands come in numerous shapes and sizes and can be fresh or dried. Noodles are used extensively in Far Eastern cuisine to accompany soups, sauces and stir-fried dishes.

Noodles are made from flour that is the staple food of the area, so they can be made from wheat flour, mung bean flour, buckwheat flour, potato flour or rice flour. Chinese egg noodles, made with wheat flour, can be used in soups, stir-fries or in sauces for dishes using shredded meats, prawns or vegetables. Mung bean flour is used to make thin bean cellophane noodles which can be served as a noodle dish with a sauce or served with rice.

Rice noodles are used in soups or in meat and vegetable sauce dishes. They're perfect store cupboard ingredients - quick to cook and very versatile.

Nori Paper-thin toasted sheets of seaweed (laver - also used in Wales, Scotland and Ireland) used in Japanese cooking for wrapping sushi. There are lots of different varieties - dark green is the most common, but it also can be black, purple or dark red and comes in varying thicknesses.

Although it's commonly used to roll sushi, it can also be crumbled over fish dishes and salads as a garnish. Nori sheets can be kept in the freezer; they thaw almost instantly when removed. Make them more pliable for rolling by laying them on damp sheets of paper towel.

Normande A term used to describe various dishes based on the cooking of Normandy or made using typical products from that region of France butter, cream, seafood, apples, cider and Calvados.

No-till farming A methodology of crop production in which the farmer avoids mechanical cultivation (i.e., only one pass over the field). The plant residue remaining on the field's surface helps to control weeds and reduce soil erosion, but it also provides sites for insects to shelter and reproduce, leading to a need for increased insect control.

Nougat A confection made from boiled honey and/ or sugar syrup mixed with beaten egg white, almonds and sometimes pistachios and preserved fruit.

It has a distinctive almond flavour and either a chewy or brittle texture, depending on how the honey or sugar syrup has been cooked. Serve it as an after-dinner sweet with coffee, crumble it over ice cream or use it in desserts and puddings. Italian torrone and Spanish turron are other forms of nougat.

Nourishment Biological and cultural process invloving the choice, preparation and consumption of one or more foods.

Noxious stimulus Stimulus that causes or has the potential to cause pain.

Nucleic acids Polymers of purine and pyrimidine sugar phosphates; two main classes: ribonucleic acid (RNA) and deoxyribonucleic acid (DNA). Collectively the purines and pyrimidines are called bases. DNA is a double-stranded polymer (the so-called 'double helix') containing the five-carbon sugar deoxyribose. RNA is a single-stranded polymer containing the sugar ribose.

They are not nutritionally important, since dietary nucleic acids are hydrolysed to their bases, ribose and phosphate, in the intestinal tract; purines and pyrimidines can readily be synthesized in the body, and are not dietary essentials.

Fig. Nucleic acids

Nutmeg Nutmeg is a spice from the nutmeg tree, which is native to several Indonesian islands.

Both nutmeg and mace come from the same plant. Nutmeg is the 'nut', while mace is the surrounding lacy 'aril'. Nutmeg has a warm, spicy aroma and flavour and can be used in sweet and savoury cooking. It's a component of the classic bıchamel sauce and is used to flavour a host of cakes, puddings and custards. Buy nutmeg whole and grate it as you need it. Avoid using ready-ground nutmeg, which quickly loses its flavour.

Nutraceuticals One term used to describe substances in or parts of a food that may be considered to provide medical or health benefits beyond basic nutrition, including disease prevention. Research indicates this term might not appeal to consumers. Also, see "functional foods."

Nutrient A substance derived from food, and is needed by the body to supply energy and maintain normal cell functioning, rεpair, and growth.

Nutrient density The term "nutrient density" has several meanings.Firstly, nutrient density is defined as a ratio of nutrient content (in grams) to the total energy content (in kilocalories). Nutrient-dense food is opposite to energy-dense food (also callec "empty calorie" food). According to the Dietary Guidelines for Americans 2005, nutrient-dense foods are those foods that provide substantial amounts of vitamins and minerals and relatively few calories. For example, fruit and vegetables are considered nutrient-dense food, while products containing added sugars, saturated fats, and alcohol are considered nutrient-poor food.

Nutrition 1. The science or practice of taking in and utilizing foods.

2. A nourishing substance, such as nutritional solutions delivered to hospitalized patients via an IV or IG tube.

Nutrition security The provision of an environment that encourages and motivates society to make food choices consistent with short- and long-term good health.

Nutrition services incentive program A program administered through the Administration on Aging at HHS that provides states with funding, in the form of cash or commodities, for the effective delivery of nutritious meals to seniors. States must use benefits under this program to provide meals in conjunction with other Administration on Aging-supported programs. At the state level, this program is administered through the State Agency on Aging or Indian Tribal Organizations.

Nutritionist According to the US Department of Labor, Dictionary of Occupational Titles, one who applies the science of nutrition to the promotion of health and control of disease, instructs auxiliary medical personnel, and participates in surveys. Not legally defined in the UK, but there is a Register of Accredited Nutritionists maintained by the Nutrition Society and Institute of Biology.

Nutrition-related diseases Terminology for a great variety of diseases that results from insufficient consumption, excessive consumption or a prolonged imbalance between the ingestion and utilization of nutritive elements that should be harmoniously combined. Various other entries describe specific situations: goiter, malnutrition, nutritional deficiences.

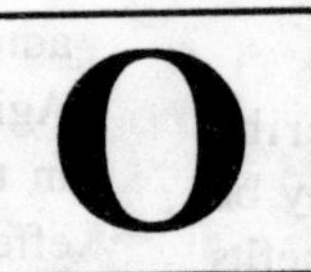

OANE Office of Analysis, Nutrition, and Evaluation. This research division within FNS at the USDA conducts program analysis and assessment of the programs under FNS' jurisdiction. The office also serves as a coordinating point for program-related nutrition policy and services.

Oats A cereal grass cultivated for its edible seed, used by both man and animals. Most commonly used to make the famous breakfast of the Scotsman - Porridge.

Obese Well above ones normal weight. A person has traditionally been considered to be obese if they are more than 20 percent over their ideal weight. That ideal weight must take into account the person's height, age, sex, and build.

Obesity Having a high amount of body fat. A person is considered obese if he or she has a body mass index (BMI) of 30 kg/m2 or greater.

Obesity, or overweight Although precise definitions vary among experts, overweight has been traditionally defined as 10 percent to 20 percent above an optimal weight for height derived from statistics. Obesity is defined as body weight being 20% above normal. Some scientists argue that the amount and distribution of an individual's body fat is a significant indicator of health risk and therefore should be considered in defining overweight. Abdominal fat has been linked to more adverse health consequences than fat in the hips or thighs. Thus, calculations of waist to hip ratio are preferred by some health experts to help determine if an individual is overweight.

Obstipation Constipation caused by a blockage, resulting in an accumulation of stool with the development of colon distension; leads to fecal impaction

Oenin An anthocyanidin from the skin of purple grapes.

Oestrogens The female sex hormones; chemically they are steroids, although non-steroidal compounds also have oestrogen activity, including the synthetic compounds stilboestrol and hexoestrol. These have been used for chemical caponization of cockerels and to increase the growth rate of cattle. See also capon.

Compounds with oestrogen activity are found in a variety of plants; collectively these are known as phyto-oestrogens.

Offal The internal organs and innards of an animal or fish, including brain, liver, kidney, tripe, and heart. It can also refer to the animal's extremities, too, such as head, tail, trotters and tongue.

Offshore farming It takes place in deep, navigable waters and involves the use of boats.

Okra Also known as gumbo, bamya, bamies, and ladies' fingers; the edible seed pods of Hibiscus esculentus. Small ridged mucilaginous pods resembling a small cucumber, grown in South America, the West Indies, and India; used in soups and stews. There are two varieties: gomba are oblong, bamya are round. A 100-g portion (raw) is a rich source of vitamin C; a good source of calcium; a source of carotene (500 Og), vitamin B 1, and folate; contains 4 g of dietary fibre; supplies 30 kcal.

Olive In neuroanatomy, a rounded oval prominence on the surface of the medulla oblongata in the brain. There are two olives, corresponding to the two olivary bodies, one on each side of the medulla oblongata. Nerve fibers in the olivopontocerebellar pathway connect the olives to the pons and cerebellum .

Olive oil Pressed from olives, this is a rich, fruity oil used for marinades, dressings, baking and shallow frying. Hundreds of varieties of olive are used to make olive oil so the range available is huge, varying in colour, flavour, aroma and character.

Produced mainly in France, Spain, Italy and Greece, olive oil is similar to wine in that it varies with the climate, country, area of origin and seasonal factors. The oil from the first pressing is pure, pale greenish-yellow in colour and is the best quality. This is sold as 'extra virgin' olive oil and is best used for salads, marinades and pasta dishes.

The pulp is then pressed again to yield a darker oil that is less flavoursome than the first pressing and sold just as 'olive oil' or 'pure olive oil'. Olive oil has many health-promoting properties because it's relatively high in monounsaturates. Picking up on this fact, food manufacturers have turned to making spreads similar to margarine but containing up to 20 per cent olive oil.

Olive oil can be bought with additions such as herbs, garlic or chilli. Store it in a cool dark place away from direct sunlight but not in the fridge or it will turn cloudy.

Omega-3 Fatty Acids Help protect the heart, help prevent stroke, lower cholesterol levels and alleviate arthritis.

Orange Citrus fruit, from the subtropical tree Citrus sinensis. Of nutritional value mainly because of its vitamin C content of 40-60 mg/ 100 g. Blood oranges are coloured by the presence of anthocyanins in the juice vesicles. One medium orange (160 g) is a rich source of vitamin C; a good source of folate; a source of vitamins A (as carotene) and B1; contains 3.2 g of dietary fibre; supplies 60 kcal.

Oregano A pungent green culinary herb with a great affinity for a variety of foods, from lamb to vegetables, stuffings and egg dishes. There are many species and varieties of the genus Origanum, each with quite different characteristics and flavours.

Oregano is closely related to marjoram. It grows wild in many parts of southern Europe and the Mediterranean and some parts of Asia. It's characteristic of many Greek dishes (particularly lamb) and in the UK is often sprinkled liberally on pizzas.

Oregano grows easily in well protected areas in the UK. Because of its high oil content, it retains its flavour and aroma when dried. You can replace dried oregano for fresh, but reduce the amount used by about half. Dried oregano is a kitchen essential, but ensure you replace it frequently, because it quickly loses its pungency. Oregano is one of the herbs in the mixture called herbes de Provence.

Organic Organic defines agricultural products that are grown using cultural, biological and mechanical methods prior to the use of synthetic, non agricultural substances to control pests, improve soil quality an/or enhance processing. The USDA is currently addressing the issue of organic products, and aims to have official rules for what may be considered organic ready for the 1999 spring planting season. Currently organic defines an agricultural process in which farmers use techniques such as crop rotation, cultivation, mulching, soil enrichment and the "encouragement" of predators and microorganisms which naturally keep pests away. The now widely accepted definition allows farmers to use natural pesticides, but nothing synthetic.

Organic food Produced by farmers who emphasize the use of renewable resources and the conservation of soil and water to enhance environmental quality for future generations. Organic meat, poultry, eggs, and dairy products come from animals that are given no antibiotics or growth hormones. Organic food is produced without using most conventional pesticides; fertilizers made with synthetic ingredients or sewage sludge; bioengineering; or ionizing radiation. Before a product can be labeled organic, a government-approved certifier inspects the farm where the food is grown to make sure the farmer is following all the rules necessary to meet USDA organic standards. Companies that handle or process organic food before it gets to your local supermarket or restaurant must be certified, too.

Osmazome Obsolete name given to an aqueous extract of meat regarded as the 'pure essence of meat'.

Osmolality The concentration of a solution expressed in osmoles of solute particles per kilogram of solvent. Infants and some children may be unable to tolerate a formula with a high osmolality.

Osteomalacia Softening of the bone because of a loss of calcium in the bone material; can be caused by inadequate vitamin D intake and/or disorders that interfere with the absorption of vitamins and minerals

Osteoporosis Osteoporosis is a skeletal disease in which the bones lose mass and density, the pores in bones enlarge, and the bones generally become fragile. Osteoporosis often is not diagnosed until a fracture occurs, most commonly in the spine, hip or wrist. The National Osteoporosis Foundation estimates that about 1.5 million such fractures occur each year in the United States, at an estimated annual cost of $14 billion in 1995.

Osteoporosis is four times more common in women, whose bones are naturally thinner and less dense, than in men. Women start losing bone mass and density at an earlier age, and the process is accelerated by menopause, causing osteoporosis to manifest itself between the ages of 50 and 60. Research has shown that in addition to regular exercise, calcium intake during childhood, adolescence and early adulthood helps build a "bone bank" of calcium stores. While bone length is established by age 20, bone strength and density continue to develop through age 30.

Ounce A measure of weight equal to 1/16th of a pound or, metrically, 28.35 grams. The abbreviation for ounce is oz. (An ounce of prevention is reputedly worth a pound of cure.)

Outcomes research A type of research increasingly used by the health industry which provides information about how a specific procedure or treatment regimen results the subject (clinical safety and efficacy), the subject's physical functioning and lifestyle, and economic considerations such as saving/prolonging life and avoiding costly complications.

Ouzo A Greek spirit flavoured with aniseed. Like French pastis, it's usually served with water which turns it whiteish and opaque.

Overweight Also defined as an excessively high amount of body fat in relation to lean body mass. However, the range for an overweight person is a Body Mass Index (BMI) from 25 to 30 kg/m2.

Oxidation The loss of electrons from a compound (or element) in a chemical reaction. When one compound is oxidized, another compound is reduced. That is, the other compound must "pick up" the electrons that the first has lost.

Oxtail Classed as offal; a 150-g portion of stewed lean meat is a rich source of iron, vitamin B 2, protein, and niacin; contains 20 g of fat and supplies 360 kcal.

Oyster A saltwater bivalve with a sea-salty flavour and a succulent texture. Aficionados insist that they're best eaten raw, perhaps with freshly ground black pepper and a squeeze of lemon juice or a drop of Tabasco sauce. However, they can be steamed, grilled or poached, too, and they make excellent canapes.

Only use oysters that are tightly shut in their shells or that close when tapped. Any oysters that stay open are dead and should be thrown away.

Oyster mushrooms An ear-shaped silvery-grey or greyish-brown mushroom that grows in clumps or clusters. It's now cultivated so it's more readily available and found in most supermarkets.

Oyster mushrooms have a subtle flavour and are often used in oriental cookery. They cook down to virtually nothing and are quite expensive, so they're often used in combination with other mushrooms.

Oyster sauce Oyster sauce is a thick, rich brown southern Chinese condiment, flavoured with extract of oysters. Spend a bit more on a good brand of oyster sauce - it will have more natural oyster flavour and less monosodium glutamate (MSG). Keep refrigerated once opened.

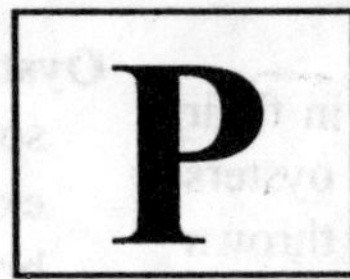

P value The p (probability) value is a calculation used in studies to determine if the results are caused by chance or not. The lower the p-value, the more likely it is that the difference between groups was caused by treatment. A p value less than 0.05 is statistically significant and indicates that the result is not due to chance.

Paella A Spanish dish of rice and saffron that usually includes tomatoes, chicken and seafood. It originated in the Valencia region of Spain and gets its name from the broad shallow pan (paella or paellera) in which it's traditionally cooked and served from.

The rice used is similar to risotto rice. Buy calasparra rice if you can, which is a Spanish short-grain rice; otherwise any risotto rice will do.

Paella is cooked differently from risotto. Rather than constantly stirring it, paella shouldn't be stirred at all once the ingredients have been mixed together. For full authenticity, cook paella outside over an open fire.

Paid meal certification A classification within the child nutrition programs where children pay most of the cost for receiving meals and snacks. Through the five child nutrition programs, the federal government pays some of the administrative costs. Children from families with incomes above 185 percent of poverty pay for meals and snacks.

Pak choi Closely related to bok choi, this leafy green Chinese vegetable belongs to the cabbage family (although it tastes nothing like cabbage!). It has long green, slightly ribbed leaf stalks and soft oval green leaves.

The leaves and stems are best suited to brief stir-frying or steaming to retain their mild flavour. Occasionally you may be able to find baby pak choi which can be cooked whole.

Palmar grasp Hand movement in which the palm (not the fingertips) is used to pick up an item; important precursor to self-feeding

Palmomental reflex A reflex in which stroking the palm of the hand causes a wrinkling of the mentalis muscle (an elevation of the angle of the mouth) on the same side of body

Pancakes Pancakes are thin cakes made from a batter of milk (or milk and water), eggs and flour which is then cooked in a frying pan or on a griddle until golden brown on both sides. You can buy special pancake pans which are shallow and non-stick with curved sides.

Pancakes are delicious eaten simply with lemon juice and sugar, but they can be filled with a variety of sweet ingredients such as maple syrup, fruit, ice cream or chocolate sauce.

They make a good base for savoury fillings too, such as fried mushrooms, cheese, spinach, seafood - anything goes, really.

Pancakes are made from a wide variety of flours and in a range of styles in many countries. French pancakes are made slightly thinner and are called crкpes. Scotch pancakes are small and thick, usually cooked on a griddle and sometimes flavoured with sultanas or raisins. American pancakes are normally served at breakfast. They tend to be light and fluffy, served in generous stacks with bacon and maple syrup. There is also the Russian blini, Chinese pancakes served with Peking duck, Italian crespelle, and so on.

Pancetta An Italian type of bacon produced from belly of pork which is seasoned, then rolled up and dry cured. Flat slabs of pancetta are also available and this is normally how you'd find it in Italy.

It can be bought in the UK pre-packed and either in cubes (cubetti di pancetta) or slices, the latter often smoked. The cubes are fried and used in soffrito (the Italian version of a mirepoix) to give a base flavour to dishes or incorporated in pasta dishes such as spaghetti carbonara.

Sliced pancetta can be served as part of a selection of cold meats, or grilled until crisp and then crumbled over pasta, rice, salads and soups. Wrap pieces of fish, chicken or meat in slices of pancetta and oven-bake them, or use it as a pizza topping. Thinly sliced, unsmoked, streaky bacon rashers will make a suitable substitute if you can't get pancetta.

Pancreas A gland that makes enzymes that help the body break down and use nutrients in food. It also produces the hormone insulin [see definition] and releases it into the bloodstream to help the body control blood sugar levels.

Panettone A large, round yeasted fruit cake from Italy, traditionally eaten at Christmas and Easter. It's baked in a special tubular mould to give it height. They're beautifully packaged in tall decorated boxes and available from Italian delis and some larger supermarkets, although they're generally only available seasonally.

Panettone can be served as a dessert, accompanied by sweet wine; it's also delicious toasted and spread with butter, or used in place of bread in a bread and butter pudding.

Panna cotta The name for this cold dessert from Italy means 'cooked cream', although not all recipes call for the cream to be actually cooked.

To make panna cotta, cream is added to gelatine and then flavoured, usually with vanilla or cinnamon but sometimes with alcohol or other flavourings. The mixture is then cooled until it sets and is served with a sweet sauce.

Pantry chef or Garde Managr The person who prepares cold savory items Boucher

Papaya Also called a paw paw, this is a large fragrant fruit that looks a bit like a large mango, with green skin and sweet orange flesh filled with round black seeds. It's delicious on its own with a squeeze of lime juice, or use it in salsas, add it to fruit smoothies or fruit salads or even savoury salads.

Paprika Paprika is the ground bright red powder from sweet and hot dried peppers. It's much milder than cayenne pepper and has a characteristic sweetness. It's a favourite ingredient in European cookery in Austria and Hungary paprika is a main flavouring in meat stews such as goulash, of which paprika is the essence.

Eastern Europeans use it to flavour venison stews and soured cabbage and other vegetable dishes. In Spain, Portugal and Mexico paprika is used to flavour chorizo.

Spanish smoked paprika, which adds a delicious smoky note to meat or vegetable dishes, is available in supermarkets in the UK. Portuguese cooks use paprika to flavour fish stews.

Use it to give spicy depth to lamb, chicken and fish dishes or try sprinkling a pinch over the yolk of a fried egg or creamy scrambled eggs.

Parenteral nutrition The slow infusion of a solution of nutrients into a vein through a catheter, which is surgically implanted. This may be partial, to supplement food and nutrient intake, or total (TPN, total parenteral nutrition), providing the sole source of energy and nutrient intake for the patient.

Pareve Jewish term for dishes containing neither milk nor meat. Orthodox Jewish law prohibits mixing of milk and meat foods or the consumption of milk products for 3 hours after a meat meal. See also milchig, fleishig.

Parmentier French; made or served with potatoes, named after Parmentier, who popularized the potato in France in the eighteenth century. Pommes parmentier are diced and fried; parmentier soup is a leek and potato soup.

Parmesan Originating from around Parma in the north-west of Italy, this is one of the world's best-known cheeses. It's stamped with the official Parmigiano Reggiano mark as a guarantee of origin. Fragrant and tangy, it has a hard, grainy texture and a buttery yellow colour. Buy fresh parmesan where possible; the taste is far superior to pre-packed cheese - and avoid ready-grated cheese at all costs.

Grate Parmesan into cooked dishes, add it to risotto, serve a generous chunk on its own with fruit after a meal, or use a potato peeler to make parmesan shavings and scatter them on pasta dishes or salads. Because Parmigiano Reggiano cheese isn't made with vegetarian rennet, strict vegetarians avoid it. However, there are good vegetarian Parmesan-style cheeses available in most supermarkets, including cheese made in the UK.

Parsley No kitchen should be without a good supply of this multi-purpose herb. It can be used as a garnish and flavouring and as a vegetable.

There are two main varieties curly leaf and flatleaf. Both can be used for the same purposes, although flatleaf parsley has a stronger flavour and tends to be favoured in Mediterranean cooking.

Parsley can be used in almost any savoury dish. It's especially good used in great quantities in fresh salads or in soups and sauces. Chop or shred it and mix with butter to melt over fish or to glaze vegetables.

There's just as much flavour in the stalk as in the leaf and both are used in bouquet garni to flavour stews and stocks. It's delicious briefly deep-fried and served as a vegetable to accompany chicken, veal or fish. Use it in marinades, stuffings, in omelettes - the list goes on!

Parsley types Three types of parsley are widely available. They are curly, flat-leafed or Italian, and Hamburg-grown for its white root. Curly parsley has a milder flavor than flat-leafed, known for its stronger flavor. The Hamburg white root is favoured by those who like parsnips. Avoid wild plants that look like parsley; they are called fool's parsley because they smell bad and are poisonous.

Paskha A Russian dessert traditionally served at Easter. It's a creamy set pudding with a similar consistency to cheesecake, made from curd, cream or cottage cheese, eggs, sugar and dried fruit and flavoured with vanilla. The sides of the cake are sometimes decorated with almonds, cherries or angelica and the mixture is moulded into a four-sided pyramid and decorated with fruits and nuts with a shape of a cross on top.

Passata Passata is made from ripe tomatoes that have been puried and sieved to remove the skin and seeds. It's sold in jars and can be smooth or chunky depending on the level of sieving.

It's useful to keep in the cupboard to use in soups, sauces, pasta dishes, casseroles, or anything that needs a concentrated tomato flavour. Passata is also great for using in drinks with a tomato base, such as Bloody Mary. Once opened a jar will keep in the fridge for up to a week.

Passion fruit Also known as parchita, granadilla, and water lemon; fruit of the tropical American vine, Passiflora spp. Purple or greenishyellow when ripe, it contains watery pulp surrounding small seeds; used in fruit drinks. A 100-g portion (four fruits, 60 g of edible flesh and pips) is a good source of vitamin C; supplies 20 kcal.

Pasta Made from a dough of durum-wheat semolina, water and sometimes eggs, which is kneaded and cut into a wide variety of shapes. There are basically two types - fresh or dried.

Fresh pasta is often made with eggs, giving it a richer flavour and texture than the dried varieties; it has the consistency of a soft dough and only needs to be cooked for a very short time compared with dried pasta.

You need to serve slightly more fresh pasta compared with dry because it doesn't absorb as much water as dried so doesn't swell up as much. It should be kept in the fridge and used within two days (or check the packet information), but it does freeze well for up to a month. You can buy filled fresh pastas with a variety of meat and vegetable fillings - they make a simple supper served with a home-made sauce. Dried pasta is convenient and widely available.

Choose good quality pasta made only from durum-wheat semolina. It will store unopened for more than a year in a cool dry cupboard and for about a month once opened. The choice of pasta these days is quite overwhelming and it's eaten around the world from Italy to China.

It can be served simply with sauces, stuffed, baked or added to soups for bulk. See individual entries for different types available farfalle, fettuccine, fusilli, gnocchi, linguine, penne, ravioli, rigatoni, tagliatelle, vermicelli. See also noodles.

Pastry chef or patissier Is responsible for cold foods, including salads and dressings, pβtιs, cold hors d'oeuvres, and buffet items.

Pate A rich paste made of liver, pork, game or other meats, cooked in a terrine or wrapped in pastry and cooked. Fish can also be used as the basis of a pβtι, combined with soft cheese, mayonnaise or soured cream.

Pate can be smooth or coarse and is delicious simply spread on warm toast or crusty bread. It can also be used as a component in main dishes such as beef Wellington in which fillet steaks are spread with duxelles and enclosed in pastry.

Pathogenesis The origin and development of a disease or disorder.

Pathogens Virus, bacterium, parasitic protozoan, or other microorganisms that cause infectious disease by invading the body of an organism know as the host. Note that infection is not synonymous with disease because infection does not always lead to injury of the host.

Pathology The study of the fundamental nature, causes, and development of abnormal conditions and the structural and functional changes that result.

Patty pan A small, round flattish summer squash, yellow, green or white in colour with pretty fluted edges. It's sometimes known as a custard squash or custard marrow and can be cooked in a similar way to courgettes. They don't need to be peeled, just washed clean and the ends trimmed.

Bake them in the oven, slice and fry them in butter or eat them raw in salads. They go well with Mediterranean ingredients - garlic, onions, tomatoes and lots of fresh summery herbs.

Peanut Also known as a groundnut or monkey nut. This edible nut is the seed of a member of the pea family, so is not a true nut. The pods mature underground and each contain two to four seeds.

Peanuts can be roasted, salted and eaten whole or used in cooked dishes. They're used a lot in South-east Asian cookery - satay is a spicy peanut sauce served with small skewers of grilled meat and chicken.

Peanut or groundnut oil is widely used in cooking and in margarine manufacture. Peanut butter is made from ground peanuts.

Pear Fruit of many species of Pyrus; cultivated varieties all descended from P. communis; The UK National Fruit Collection has 495 varieties of dessert and cooking pears, and a further 20 varieties of perry pears. A 200-g portion (an average fruit) is a source of vitamins B6 and C and copper; contains 4-5 g of dietary fibre; supplies 80 kcal (340 kJ). See also poire williams.

Pecan Also known as a hickory nut, the pecan is related to the walnut and grown mainly in North America. It's a delicious nut with a toffee-like taste that's perfect for just eating as it is. In cooking it's probably best known as the basis for pecan pie, but it can be used in all kinds of cake recipes, in sweets and in savoury dishes.

Pectin A natural gelling agent found in ripe fruit. Pectin is an important ingredient in making jams and jellies. The levels of pectin vary from fruit to fruit. Some fruits, such as citrus fruit, blackberries, apples and redcurrants have high pectin levels. Others are low in pectin such as strawberries - so lemon juice is added to strawberry jam to help it set. It's possible to buy pectin as a liquid extract or in powdered form. On ready-made jams and jellies it's labelled as E440.

Pediatric Pertaining to children.

Pelvic Having to do with the pelvis (the lower part of the abdomen located between the hip bones).

Peptic ulcer A sore in the lining of the esophagus, stomach, or duodenum, usually caused by the bacterium Helicobacter pylori (H. pylori). An ulcer in the stomach is a gastric ulcer; an ulcer in the duodenum is a duodenal ulcer.

Percutaneous endoscopy One method of placing a feeding tube, where the feeding tube is placed using an endoscope

Perineum The area of the body between the anus and the vulva in females, and between the anus and the scrotum in males.

Peristalsis Rhythmic, wavelike contraction of smooth muscle in intestines or other tubular structures; circular contraction and relaxation of the tube propels its contents

Peristalsis Synchronized or coordinated contraction of the muscles that propel food content through the gastrointestinal (GI) tract to facilitate normal digestion and the absorption of nutrients. Peristalsis is dependent upon the coordination between the muscles, nerves, and hormones in the digestive tract.

Permeability Permeability, permeable and semipermeable have several meanings:Permeability (electromagnetism), in electromagnetism, is the degree of magnetisation of a material in response to a magnetic field.Permeability (fluid), in earth sciences, is a measure of the ability of a material to transmit fluids. Semipermeable membrane, a membrane which will allow certain molecules or ions to pass through it by diffusion.Permeability tensor, permeability in an anisotropic medium.Vascular permeability, the movement of fluids and molecules between the vascular and extravascular compartments.

Perry An alcoholic drink, similar to cider, made from specially grown varieties of pears. Look out for single variety perry, which is still made in small amounts by artisan producers; otherwise, sparkling perry is available in supermarkets. A subtly flavoured vinegar is made from perry. Use it in salad dressings and marinades. Cider and cider vinegar are suitable substitutes.

Pesticide A broad class of crop protection chemicals including four major types insecticides used to control insects; herbicides used to control weeds; rodenticides used to control rodents; and fungicides used to control mold, mildew and fungi.

In addition consumers use pesticides in the home or yard to control termites and roaches, clean mold from shower curtains, stave off crab grass on the lawn, kill fleas and ticks on pets and disinfect swimming pools, to name just a few "specialty" pesticide uses.

Pesto An Italian dark green sauce for pasta originating in Genoa. It's made from pine nuts blended with fresh basil, parmesan or pecorino cheese, garlic and olive oil.

Red pesto is made similarly but is based on either sun-dried tomatoes or grilled red peppers. It's uncooked and can be bought preserved in jars or fresh in tubs. The contents of jars, once opened, should be kept in the fridge and used within a couple of weeks. Keep the surface covered with oil. Fresh pesto in tubs should be used within two to three days. It can easily be made at home but you do need a generous amount of basil leaves to make just a small portion of pesto.

Variations include using rocket, watercress or parsley instead of basil and nuts such as walnuts, hazelnuts or pistachios instead of pine nuts.

The sauce can be stirred into freshly cooked pasta, spooned onto thick soups, spread on bruschetta, fillets of fish or chicken before grilling, or added to mayonnaise and salad dressings.

Petit fours A small French fancy biscuit or cake often served at the end of a meal. Strictly speaking they're oven-baked little cakes ('four' is French for oven) and were classically made with choux pastry or flan pastry. However, a selection of petits fours these days can cover a wide variety of sweet things, not necessarily cooked, and made possibly with meringue, marzipan, chocolate, and so on.

Pharmaceutical products The term is used in this document to designate pharmacological preparations in medication from that are based on specific nutrients, such as vitamins, iron, iodine, zinc, etc.

Pharmacokinetics How the body handles a drug, including how it is absorbed, circulated, transformed, and eliminated.

Pharmacology Pharmacology meaning drug, and logos is the study of how substances interact with living organisms to produce a change in function. If substances have medicinal properties, they are considered pharmaceuticals. The field encompasses drug composition and properties, interactions, toxicology, therapy, and medical applications and antipathogenic capabilities.

Phasic activity Activity which is demonstrated in various phases.

Phospholipid Phospholipids are a class of lipids formed from four components: fatty acids, a negatively-charged phosphate group, nitrogen containing alcohol and a backbone. Phospholipids with a glycerol backbone are known as glycerophospholipids or phosphoglycerides. There is only one type of phospholipid with a sphingosine backbone; sphingomyelin. Phospholipids are a major component of all biological membranes, along with glycolipids and cholesterol.

Phenylketonuria An inherited (autosomal recessive) metabolic disorder, marked by the deficiency of the enzyme that converts phenylalanine (an amino acid) to tyrosine; accumulation of phenylalanine in the blood can lead to mental retardation and other neurologic problems; treatment includes a low-phenylalanine diet and a phenylalanine-free medical food

Pheromones "Sex perfume" traps used to disrupt insect reproduction cycles.

Phosphatase test A test for the adequacy of pasteurization of milk. The enzyme phosphatase, normally present in milk, is denatured at a temperature slightly greater than that required to destroy the tubercle bacillus and other pathogens; therefore the presence of detectable phosphatase activity indicates inadequate pasteurization. The test can detect 0.2% raw milk in pasteurized milk.

Phosphatidic acid Glycerol esterified to two molecules of fatty acid, with the third hydroxyl group esterified to phosphate; chemically diacylglycerol phosphate; intermediates in the metabolism of phospholipids.

Phospholipids Glycerol esterified to two molecules of fatty acid, one of which is commonly a polyunsaturated fatty acid. The third hydroxyl group is esterified to phosphate and one of a number of water-soluble compounds, including serine (phosphatidylserine), ethanolamine (phosphatidylethanolamine), choline (phosphatidylcholine, also known as lecithin), and inositol (phosphatidylinositol).

Cell membranes are a double layer of phospholipids with the fatty acid side-chains on the inside and the water-soluble compound esterified to the phosphate interacts with water. This is why phospholipids can be used to emulsify oils and fats in water and are commonly used in food manufacture as emulsifiers.

From the energy point of view they can be regarded as being equivalent to simple fats (triacylglycerols); they also provide a dietary source of choline and inositol, neither of which is a dietary essential.

Phosphoproteins Proteins containing phosphate, other than as nucleic acids (nucleoproteins) or phospholipids (lipoproteins), e.g. casein from milk, ovovitellin from egg yolk.

Phosphoric acid May be one of three types: orthophosphoric acid (H3PO4), metaphosphoric acid (HPO_3), or pyrophosphoric acid ($H_4P_2O_7$). Orthophosphoric acid and its salts are E-338-341, used as acidity regulators and in acid-fruit-flavoured beverages such as lemonade.

OH
|
O═P—OH
|
OH

Fig. Phosphoric acid

Phosphorus An essential element, occurring in tissues and foods as phosphate (salts of phosphoric acid), phospholipids, and phosphoproteins. In the body most (80%) is present in the skeleton and teeth as calcium phosphate (hydroxyapatite); the remainder is in the phospholipids of cell membranes, in nucleic acids, and in a variety of metabolic intermediates, including ATP. The parathyroid glands control the concentration of phosphate in the blood, mainly by modifying its excretion in the urine.

Human dietary needs (about 1.3 g per day) are always met; a deficiency never occurs in man. The calcium to phosphate ratio of infant foods is, however, important. Phosphate deficiency is common in livestock and gives rise to osteomalacia (also known as sweeny or creeping sickness).

Physical activity Any form of exercise or movement. Physical activity may include planned activity such as walking, running, basketball, or other sports. Physical activity may also include other daily activities such as household chores, yard work, walking the dog, etc. It is recommended that adults get at least 30 minutes and children get at least 60 minutes of moderate physical activity most days of the week. Moderate physical activity is any activity that requires about as much energy as walking two miles in 30 minutes.

Physiology The study of the functions or vital processes of living things.

Phytate A chemical complex (large molecule) substance that is the dominant (i.e., 60 to 80%) chemical form of phosphorous within cereal grains, oilseeds, and their by products. Monogastric animals (e.g., swine) cannot digest and utilize phosphorus within phytate, because they lack the enzyme known as phytase in their digestive system, so that phosphorus (phytate) is excreted into the environment. When phytase enzyme is present in the ration of a monogastric animal, at a high enough level, the monogastric animal is then able to digest the phytate (thereby releasing that phosphorus for absorption by the animal).

Phytochemical Phytochemicals are substances found in edible fruits and vegetables that may be ingested by humans daily in gram quantities and that exhibit a potential for modulating the human metabolism in a manner favourable for reducing risk of cancer.

Phytonutrients/Phytochemicals Reducing risks of diseases of aging such as Alzheimer's, osteoporosis, cancer and heart disease. Plant foods, including soy products and fruits and vegetables, cruciferous vegetables such as Brussels sprouts, cabbage, broccoli, kale, bok choy and cauliflower.

Pickles Pickles fermented in a mixture of brine, dill weed, mixed spices, and vinegar.

Pigeon Columbia livia; young about 4 weeks old is a squab. A 150-g portion is an extremely rich source of iron, a rich source of protein, niacin, and vitamins B1 and B2; contains 20 g of fat; supplies 350 kcal.

Pilchard An adult sardine, pilchards are an oil-rich fish. They're rarely available fresh and are mainly sold processed and canned. You're most likely to find them fresh during the summer months. If you do, cook them as you would sardines. They're particularly delicious barbecued and served with a rich tomato sauce or just butter and lemon.

Pine nut Also called pine kernels, pine nuts are the edible seed of about a dozen species of pine trees. The cones are sun-dried, then threshed to shake out the seeds, which are then hulled. Pine nuts are oily and rich in protein, so they tend to go rancid quite quickly; store them in the fridge and they'll keep longer.

The longer, thinner Asian varieties are higher in oil than American or Mediterranean types. Pine nuts have a rich buttery, resinous flavour and are used in many savoury dishes, especially vegetarian ones, but are particularly associated with Mediterranean cooking. They're a key ingredient in pesto and appear in lots of pasta dishes.

Pineapple Fruit of the tropical plant Ananas sativus, one of the bromeliad family. The fruit contains the proteolytic enzyme bromelain, which has been used (like papain) to tenderize meat. A 100-g portion is a rich source of vitamin C; a source of copper; provides 0.8 g of dietary fibre; supplies 30 kcal.

Piri-piri Piri-piri is an African word for chilli and also a hot chilli sauce used in Portuguese, African and Brazilian cookery. The Portuguese introduced chillies to their African colonies after discovering them in Brazil, so piri-piri plays a major part in the fiery food of Mozambique - chicken, fish, seafood and vegetables are all cooked with piri-piri. It's available in bottles from delis and supermarkets.

Pithaya The fruit of a Central and South American cactus, the pitahaya has a knobbly yellow skin and a deep-pink, dense flesh. The fruit can be cut in half and the flesh, which has a mild, sweet flavour, eaten with a spoon (along with the seeds) - a squeeze of lemon or lime juice will help it along. Add the bright pink flesh to a fruit salad for a splash of brilliant colour.

Placebo For the band Placebo go to Placebo (band)A placebo, from the Latin for "I will please", is an inactive substance (pill, liquid, etc.), which is administered as if it were a therapy, but which has no therapeutic value other than the placebo effect.

Plaice An orange-spotted flat sea fish. It's available fresh or frozen, whole or in fillets and has a mild sweet flavour. Fry or grill it on the bone, poach whole fish or fillets and use the poaching liquor to make a sauce, or coat fillets of plaice in egg and breadcrumbs and pan-fry in butter and a little oil. Sole or brill can be used instead of plaice.

Plaque The word plaque or placque may mean: Dental plaque, a yellowish film that builds up on the teethAtheromatous plaque, a buildup of fatty deposits within the wall of a blood vesselMucoid plaque, a supposed thick coating of abnormal mucous material in the colonCommemorative plaque, a flat ornamental plate or tablet fixed to a wall, used to mark a significant event, person, etc.Viral plaque, a visible structure formed by virus propagation within a cell cultureAmyloid plaque, an extracellular protein buildup implicated in various diseases (Alzheimer's disease, Parkinson's disease).

Polenta A golden-yellow Italian cornmeal made from ground maize, and also the name given to the savoury cornmeal porridge that's made from it.

Polenta can be coarse or fine. The type most widely available in the UK is the instant or quick-cook powdered variety, which can be made in minutes. The dish itself is the traditional staple of northern Italy and is made by simply mixing the cornmeal with water and simmering and stirring until it thickens. It can be served hot - known as wet polenta - or left to cool and set in a dish and then cut into squares or slices which are fried or grilled to give a light crust.

Ready-to-eat polenta is also available, sold in rubbery looking blocks. Wet polenta can be bland so tends to be mixed with flavourings such as butter, cheese, herbs, cooked onions or mushrooms. It's also used as a side dish to accompany meat dishes, stews or casseroles. Fried or grilled polenta slices also make a good accompaniment to dishes such as stews, or can be topped with cheese and grilled. Polenta meal can also be used in baking.

Polony Italian smoked pork and veal sausage, ready to slice and eat; also known as bologna. A 150-g portion is a good source of protein, vitamin B 1, and niacin; a source of iron; contains 30 g of fat and 1200 mg of sodium; supplies 320 kcal (1280 kJ).

Polyols A type of sweetener used in reduced calorie foods. They differ from intense sweeteners in that they are considered nutritive; that is, they do contribute calories to the diet. Polyols are incompletely absorbed and metabolized, however, and consequently contribute fewer calories than sucrose. The polyols commonly used in the United States include sorbitol, mannitol, xylitol, maltitol, maltitol syrup, lactitol, erythritol, isomalt and hydrogenated starch hydrolysates. Most are approximately half as sweet as sucrose; maltitol and xylitol are about as sweet as sucrose. Polyols are found naturally in berries, apples, plums and other foods. They also are produced commercially from carbohydrates such as sucrose, glucose, and starch for use in sugar free candies, cookies and chewing gum. Along with adding a sweet taste, polyols perform a variety of functions such as adding bulk and texture, providing a cooling effect or taste, preventing the browning that occurs during heating and retaining the moisture in foods.

Polysaccharide Polysaccharides (sometimes called glycans) are relatively complex carbohydrates.They are polymers made up of many monosaccharides joined together by glycosidic linkages. They are therefore very large, often branched, molecules. They tend to be amorphous, insoluble in water, and have no sweet taste.When all the constituent monosaccharides are of the same type they are termed homopolysaccharides; when more than one type of monosaccharide is present they are termed heteropolysaccharides.

Polyunsaturated fat A highly unsaturated fat that is liquid at room temperature. Fats that are in foods are combinations of monounsaturated, polyunsaturated, and saturated fatty acids. Polyunsaturated fats are found in greatest amounts in corn, soybean, and safflower oils, and many types of nuts. They have the same number of calories as other types of fat, and may still contribute to weight gain if eaten in excess.

Pomes Botanical name for fruits such as apple or pear, formed by the enlargement of the receptacle which becomes fleshy and surrounds the carpels.

Pond culture It is the most widely used method of fish farming. All catfish farming is pond raised. The farming is done in man-made ponds that are drainable and often incorporate a system of dikes for harvesting.

Portobello mushrooms Also known as field mushrooms (and spelled 'portabella', 'portobella', and 'portabello'), these are flat, dark open-capped mushrooms which can be 8cm to 10cm (3in to 4in) wide. They have a robust meaty texture making them good for roasting, baking and stuffing.

They're great for barbecuing, too - just dot with butter, crushed garlic, herbs and seasoning and cook for a few minutes until the juices run, or slice thickly and sautı with onions and garlic.

Post harvest waxes After a fruit or vegetable is picked, it continues to need moisture to stay fresh and edible. To help retain moisture, certain varieties of fresh produce are given new wax coating to replace the natural wax the fruit or vegetable loses during harvest and shipping. If a fungicide is mixed with the wax to prevent molding, retail stores must label the waxed produce.

Post transcriptional changes Changes to a protein that occur after DNA has been copied to form messenger RNA and this has been translated to produce protein - for example, to facilitate excretion of the protein from the cell.

Prevalence In epidemiology, the prevalence of a disease in a statistical population is defined as the total number of cases of a given disease in a specified population at a specified time and/ orthe ratio of the number of cases of a disease present in a statistical population at a specified time and the number of individuals in the population at that specified time.

Potassium The major positive ion (cation) found inside of cells. The chemical notation for potassium is K^+.

Potato crisps Flavoured, thin slices of potato, deep-fried and eaten cold, sometimes as an accompaniment to meals, more commonly as a snack. Called chips in the USA. A 30-g portion (1 oz bag) of conventional crisps, ten crisps, is a source of niacin and vitamin C; contains 11 g of fat, of which 30% may be saturated and 40% mono-unsaturated; 180-450 mg of sodium; supplies 165 kcal (700 kJ). The same portion of low-fat crisps is a source of niacin; may contain 6 g of fat; 180-450 mg sodium; supplies 145 kcal (610 kJ). A large bag of conventional crisps (75 g) is a rich source of vitamin C; a good source of niacin; a source of iron; contains 20 g of fat; provides 4 g of dietary fibre; 450-1100 mg of sodium; supplies 410 kcal (1700 kJ). The same portion of low-fat crisps is a good source of niacin; a source of vitamins B 1 and C, and iron; contains 16 g of fat; provides 5 g of dietary fibre; 450-1100 mg of sodium; supplies 360 kcal (1500 kJ).

Potato starch Also called farina. Prepared from potato tuber and widely used as a stabilizing agent when gelatinized by heat.

Potato, irish The 'ordinary' potato, tuber of Solanum tuberosum. A 200-g portion is a rich source of vitamin B6; a good source of vitamins B 1 and C (new potatoes are a rich source of vitamin C), and folate; a source of niacin; provides 2.5 g of dietary fibre, 560 mg of potassium; supplies 140 kcal (590 kJ).

Potato, sweet Tubers of the herbaceous climbing plant Ipomoea batatas, known in Britain before the Irish potato. The flesh may be white, yellow, or pink (if carotene is present); the leaves are also edible. A 200-g portion is a rich source of vitamins A (as carotene if pink) and C; a source of iron and vitamin B1; provides 4.5 g of dietary fibre; contains 0.4 g of fat of which 16% is saturated; supplies 170 kcal (700 kJ).

Pottage Thick, well-seasoned meat or vegetable soup, usually containing barley or other cereal or a pulse (e.g. lentils).

Poussin A small, immature chicken, sometimes called a spring chicken, and weighing about 400g to 500g. Because the bird is only four to six weeks old, the flavour hasn't developed and there isn't much flesh on the bones, but one bird is perfect for a single serving. Poussins benefit from a rich stuffing to add flavour. A good way to cook them is spatchcocked (split open down the back and flattened out) on the barbecue.

Praline A brittle sweet made of almonds and caramelised sugar. It can be eaten as a sweet, served as an after-dinner treat with coffee, or crumbled or ground and used in desserts as an ingredient, filling or crunchy topping.

Prawn A type of shellfish. Called shrimp in the US, prawns are available fresh or frozen, in or out of their shells. In the UK, the prawns seen most commonly in supermarkets are small and pink. These have already been cooked. Fresh, raw prawns are grey and have a better texture than frozen prawns. If you buy whole prawns, the shells and heads are excellent for making stock. Prawns are used a great deal in Asian cooking, in stir-fries and curries. Prawns can be boiled, steamed or fried and are perfect for the barbecue. Look out for North Atlantic prawns, which are more likely to be sustainably fished.

Prescreening tool A computer program that estimates an individual's eligibility for various income support programs, such as Food Stamps. Information about an individual's household and income is entered into the computer program, which then estimates Food Stamp Program eligibility and approximate benefit levels. Some prescreening tools are web-based, while others are utilized by outreach workers on laptop computers.

Preservation Protection of food from deterioration by micro-organisms, enzymes, and oxidation: by cooling, destroying the micro-organisms and enzymes by heat treatment or irradiation, reducing their activity through dehydration or the addition of chemical preservatives, and by smoking, salting, and pickling.

Prevalence The number of existing cases of a disease in a defined population at a specified time.

Prickly pear The fruit of a type of cactus and also called a Barbary pear, cactus pear, Indian pear or Indian fig. The fruit contains yellow or red flesh with a sweet mild flavour that's similar to watermelon. The prickles are usually removed before they're sold but if they're not, take care when handling them because the needles can stick into your hands. To eat it just cut the pear in half and scoop out the flesh (don't eat the seeds). A squeeze of lemon or lime juice helps bring out the flavour.

Primary lactase deficiency When a person is born with the inability to digest lactose, a sugar found in milk and milk products. Lactose can't be digested because there is not enough of an enzyme, called lactase, in the body. Consuming milk and dairy products causes diarrhea, bloating, gas, and discomfort. This deficiency can also develop over time, as the amount of lactase in the body decreases with age.

Prion The infective agent(s) believed to be responsible for KreutzfeldJacob disease, kuru and possibly other degenerative diseases of the brain in human beings, scrapie in sheep, and bovine spongiform encephalopathy (BSE). They are simple proteins, and unlike viruses do not contain any nucleic acid. Transmission occurs by ingestion of infected tissue.

Proanthocyanidins A type of tannin found in cranberries, cranberry products, cocoa and chocolate which may provide the health benefits of improving urinary tract health and of reducing the risk of cardiovascular disease.

Probiotics Microbial cell preparations or components of microbial cells that have a beneficial effect on the health and well being of the host.

Proceedings A collection of current research reports, usually presented as brief abstracts, from a scientific meeting.

Progressive muscle relaxation Voluntary relaxation through systematic tensing and relaxing of different muscle groups.

Prokinetic Drugs that enhance propulsion of contents through the gut.

Proline A non-essential amino acid.

Pronutro Protein-rich baby food (22% protein) developed in South Africa; made from maize, skim-milk powder, groundnut flour, soya flour, and fish protein concentrate with added vitamins.

Proof spirit An old method of describing the alcohol content of spirits; originally defined as a solution of alcohol of such strength that it will ignite when mixed with gunpowder. Proof spirit contains 57.07% alcohol by volume or 49.24% by weight in the UK. In the USA it contains 50% alcohol by volume. Pure (absolute) alcohol is 175.25° proof UK or 200° proof USA.

Spirits were described as under or over proof; a drink 30° over proof means that 100 volumes contains as much alcohol as 130 volumes of proof spirit; 30° under proof means that 100 volumes contains as much alcohol as 70 volumes of proof spirit.

Nowadays alcohol content is usually measured as % alcohol by volume.

Prophylactic treatment Treatment performed to prevent diseases or nutritional damages.

Propionates Salts of propionic acid, CH_3 CH_2 COOH, a normal metabolic intermediate. The free acid and salts are used as mould inhibitors, e.g. on cheese surfaces, and to inhibit rope in bread and baked goods.

Prospective study A study in which the study population is characterised at the start of the study and followed into the future. A population of people who do not (yet) have the disease under investigation is identified, and information is collected on the subjects' exposure to risk factors generally including nutritional factors. The frequency of the disease among subjects exposed to a particular risk factor during the follow up period is compared with the frequency among those who were not exposed.

Prostaglandin A prostaglandin is any member of a group of lipid compounds that are derived enzymatically from fatty acids and have important functions in the animal body. Every prostaglandin contains 20 carbon atoms, including a 5-carbon ring. They are mediators and have a variety of strong physiological effects; although they are technically hormones, they are rarely classified as such.

Prospective study Epidemiological research that follows a group of people over a period of time to observe the potential effects of diet, behaviour and other factors on health or the incidence of disease. In general, this is considered a more valid research design than retrospective research.

Proteans Slightly altered proteins that have become insoluble, probably an early stage of denaturation.

Protease Proteases (proteinases, peptidases, or proteolytic enzymes) are enzymes that break peptide bonds between amino acids of proteins. The process is called proteolytic cleavage, a common mechanism of activation or inactivation of enzymes, especially those involved in blood coagulation or digestion. They use a molecule of water for this and are thus classified as hydrolases.

Protein Chemically, a protein is a complex nitrogenous compound made up of amino acids in peptide linkages. Dietary proteins are involved in the synthesis of tissue protein and other special metabolic functions. In anabolic processes they furnish the amino acids required to build and maintain body tissues. As an energy source, proteins are equivalent to carbohydrates in providing 4 calories per gram. Proteins perform a major structural role in all body tissues and in the formation of enzymes, hormones and various body fluids and secretions. Proteins participate in the transport of some lipids, vitamins and minerals and help maintain the body's homeostasis.

Protein milk Partially skimmed lactic acid milk plus milk curd (prepared from whole milk by rennet precipitation); richer in protein and lower in fat than ordinary milk, and supposed to be better tolerated in digestive disorders. Also known as albumin milk and eiweiss milch.

Protein rating Used in Canadian Food Regulations to assess the overall protein quality of a food. It is Protein Efficiency Ratio multiplied by the protein content of food (per cent) multiplied by the amount of food that is reasonably consumed. Foods with a rating above 40 may be designated excellent dietary sources; foods with a rating below 20 are considered to be insignificant sources; 20-40 may be described as good sources.

Protocol An action plan for a clinical trial. The plan states what the study will do, how, and why. It explains how many people will be in it, who is eligible to participate, what study agents or other interventions they will be given, what tests they will receive and how often, and what information will be gathered.

Proton pump inhibitor (PPI) A drug that limits acid secretion in the stomach.

Protopectinase The enzyme in the pith of citrus fruits which converts protopectin into pectin with the resultant separation of the plant cells from one another. Also known as pectosinase and pectosase.

Prunus Genus of plants including plums, peaches, nectarines, cherries, and almonds.

Pseudo-obstruction A motility disorder with symptoms like those of a bowel blockage, but with no physical evidence of blockage or obstruction. Symptoms may include cramps, stomach pain, nausea, vomiting, bloating, fewer bowel movements than usual, and loose stools.

Psychophysics Psychophysics is a subdiscipline of psychology dealing with the relationship between physical stimuli and their subjective correlates, or percepts. Gustav Theodor Fechner founded psychophysics in 1860 with the publication of Elemente der Psychophysik. He described research relating physical stimuli with how they are perceived and set out the philosophical foundations of the field. Fechner wanted to develop a theory that could relate matter to the mind, by describing the relationship between the world and the way it is perceived (Snodgrass, 1975). Fechner's work formed the basis of psychology as a science. Wilhelm Wundt, the founder of the first laboratory for psychological research, built upon Fechner's work.

Public charge Immigrants who become primarily dependent on the government for subsistence may be denied adjustment to permanent resident status or may be deported on the grounds they have become a "public charge." Nutrition programs have been specifically excluded from consideration in public charge determinations. This includes Food Stamps, the Special Supplemental Nutrition Program for Women, Infants, and Children (WIC), school meals programs, and other supplementary and emergency food assistance programs. Confusion about public charge keeps some immigrants from accessing nutrition benefits for which they or other household members are eligible. For additional information.

Pudding A baked or steamed sponge or suet dish, usually sweet and served as a dessert, but also savoury suet puddings (e.g. steak and kidney). Also milk puddings, made by baking rice, semolina, or sago in milk.

Purifies water Bottled water produced by distillation, reverse osmosis, deionization or suitable processes that meet governmental standards.

Purines Nitrogenous compounds (bases) that occur in nucleic acids (adenine and guanine) and their precursors and metabolites; inosine, caffeine, and theobromine are also purines. They are not dietary essentials; both dietary and endogenously formed purines are excreted as uric acid.

Sweetbread (pancreas) is rich in purines, as is fish roe; there are moderate amounts in sardines and anchovies, lesser amounts in other fish and meat; little in vegetables, fruits, and cereals.

Puy lentils A small slate-green lentil with a delicate blue marbling. Puy lentils are considered by many to be the best lentil because of their unique peppery flavour and the fact they hold their shape during cooking. They're the only lentil to be identified by area of cultivation - grown in the Le Puy region of France. Serve them hot or cold as a salad starter or as an accompaniment to poultry, meat or fish dishes, or use them in soups or casseroles. Available from delis and some supermarkets, they will keep for up to a year in a cool dry cupboard.

Pyloric sphincter A circular layer of muscle that separates the stomach from the duodenum of the small intestine

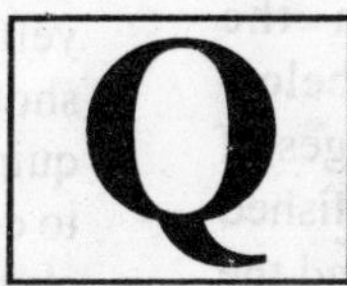

Quail Formerly a game bird, now so endangered in the wild that shooting is prohibited, but farmed to some extent. Two main species, Bonasa umbellus and Colinus virginianus; Californian quail is Lophortyx californica. The small eggs are much prized as a delicacy. A 150-g portion (whole bird) is a rich source of protein and niacin; a good source of vitamins B1 and B2; contains 3 g of fat and supplies 180 kcal (760 kJ).

Qualified immigrants Refers to legal immigrants and their eligibility for federal public benefits. Most qualified immigrants entering the United States after August 22, 1996, are barred from receiving federal benefits, including food stamps, for five years. Eligibility for food stamps has been restored to immigrant children, disabled, and some elderly immigrants. The term qualified immigrants was created in the 1996 welfare reform legislation, P.L. 104-193, and refers specifically to: lawful permanent residents, refugees, Cuban and Haitian entrants, asylees, aliens paroled into the United States for a period of at least one year, aliens granted withholding of deportation, aliens granted conditional entry into the United States, and certain battered alien spouses and children.

Quality The totality of features and characteristics of a product or service that bear on its ability to satisfy stated or implied needs. Not to be mistaken for "degree of excellence" or "fitness for use" which meet only part of the definition.

Quality assurance Quality Assurance (or QA) covers all activities from design, development, production, installation, servicing and documentation. It introduced the sayings "fit for purpose" and "do it right the first time". It includes the regulation of the quality of raw materials, assemblies, products and components; services related to production; and management, production, and inspection processes.

Quality control In engineering and manufacturing, quality control and quality engineering are involved in developing systems which ensure that products or services are designed and produced to meet or exceed customer requirements and expectations. These systems are often developed in conjunction with other business and engineering disciplines using a cross-functional approach.

Quality management All activities of the overall management function that determine the quality policy, objectives and responsibilities and that implement them by means such as quality planning, quality control, quality assurance and quality improvement within the quality system.

Quality management system A quality management system (QMS) is a system that outlines the policies and procedures necessary to improve and control the various processes that will ultimately lead to improved business performance. One of their purposes is quality control in manufacturing.Although it may seem obvious that quality systems are necessary, many small or start-up companies function, or attempt to function, with only some areas covered. A survey performed in 1988 indicates the breadth of the systems established within the biopharmaceutical industry. The table below summarizes the systems and the percentages of the respondent companies that had established these systems. The age of the company and the industry had some effect on the extensiveness of the quality function activities . It is clear that testing is the primary emphasis. This supports the observation that testing or QC is perceived, at least in the beginning, as the emphasis of the quality function.

Quenelle A fine minced fish or meat mixture formed into small portions and poached in stock and served in a sauce, or as a garnish to other dishes. The term quenelle is also used to describe the decorative shape of the portions - a neat, three-sided oval (a bit like a mini rugby ball!) formed by smoothing the mixture between two dessertspoons. A quenelle can be formed from other foods such as chocolate mousse.

Quiche An open flan or tart with a savoury custard filling, usually of egg and milk with other ingredients added to taste - fish, meat or vegetables. Originally from the Lorraine region of north-east France (hence quiche Lorraine with bacon, onion and cheese), the quiche has become a classic of French cuisine but is eaten across Europe and in many other countries.

Quince Quince (Cydonia oblonga) belongs to the same family as apples and pears. It has a shape that's similar to a pear, but larger. It has lumpy yellow skin and its hard flesh is quite bitter so it shouldn't be eaten raw. When fully ripe, the quince has a wonderful perfume. It can be added to cooked apple and pear dishes or used to make quince sauce, and it makes excellent preserves, especially marmalade. Quince paste or 'membrillo' is a popular accompaniment to cheese in Spain.

Quinoa Dating back to the Incas, this grain is still grown in Bolivia and Peru. It's extremely rich in complete protein, so is excellent for vegetarians.

The small round grains look similar to millet but are pale brown in colour. The taste is mild, and the texture firm and slightly chewy. It can be cooked like millet and absorbs twice its volume in liquid. When cooked, the grains sweeten and become translucent, ringed with white.

Use it in place of rice in cooked dishes, serve it as an accompaniment, in salads or as a stuffing. Or, try it as a porridge, served hot with cream, dried fruit and brown sugar.

R

Radiation proctitis Bleeding, mucous and bloody discharge, spasm of the rectal wall, urgency, and incontinence due radiation-induced damage to the rectum. Late symptoms result from scarring of the rectal and anal muscles with loss of some of the small blood vessels. The rectum becomes stiff and noncompliant (nonstretchable) and abnormal blood vessels may develop.

Radicchio A member of the chicory family sometimes known as red chicory, radicchio has distinctive pink-red leaves with white veins and a bitter peppery taste. It's generally used in salads mixed with other salad leaves.

Ragout A French stew of meat, poultry, fish or vegetables. 'Ragout' (ragɷ in Italian) is French for stew but the term can also refer to a sauce.

Raised pie A pork, ham or game pie moulded entirely from hot water crust pastry - top crust, walls and bottom. It can be served hot or cold and is ideal for taking on picnics.

Rambutan A relation of the lychee, but slightly bigger in size, this exotic fruit has a brown leathery skin with soft red spines and a white, translucent flesh that resembles the lychee in taste and texture.

Random allocation A method where all participants in a study have the same chance of being assigned to a study group, rather than allocation being assigned by the investigators, clinicians, or participants.

Random sample A random sample is a procedure to select subjects for a study in which all individuals in a population being studied have an equal chance of being selected. using a random sample allows the results of the study to be generalized to the entire population. The term random also applies to assignments within controlled studies, or the division of subjects into groups. Random assignment ensures that all subjects have an equal chance of being in the experimental and control groups, and increases the probability that any unidentified variable will systematically occur in both groups with the same frequency. Randomization is crucial to control for variables that researchers may not be aware of or cannot adequately control, but which could affect the outcome of an experimental study.

Randomization, or random assignment A process of assigning subjects to experimental or control groups in which the subjects have an equal chance of being assigned to each group. Randomization is used to control for known, unknown and difficult to control for variables. random sample A random sample is a procedure to select subjects for a study in which all individuals in a population being studied have an equal chance of being selected. using a random sample allows the results of the study to be generalized to the entire population.The term random also applies to assignments within controlled studies, or the division of subjects into groups. Random assignment ensures that all subjects have an equal chance of being in the experimental and control groups, and increases the probability that any unidentified variable will systematically occur in both groups with the same frequency.

Randomization is crucial to control for variables that researchers may not be aware of or cannot adequately control, but which could affect the outcome of an experimental study. random sampling A method by which subjects are selected to participate in a study in which all individuals in a population have and equal chance of being chosen. This helps to ensure the generalizability of the study results.

Randomized controlled trial A study in which people are allocated at random to receive one of several clinical interventions. One intervention is regarded as a standard of comparison or control.

Rape Brassica napus, also known as cole, coleseed, or colza. Grown for its seed, as source of oil for both industrial and food use. Varieties low in erucic acid are termed '0' or single low; varieties also low in glucosinolates are termed '00' or double low, both these being undesirable constituents of ordinary rapeseed. Oil is very rich in monounsaturates (60%), contains 33% polyunsaturates, and only 7% saturates.

Rapid assays These diagnostic tests use emerging technology to identify and remove impurities from foods before they reach the consumer. There are two major types of rapid assays. Antibody based assays link a "familiar" characteristic on a pathogen's surface (the antigen) to a substance known as an antibody. When this connection is made, the test registers "success." Similarly, nucleic acid based assays use the unique genetic materials of the cells to detect a pathogen.

Ras-el-hanout A Moroccan dried-spice mixture. The mixture can be used in couscous, rice, meat and vegetable dishes; as with garam masala, the mixture of spices in ras-el-hanout depends on the maker and the spices available, but may include a wide variety of spices, such as cardamom, cayenne, aniseed, nutmeg, mace, ginger, galangal and dried ground rosebuds.

Ratafia biscuits Light biscuits made with almond essence, very similar to the Italian amaretti biscuit but usually smaller and a little darker in colour. They can be used in trifles or crumbled into puddings or served after dinner with coffee.

Ratatouille A rich vegetable Provenηal stew, made from aubergines, courgettes, sweet peppers, tomatoes, onions and garlic simmered in olive oil with herbs. It can be eaten hot or cold, as a main course or served as an accompaniment to meat dishes. It also makes a good filling for other vegetables or a stuffing for chicken.

Ratio scaling Method for quantification of effects through magnitude estimation of how many times the effect of a sample is compared to a standard.

Reactive oxygen species Reactive oxygen species (ROS) include oxygen ions, free radicals and peroxides both inorganic and organic. They are generally very small molecules and are highly reactive due to the presence of unpaired valence shell electrons. ROSs form as a natural byproduct of the normal metabolism of oxygen and have important roles in cell signaling. However, during times of environmental stress ROS levels can increase dramatically which can result in significant damage to cell structures. This cumulates into a situation known as oxidative stress. Cells are normally able to defend themselves against ROS damage through the use of enzymes such as superoxide dismutases and catalases. Small molecule antioxidants such as Ascorbic acid (vitamin-C),uric acid, and glutathione also play important roles as cellular antioxidants. Similarly, Polyphenol antioxidants assist in preventing ROS damage by scavenging free radicals. In contrast, the antioxidant ability of the extracellular space in relatively less. E.g., the most important plasma antioxidant in humans is probably uric acid.

RDA Nutrient intake recommendations from the Institute of Medicine, an arm of the American Academy of Sciences. RDAs are safe levels of intake for essential nutrients, based on current scientific knowledge. They are set to meet the known nutrient needs or practically all healthy people. RDAs have been around and updated regularly for more than 50 years. RDAs are gradually being replaced by revised guidelines called Dietary Reference Intakes or DRIs.

Receptor A structure in each cell that selectively receives and binds a specific substance, such as a neurotransmitter.

Recombinant DNA (rDNA) The DNA formed by combining segments of DNA from different organisms. reliability Whether a test or instrument used to collect data, such as a questionnaire, gives the same results if repeated on the same person several times. A reliable test gives reproducible results.

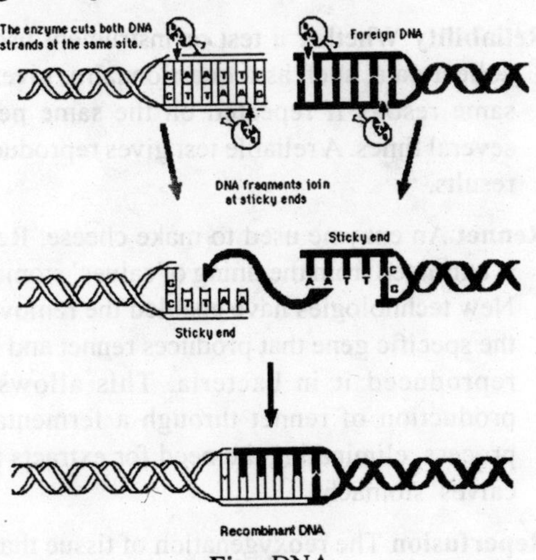

Fig. rDNA

Recombinant organism An organism in which the DNA has been made by joining together segments of DNA using the techniques of genetic modification.

Recommended daily intake Recommended Daily Intakes for vitamins and mineral nutrients is a reference standard created for use in the nutrition labelling of foods in Canada. It is based on the Recommended Nutrient Intakes for Canadians, and corresponds to the highest recommended intake of each nutrient for each age/sex group, excluding supplemental requirements for pregnancy and lactation.

Red cooking Chinese method of cooking; meat or poultry is first stir fried, then simmered in broth or water with soy sauce, herbs, and spices.

Red herrings Herrings that have been well salted and smoked for about ten days. Bloaters are salted less and smoked for a shorter time; kippers lightly salted and smoked overnight. Also called Yarmouth bloaters.

Red tide Sudden, unexplained increase in numbers of toxic organisms (dinoflagellates) in the sea which cause fish and shellfish feeding on them to become seasonally toxic.

Redcurrants Fruit of Ribes sativum (same species as whitecurrants); the UK National Fruit Collection contains 78 varieties. An 80-g portion is a rich source of vitamin C; a source of copper; supplies 5.6 g of dietary fibre; 15 kcal.

Reduce To evaporate by fast boiling a flavoured liquid, such as a sauce or syrup, in order to concentrate the flavour or to thicken it.

Reduced-price Meal Certification A classification within the child nutrition programs indicating that a child is able to receive reduced cost meals and snacks. Students can not be charged more than $0.40 for reduced-cost lunches or $0.30 for reduced-cost breakfasts. Children from families with income between 130 percent and 185 percent of the Federal Poverty Level are certified for reduced-price meals. In the 2005 2006 school year, a family of four with an annual income between $25,155 and $35,798 would qualify for reduced-price meals.

Reducing sugars Sugars that are chemically reducing agents, including glucose, fructose, lactose, pentoses, but not sucrose.

Reduction The opposite of oxidation; chemical reactions resulting in a gain of electrons, or hydrogen, or the loss of oxygen.

Reference man An arbitrary physiological standard; defined as a man aged 25, weighing 65 kg, living in a temperate zone of a mean annual temperature of 10°C, performing medium work, and assumed to require an average daily intake of 3200 kcal.

Reform sauce An English sauce based on poivrade sauce (which contains shallots, red wine, herbs and vinegar). Reform sauce has the rich combination of port, gherkins, tongue, mushrooms and hard-boiled egg whites, and is best served with either lamb or game.

Refractive index Measure of the bending or refraction of a beam of light on entering a denser medium (the ratio between the sine of the angle of incidence of the ray of light and the sine of the angle of refraction). It is constant for pure substances under standard conditions. Used as a measure of sugar or total solids in solution, purity of oils, etc.

Refreshing A process used by cooks when preparing vegetables. After the vegetables have been cooked, cold water is poured over them to preserve the colour; they are then reheated before serving.

Refrigerants Cooling agents in refrigerators and freezers, originally ammonia or carbon dioxide were used, subsequently replaced by chlorofluorocarbons (CFCs), trade names Freon and Arcton. Because of the persistence of CFCs in the upper atmosphere, where they destroy the protective ozone layer, they are considered an environmental hazard, and alternative refrigerants are being developed.

Registered Dietitian (R.D.) A health professional who is a food and nutrition expert. A person who has studied diet and nutrition at an American Dietetic Association (ADA) approved college program and passed an exam to become a registered dietitian.

Relative risk In statistics and mathematical epidemiology, relative risk (RR) is the risk of an event (or of developing a disease) relative to exposure. Relative risk is a ratio of the probability of the event occurring in the exposed group versus the control (non-exposed) group. For example, if the probability of developing lung cancer among smokers was 20 nd among non-smokers 10%, then the relative risk of cancer associated with smoking would be 2. Smokers would be twice as likely as non-smokers to develop lung cancer.

Relax In pastry-making, this means to set aside the pastry in a cool place after rolling to allow the gluten to contract (because it will have expanded during rolling). This reduces the danger of the pastry shrinking in the oven. It's also a term used to refer to batter mixes - meaning to set the batter aside to allow the starch cells to swell, which will give a lighter result when it's cooked.

Release agents Substances applied to tinned or enamelled surfaces or plastic films to prevent the food adhering, e.g. fatty, acid amides, microcrystalline waxes, petrolatums, starch, methyl cellulose.

Reliability Whether a test or instrument used to collect data, such as a questionnaire, gives the same results if repeated on the same person several times. A reliable test gives reproducible results.

Rennet An enzyme used to make cheese. Rennet is extracted from the lining of calves' stomachs. New technologies have enabled the removal of the specific gene that produces rennet and have reproduced it in bacteria. This allows the production of rennet through a fermentation process, eliminating the need for extracts from calves' stomachs.

Reperfusion The reoxygenation of tissue that has been deprived of adequate oxygen (ischaemia) as a result of either surgical procedures or physiological dysfunction. Vital organs can tolerate only a brief period of oxygen deprivation before cell injury and death occur. Subsequent reperfusion, however, can also cause tissue damage. Ischaemia reperfusion damage can be prevented or decreased in the presence of antioxidants.

Research design How a study is set up to collect information, or data. For valid results, the design must be appropriate to answer the question or hypothesis being studied.

Residual confounding The effect that remains after one has attempted to statistically control for variables that cannot be measured perfectly. A particularly important concept in epidemiological studies because knowledge of human biology is still developing. Unknown variables could exist that could significantly change conclusions made on the basis of epidemiological research.

Resveratrol Inhibits tumor formation and breaks down "bad," LDL cholesterol; lowers risk of atherosclerosis. Found in grapes (particularly red) and wine, as well as peanuts, cranberries and mulberries

Retrospective study Research that relies on recall of past data, or on previously recorded information. Often this type of research is considered to have limitations, because the number of variables that cannot be controlled, and because memory is not infallible.

Rett syndrome An X-linked disorder marked by progressive neurological deterioration, seizures and cognitive impairment

Reuptake A process in which chemical neurotransmitters, after transmitting their message, are taken up again by nerve endings, broken down, and inactivated.

Rheology Study of deformation and flow of materials; in food technology it involves plasticity of fats, doughs, milk curd, etc. It provides a scientific basis for subjective measurements such as mouth feel, spreadability, pourability.

Rhodopsin The pigment in the cone cells of the retina of the eye, also known as visual purple, consisting of the protein opsin and retinaldehyde, which is responsible for the visual process. In rod cells of the retina the equivalent protein is iodopsin. See vitamin A; dark adaptation; vision.

Ribose A pentose (five-carbon) sugar which occurs as an intermediate in the metabolism of glucose; especially important in the nucleic acids and various coenzymes: occurs widely in foods.

Fig. Digram of Ribose

Rice Grain of Oryza sativa; major food in many countries. Rice when threshed is known as paddy, and is covered with a fibrous husk comprising nearly 40% of the grain. When the husk has been removed, brown rice is left. When the outer bran layers up to the endosperm and germ are removed, the ordinary white rice of commerce or polished rice is obtained (usually polished with glucose and talc).

A 200-g portion of boiled brown rice is a good source of niacin and copper; a source of protein, vitamin B 1, and selenium; provides 1.6 g of dietary fibre; supplies 280 kcal (1180 kJ). A 200-g portion of boiled white rice is a source of niacin and protein; supplies 280 kcal.

Rice vinegar Wine vinegar made from rice used in Chinese and Japanese cookery. Rice vinegar, whether of the red or black variety, tends have a mild taste and is relatively low in acidity. If you can't find rice vinegar, use wine vinegar but dilute with water, using three parts vinegar to one part water (unless you're making sushi, in which case you'd need to use rice vinegar to get the desired result).

Rice wine An essential ingredient in Chinese cooking and other oriental cuisines. Rice wine is made by fermenting freshly steamed glutinous rice with yeast and spring water. It's relatively low in alcohol and, as well as being drunk, it's used in cooking and in marinades and glazes. Rice wine is widely available in Asian markets and some supermarkets, often labelled as Shaoxing wine.

It's often confused with sakι and mirin but sakι (a Japanese rice-based brewed alcohol) is far more delicate in taste. Mirin is sweetened sakι, made for cooking. Substitute dry pale sherry for rice wine if you can'Ht find it.

Ricotta A soft Italian curd cheese made from whey which is drained and then lightly cooked. It's light and creamy with a slightly grainy texture. It has a delicate flavour and is quite low in fat, making it a good substitute for mascarpone. Ricotta can be used on its own or in sweet and savoury dishes. It's used in many Italian dishes, especially as a stuffing for ravioli or in pastries such as cannoli.

Rigatoni Large ribbed pasta tubes cut straight across (rather than diagonally like penne). Rigatoni is a good pasta to serve with fairly thick creamy or tomato-based sauces, as its shape holds the sauce well. It's also good for using in pasta bakes. Penne makes a good substitute.

Rigor mortis Stiffening of muscle that occurs after death. As the flow of blood ceases, anaerobic metabolism leads to the formation of lactic acid and the soft, pliable muscle becomes stiff and rigid. If meat is hung in a cool place for a few days ('conditioned'), the meat softens again. Fish similarly undergo rigor mortis but it is usually of shorter duration than in mammals. See also DFD meat; meat conditioning.

Rillettes A kind of pβtι made from meat, such as pork, rabbit, goose or duck, which is cooked in seasoned lard, shredded and pounded to a smooth paste. It's then packed into a terrine or into ramekins and served as a cold hors d'oeuvre, spread on toast or bread.

Rillettes are usually topped with a thin layer of fat and can be stored in the fridge for several weeks this way (but eat immediately once the fatty seal has been cut into).

Risk A term encompassing a variety of measures of the probability of an outcome. It's usually used in reference to unfavourable outcomes such as illness or death. Be certain to distinguish between absolute and relative risk.

Risk analysis A process consisting of three components: risk assessment, risk management and risk communication.

Risk factor A risk factor is anything statistically shown to have a relationship with the incidence of a disease, however it does not necessarily infer cause and effect.

Risotto An Italian dish that was originally eaten by peasants for breakfast, but which has risen in stature to become a highly regarded restaurant dish. It's simple to make at home, but requires a bit of attention.

Risotto is made from risotto rice cooked with stock. Other ingredients (such as vegetables, shellfish or meat) are then added, and the dish is usually finished off with a knob of butter and some Parmesan cheese, which is stirred through at the end of cooking.

The key to a successful risotto is the rice and the stirring. There are three main types of Italian risotto rice - arborio, carnaroli and vialone nano. Essentially they're all starchy short-grain rices. The stock is added bit by bit to the rice and stirred frequently resulting in the classic creamy texture of a risotto. It shouldn't be overcooked, but should still retain its characteristic al dente bite.

Classic risottos include mushroom risotto, often made with a combination of fresh and dried mushrooms, and Risotto alla Milanese which contains saffron and is usually served as an accompaniment to osso bucco. Arancini ('little oranges') are classic Italian rice balls made from leftover saffron risotto.

Rissole Savoury little patties made from chopped meat or fish mixed with breadcrumbs, shaped into balls or cakes and shallow-fried.

RNA Abbreviation for ribonucleic acid, the molecule that carries out DNA's instructions for making proteins.

Roast cook or rotisseur Prepares roasted and braised meats and their gravies, and broils meats and other items to order. A large kitchen may have a separate broiler cook or grillardin (gree-ar-dan) to handle the broiled items. The broiler cook may also prepare deep-fried meats and fish.

Roast Originally meant to cook meat over an open fire on a spit; now refers to cooking in. an enclosed oven, and so is 'dry heating'. With meat the juices are squeezed out and evaporate on the surface, producing the Maillard complex characteristic of roasted meat.

Rock salt Salt crystals derived from the huge seams of impacted salt that have formed below dried-out, underground saline lakes. The crystals are quite large and hard so are best used in a salt mill.

Cooking salt is refined rock salt and table salt is finely ground and refined rock salt with magnesium carbonate added to make it free-running and damp-resistant. Salt-baking, cooking food - usually fish - in a crust of salt is a traditional way of cooking fish in some Mediterranean countries.

Rocket This peppery green leaf is used in salads and as a vegetable. It's known as arugula in the US. The leaves have a slightly bitter, peppery flavour and are best gathered when they're young. Rocket is a rich source of iron as well as vitamins A and C. It makes a delicious addition to salads but can also be used to make soups and rocket pesto. A bed of rocket is a good base for serving grilled poultry or fish.

Roller mill Pairs of horizontal cylindrical rollers, separated by only a small gap and revolving at different speeds. The material is thus ground and crushed in one operation. Used in flour milling.

Rome Criteria Lists of symptoms among which a specified minimum number allows a diagnosis of a functional gastrointestinal disorder.

Rooting reflex A reflex present in newborns; when an infant's cheek is touched or stroked, he turns his head toward the touched side and begins to suck

Rope Spore-forming bacteria (Bacillus mesentericus and B. subtilis) occurring on wheat and hence in flour. The spores can survive baking and then are present in the bread. Under the right conditions of warmth and moisture the spores germinate and the mass of bacteria convert the bread into sticky, yellowish patches which can be pulled out into ropelike threads, hence the term 'ropy' bread. The bacterial growth is inhibited by acid substances. Can also occur in milk, called long milk in Scandinavia.

Rose water Rose Water is a clear liquid, distilled from fresh rose petals. It is a flavoring that can be subtle when used lightly or soapy when added with a heavy hand.

Rose essence is a more concentrated form of rose flavoring and should be added more sparingly to dishes than rose water.

Rosemary Rosemary is a most versatile herb with a flavour that complements a wide variety of dishes and ingredients. Native to the Mediterranean, its bittersweet green leaves look similar to pine needles. The plant is an evergreen shrub, so the leaves are available fresh all year round. (If fresh isn't available then dried rosemary is useful to have in the store cupboard, but replace it often because it loses its potency and flavour after a few weeks.)

When used sparingly, the flavour of rosemary goes well in subtle and delicate dishes such as ice creams, sorbets, fools and fruit salads. The robust and highly aromatic flavour of rosemary can also be used as part of a bouquet garni in soups, stews and casseroles.

Whole sprigs can be added to flavour roasted vegetables. Meat, poultry and game can be spiked with rosemary and it can be chopped and used in stuffings and sauces for fish, lamb or chicken. Some Italian breads are flavoured with rosemary leaves.

Remove leaves or sprigs after cooking; it's also a good idea to crush dried rosemary before adding it to your dish because the sharp leaves can be difficult to remove after cooking.

Rosti A Swiss potato cake made from layers of sliced or grated potatoes, fried until 'crisp and golden' which is exactly what 'røsti' means in Switzerland. The term røsti can be used for all kinds of shredded or sliced and crisply fried ingredients, such as other vegetables or potatoes and fish mixtures.

Rouille A pungent Provenηal sauce often served with fish stews such as bouillabaisse, made from a garlic and olive oil emulsion pounded with chillies and breadcrumbs.

Roux A roux is a mixture of equal quantities of melted butter and flour that is cooked in a pan and used as the base for thickening sauces such as white sauce and bιchamel.

Rump A tender cut of beef from the lower back of the cow, sold as roasting joints and steaks. It's slightly less tender than sirloin but still only needs quick cooking. Rump steaks can be grilled or fried and accompanied with a sauce such as peppercorn or red wine sauce. It's also good for stir-fries and kebabs.

Russell-Silver syndrome An inherited condition characterized by short stature, skeletal asymmetry, cafι au lait spots, and a small triangular face

Ryle tube A narrow rubber tube with a blind end containing a lead weight, with holes above this level, for removing samples of the contents of the stomach at intervals after a test meal.

S

Saccharin Saccharin, the oldest of the non nutritive sweeteners, is currently produced from purified, manufactured methyl anthranilate, a substance occurring naturally in grapes. It is 300 times sweeter than sucrose, heat stable and does not promote dental caries. Saccharin has a long shelf life, but a slightly bitter aftertaste. It is not metabolized in the human digestive system, is excreted rapidly in the urine and does not accumulate in body.

SAD Seasonal affective disorder, a form of depression that tends to occur as the days grow shorter in the fall and winter. It is believed that affected persons react adversely to the decreasing amount of light and the colder temperature as autumn and winter progress.

Safety policy The overall intentions and direction of an organisation with regard to safety as formally expressed by top management.

Safflower oil Vegetable oil extracted from the seeds of Carthamus tinctoria, 75% polyunsaturated fatty acids. See also saffron, Mexican.

Saffron The most expensive spice in the world fortunately goes a long way! It's derived from the stigmas of the saffron crocus (Crocus sativa), which can only be picked by hand. It takes 250,000 stigmas to make just half a kilo of saffron.

Saffron can be bought whole in threads or strands (stigmas), which should be crushed just before using, or in powdered form. Spanish and Kashmiri saffron are reputed to be among the best quality. Saffron gives a distinctive aroma and flavour and a yellow colour to Spanish paella and Italian risotto. Saffron is also a classic ingredient in the French fish soup bouillabaisse.

Sage Sage (Salvia officinalis) is native to the Mediterranean. The colour of the downy leaves and the flavour varies but, in essence, it's a very strong aromatic herb with a slight bitterness that can withstand long cooking times and still retain flavour.

Sago Sago is a starch from the pith of the sago palm. It's processed into sago flour, slightly coarser sago meal or pearl sago - small grains similar to tapioca. It's used in baking, to make puddings or as a thickener for desserts.

Salad Originally derived from the Latin sal for salt, meaning something dipped into salt. Now normally a dish of uncooked vegetables; either a mixed salad or just one item (commonly lettuce or tomato). In France it can mean a small, hot, savoury dish, e.g. of chicken liver, etc.

Salamander A salamander is a huge commercial grill that can be heated to very high temperatures. It's used by professional cooks for glazing, browning or caramelising savoury or sweet dishes.

Salami Salami is the Italian name for a family of 'cut-and-keep' sausages made from a mixture of raw meat, such as pork, beef or veal and flavoured with spices and herbs. Innumerable varieties are made around the world. Salami can be salted, smoked or air-dried. Salami makes great sandwich fillers, pizza toppings or salad ingredients, particularly in potato salads.

Some salamis are good for cooking with - add them to risottos, pasta sauces and other meat and vegetable dishes. Salami can be bought sliced and pre-packed or freshly sliced at deli counters.

Salmonella Salmonella is a Gram-negative bacterium, occurring in many animals, especially poultry and swine. In the environment, salmonella can be found in water, soil, insects, factory and kitchen surfaces, animal fecal matter, and raw meats, poultry (including eggs) and seafood.

Acute symptoms of the illness caused by the Salmonella species include nausea, vomiting, diarrhea, abdominal cramps, headache and fever.

Salsa A spicy relish or dip served cold and made from chopped tomatoes, onions, chillies and peppers. 'Salsa' means 'sauce' in Spanish.

Most supermarkets sell fresh salsa as well as mild or hot salsa in jars, but the flavour is never as good as homemade. It's easy to make either a coarse salsa with just a knife and chopping board, or to whizz the ingredients in a blender for a smooth salsa.

Serve salsa with other dips such as guacamole and soured cream with tortilla chips or use it as a sauce or a topping for pasta. Fruit salsas using mango or pineapple go well with grilled fish or chicken.

Salsify One of the lesser known root vegetables, salsify is also known as oyster plant because it tastes slightly of oysters. It has a beige-white skin and looks similar to a long carrot in shape. It can be used in a similar way to any other root vegetable in soups, stews or mashed. It's easier to peel after boiling.

Try adding grated cooked salsify to a salad to add a crisp, delicate flavour. Salsify is related to the black-skinned root vegetable scorzonera.

Salt cod Salt cod is dried, salted cod. It looks pretty unappetising - a bit like a dried-up leather shoe - until it's rehydrated, after which it softens and tastes delicious when cooked. Salt cod is widely used in Mediterranean countries, particularly France, Italy, Spain and Portugal, as well as in tropical countries where it keeps well despite the hot temperatures.

It's called bacalhau in Portugal and, served with potatoes, is considered the national dish. In Italy it's called baccalû and is traditionally eaten on Christmas Eve in some parts of the country. In France, salt cod is the basis for a dish called brandade - salt cod mixed with potato and garlic. To rehydrate it, salt cod should be soaked in cold water for 24 to 48 hours and the water should be frequently changed. It can then be poached or baked, used in stews, fishcakes or fish mousses.

Salt or Sodium (Sodium Chloride) While there are many types of salts, the commonly used terms salt and sodium generally refer to sodium chloride, or table salt. Sodium is necessary for the regulation of fluid balance, to maintain heart rhythm, and for muscle contraction and relaxation. Combined with chloride, sodium chloride, or salt, is used as a seasoning and a preservative.

Salted butter The most popular kind of butter in the U.S. is made from fresh cream with no less than 80 percent butterfat. This butter is lightly salted. Salted butter lasts longer than unsalted butter. When used for frying, salted butter scorches much more easily than unsalted

Saltimbocca A dish consisting of thin slices of veal or poultry, flavoured with fresh sage and topped with a slice of prosciutto, then sautied in butter and olive oil and braised in white wine. The meat can be rolled and secured with toothpicks before cooking. The word comes from the Italian for 'leap into the mouth'.

Sambuca Italian;liqueur flavoured with liquorice and elderberry (Sambucus nigra). Traditionally served with coffee beans in the glass, and set alight.

Samosa A deep-fried Indian pastry stuffed with spiced vegetables or meat, usually triangular in shape. Samosas can also be baked. Savoury samosas are more common, but sweet fillings can also be used.

Samphire Marsh samphire (Salicornia europaea), also known as glasswort or pickle-plant, is a fleshy-leaved green plant that grows on seaside marshes. It has a sea-salty flavour and a crisp, interesting texture.

Use it fresh in salads or serve it with fish, simply boiled and dipped in melted butter and eaten like asparagus.

Sanatogen Trade name for a preparation of casein and sodium glycerophosphate for consumption as a beverage when added to milk.

Sandwich Two slices of bread enclosing a filling (meat, cheese, fish, etc.). Invention attributed to the 4th Earl of Sandwich (1718-1792) who spent long periods at the gaming table and carried a portable meal of beef sandwiched with bread.

Sangria A Spanish punch drink made with red wine, sliced fruit and fruit juices, sugar, soda water and sometimes a splash of brandy. This popular blood-red drink (from which its name derives) is served over ice and is great with tapas.

Saponins The functional component of soybeans, soy foods and soy protein containing food which may lower LDL cholesterol and may contain anti cancer enzymes.

Saran Generic name for thermoplastic materials made from polymers of vinylidene chloride and vinyl chloride. They are clear, transparent films (cling film) used for wrapping food; resistant to oils and chemicals; can be heat-shrunk on to the product.

Sarcosine An intermediate in the metabolism of choline, chemically N-methylglycine. Found in relatively large amounts in starfish and sea urchins, used as an intermediate in the synthesis of antienzyme agents in toothpaste.

Sardine Sardines are baby pilchards. They're an oil-rich fish, usually sold whole, whether fresh, frozen or tinned. Bought fresh and whole, sardines are ideal fish for grilling and barbecuing. Cook them until the skin is crisp and charred and the flesh comes away from the bone easily. They go well with robust tomato sauces to counteract the oiliness of the fish, or dressed with lemon and fresh herbs and served with potatoes.

It's worth paying a premium for good-quality tinned sardines. Those from Portugal, Spain and France are particularly good.

Sassafras tea The Food and Drug Administration banned the sale of sassafras tea in 1976. Aromatic sassafras tea, once popular as a stimulant and blood thinner and as a reputed cure for rheumatism and syphilis, causes cancer in rats when taken in large amounts. Oil of sassafras and safrole, major chemical components of the aromatic oil in sassafras root bark, were taken out of root beer more than 30 years ago. Sassafras bark was banned from use in all food. Safrole-free extract, however, is allowed in food.

Satay This is a South-east Asian speciality eaten across much of Indonesia (from where it originates), Thailand and Malaysia. Small pieces of marinated meat or fish are skewered on small wooden sticks and grilled or barbecued. Satay is usually served with spicy peanut sauce. It's essentially a street food, but is good served as a starter or main course with rice.

Satiation The term for the physiologic processes that bring eating a meal to an end and control meal size.

Saturated fat Saturated fats are those in which all carbons contain a hydrogen, and therefore, no double bonds exist. In general, fats that contain a majority of saturated fatty acids are solid at room temperature, although some solid vegetable shortenings are up to 75 percent unsaturated. Some common fatty acids in foods include palmitic, stearic and myristic acids. Saturated fatty acids are more stable than unsaturated fatty acids because of their chemical structure. Stability is important to prevent rancidity and off flavors and odors. selective breeding This process allows for the transfer of only one or a few desirable genes, thereby permitting scientists to develop crops with specific beneficial traits and those without undesirable traits. Current technology allows scientists to alter one plant characteristic at a time, thereby not spending years trying to develop the tastiest and hardiest plants.

Sauce Used to flavour, coat, or accompany a dish, or may be used in the cooking to bind ingredients together; may be sweet or savoury. Thick sauces may be: 1. roux sauces based on flour heated with fat;

2. thickened with starch (arrowroot, cornflour, custard powder) or modified starch (gravy granules, thickening granules);

3. thickened with egg (Hollandaise sauce, custard);

4. Thickened by reduction.

Sauce chef or saucier The person responsible for sautıed items and many different sauces. Traditionally, it is the third person in command. This is usually the highest position of all the stations:

Savory The herbs summer savory (Satureja hortensis) and winter savory (S. montana) are both related to the mint family. Both are highly aromatic and can be used to season a variety of meat, poultry, egg dishes, soups or sauces. Both types of savory are particularly useful in stuffings. Winter savory tends to be more strongly flavoured.

Scallop An expensive but delicious shellfish with a delicate taste, available in a range of sizes.

Scallops have two fan-shaped shells which contain rounds of firm white flesh. The edible orange coral (or roe) is sometimes left attached. Scallops can be bought in or out of their shells. The two main types available in the UK are the larger king scallop and the tiny queen scallop. You'll need about four to five king scallops a person for a main meal or about a dozen queen scallops.

Scallops can be steamed, fried or grilled but should be cooked gently and only for a very short time or the delicate flavour and texture will be spoiled. Poach them in wine, wrap them in prosciutto and grill or fry for a few minutes, or pan-fry them in butter with ginger and fresh coriander. Scallops also go well with Asian ingredients.

School breakfast program (SBP) This USDA program helps public and private schools provide nutritious breakfasts to all students. Low-income students are able to receive free or reduced-price meals through the program.

Scientific knowledge The current set of peer-evaluated consensus models about how natural phenomena work, which often differ between groups of researchers at the research frontier.

Scientific progress The cumulative growth of a system of knowledge over time, in which useful features are retained and nonuseful features are abandoned, based on the rejection or confirmation of testable knowledge.

Scintigraphy An imaging method in which a mild dose of a radioactive substance is swallowed to show how material moves through the GI tract.

Scone A small round teacake made from a soft dough and cooked in a hot oven. Scones can be sweet or savoury. Sugar, fruit and spices are often added to sweet scones and they're often served with clotted cream and jam.

Savoury scones might incorporate cheese, herbs or potato. A drop scone isn't a scone at all - it's more of a small thick pancake.

Scrag The scrag or scrag end is an inexpensive cut of lamb from the neck. It contains a lot of bone and is best used in casseroles, soups and stews.

Sea bream A firm-fleshed white fish. There are numerous species available, known by a variety of names, which can be confusing. Sea bream is sold whole or as fillets. It has succulent flesh that's ideal for grilling, baking and frying. Red snapper or sea bass make good substitutes.

Sea salt Sea salt is the compound remaining when sea water is evaporated. It contains some elements in addition to sodium and chloride. It may contain trace amounts of copper, manganese, nickel, flourine, tin, and iodine. The mineral content varies depending upon the source of the sea water.

Selective breeding This process allows for the transfer of only one or a few desirable genes, thereby permitting scientists to develop crops with specific beneficial traits and those without undesirable traits. Current technology allows scientists to alter one plant characteristic at a time, thereby not spending years trying to develop the tastiest and hardiest plants.

Selenium Works with vitamin E as an antioxidant and binds with toxins in the body, rendering them harmless. Lobster, clams, crabs, whole grains, Brazil nuts and oysters.

Self fixer The innate ability of legumes like soybeans to "fix" nitrogen, which means to use the natural nitrogen in the soil and air. These natural nitrogen fixers replenish the nitrogen supply in the soil from which they were harvested. Breeders desire to develop other crops that can "fix" their own nitrogen which would thereby decrease farmers' use of synthetic fertilizers while maintaining bountiful yields.

Seltzer water Flavorless natural mineral water with carbonation, originally from the German town of Nieder Selters.

Semolina A coarse pale-yellow flour ground from hard durum wheat used to make traditional pasta. Semolina can also be used to make pizza, bread and gnocchi and is added to biscuits to give a lovely texture. The term also refers to a British milk pudding of the same name. The semolina is cooked slowly in milk and sweetened with sugar. It can be served like porridge with a spoonful of honey or jam stirred through or topped with fresh or dried fruit.

Semolina isn't widely available but some supermarkets and health-food shops stock coarser varieties (sometimes labelled 'pudding semolina').

Senior farmers market nutrition program A USDA program that provides fresh, locally grown fruits, vegetables and herbs to low-income seniors, as well as increases the consumption of fresh fruits and vegetables. The program was first authorized in the 2002 Farm Bill. The program does not operate in all states.

Sensitization Enhancement of a response by an organism that is produced by delivering a strong, generally noxious, stimulus. A neuron becomes more excitable or responsive; it may respond more intensely to naturally occurring stimuli, either peripherally (in the viscera) or centrally (in the brain).

Sequence characterisation Determination of the order in which the nucleic acids making up a DNA molecule, or the amino acids making up a protein molecule, are linked together.

Short-chain fatty acids Fatty acids with chain lengths of two to six carbon atoms.

Specificity of gene expression A measure of the extent to which the ability of an organism to produce a particular gene product is determined by factors affecting the cell, for example, its function, phase of growth or environmental pressures.

Stem cell Stem cells in people are primal undifferentiated cells that retain the ability to produce an identical copy of themselves when they divide (clone) and differentiate into other cell types. In higher animals this function is the defining property of the deleted cells. Stem cells have the ability to act as a repair system for the body, because they can divide and differentiate, replenishing other cells as long as the host organism is alive.

Serotonin (5-hydroxytryptamine, or 5-HT) A chemical neurotransmitter (a chemical that acts on the nervous system to help transmit messages along the nervous system). It is found in the intestinal wall and the central nervous system. It is now widely understood that 95% of the serotonin in the body resides in the gut.

Serving size 1. The portion of food used as a reference on the nutrition label of that food.

2. The recommended portion of food to be eaten.

Shaoxing wine An essential ingredient in Chinese cooking and other oriental cuisines. This sweet wine is made by fermenting freshly steamed glutinous rice, yeast and spring water. It's low in alcohol and as well as being drunk like wine, it's used in cooking, marinades and glazes.

Shaoxing wine is widely available in Asian markets and some supermarkets. It's often confused with sakı and mirin but sakı (a Japanese rice-based brewed alcohol) is far more delicate in taste. Mirin is sweetened sakı, made for cooking. Substitute dry pale sherry if you can't find it.

Shin One of the cheapest cuts of beef, shin comes from the foreleg. It needs long slow cooking but has a superb flavour. Use it in casseroles and stews - it makes the most delicious gravy because the connective tissue in it turns to gelatine, thickening and flavouring the sauce.

Shortbread A sweet Scottish biscuit made with sugar, flour and a generous amount of butter, which gives it its melt-in-the-mouth texture. Shortbread, which is pale golden in colour and quite crumbly, is traditionally baked in a round, flat shape, pricked with a fork and sprinkled with caster sugar. It can be eaten on its own or used as a base for tarts.

You can buy good quality packets or tins of individual shortbread biscuits - either plain or with additions such as pieces of chocolate or stem ginger. Make strawberry shortcakes by serving a sandwich of shortbread filled with whipped cream and fresh strawberries.

Shortcrust pastry Probably the most useful and versatile pastry, shortcrust is a crumbly pastry that's ideal for pies and tarts. The degree of 'shortness', or crisp crumbliness, depends on the amount and type of fat incorporated into the flour and the way in which the pastry is handled.

Shuck To 'shuck' means to open an oyster shell using a stubby, thick-bladed knife. It's a skill that takes a little while to master but is easy once you know how.

You can find out more about shellfish, including ways of cooking and preparing them, in our Back to basics section.

Sichuan pepper Sichuan pepper isn't actually pepper, but the dried red-brown berries of a type of ash tree. The berries are dried and then sold whole or crushed to a powder.

Try to buy the freshest berries you can find, because they quickly lose their lemony, peppery pungency. Sichuan pepper has a characteristic mouth-numbing quality that's typical of many Sichuan dishes. Sichuan pepper is also one of the spices in Chinese five-spice powder.

Sigmoid colon The S-shaped section of the colon that connects to the rectum.

Sigmoidoscopy Examination of the inside of the sigmoid colon and rectum using an endoscope — a thin, lighted tube (sigmoidoscope). Samples of tissue or cells may be collected for examination under a microscope. Also called proctosigmoidoscopy.

Significant or statistically significant A statistical term indicating that the results of a study are stronger than would be expected from chance alone.

Silverside A cheaper cut of beef from the rear of the animal. It's very lean and contains no bone, making it a good cut for braising or for using in stews and casseroles - or to make mince.

Simnel cake Now an Easter speciality, this cake was originally given by servant girls to their mothers when they went home on Mothering

Sunday. A fairly rich fruit cake, it's covered with almond paste or marzipan, stamped with the figure of Christ and decorated with 11 marzipan balls to represent the 11 apostles (excluding Judas).

Simplified summer food service program In nineteen states and Puerto Rico this program streamlines reimbursement and paperwork in the Summer Food Service Program (SFSP) by eliminating cost-based accounting. Reimbursement for SFSP sponsors is calculated by "meals times rates," providing the maximum reimbursement. This program was originally called the Lugar Pilot Program. The Simplified Summer Food Service Program currently operates in: Alaska, Arkansas, Colorado, Idaho, Indiana, Iowa, Kansas, Kentucky, Louisiana, Michigan, Mississippi, Nebraska, New Hampshire, North Dakota, Ohio, Oklahoma, Oregon, Texas, Wyoming and Puerto Rico.

Simply dissolving sugar in water makes Candy candy The different heating levels determine the types of candy: Hot temperatures make hard candy, medium heat will make soft candy and cool temperatures make chewy candy. Cavemen who ate honey from beehives first invented the idea of a sweet treat. During ancient times the Egyptians, the Arabs and the Chinese prepared confections of fruit and nuts candied in honey. In Europe during the Middle Ages, the high cost of sugar made sugar candy a delicacy available only to the wealthy. Boiled sugar candies were enjoyed in the seventeenth century in England and in the American colonies. Sweet making developed rapidly into an industry during the early 19th century through the discovery of sugar beet juice and the advance of mechanical appliances. Homemade hard candies, such as peppermints and lemon drops became popular in America during that time. By the mid-1800s, over 380 American factories were producing candy — primarily "penny candy," which was sold loose from glass cases in general stores.

Sirloin A prime cut of beef from the back, sold as roasting joints, either on or off the bone, and as sirloin steaks.

Sitting height Length between a child's head and buttocks, sometimes used as an estimator of height

Skin The skin is the body's outer covering. It protects us against heat and light, injury, and infection. It regulates body temperature and stores water, fat, and vitamin D. Weighing about 6 pounds, the skin is the body's largest organ. It is made up of two main layers; the outer epidermis and the inner dermis.

Skinfold thickness A measure of the amount of fat under the skin; the measurement is made with a caliper and used to estimate body fatness

Slake To mix a thickening agent with liquid, such as cornflour or arrowroot.

Small intestine The part of the digestive tract that is located between the stomach and the large intestine.

Smith-Lemli Opitz syndrome An autosomal recessive condition characterized by dysmorphic features, short stature, abnormal facies, psychomotor retardation, and genital anomalies in males

Smoothie A non-alcoholic cold drink made up of a mixture of the juices and pulp of fruit or vegetables mixed into a smooth drink using a blender. Other ingredients such as milk, yoghurt or honey can be added to thicken and flavour.

Smoothies make a great breakfast and are an excellent way to help get your recommended 'five a day'.

Smorgasbord An assortment of hot and cold dishes served in Sweden as hors d'oeuvres or as a full buffet meal. The name translates as 'buttered bread table'. A smorgasbord can include all kinds of things, such as potato-based dishes, salads, meats and cheeses, marinated salmon, meatballs, etc. A selection of herring specialities - fresh, salted, smoked and pickled - is a classic part of a smorgasbord.

Soba noodles Thin grey-brown Japanese noodles made from buckwheat (which is gluten-free).

Available dried, they're long and straight and look similar to spaghetti. They're used mostly in soups and can be used in stir-fries, although you must stir them carefully because they break apart easily.

Social services block grant (SSBG) A capped entitlement that provides funds to states to assist with the provision of social services to adults and children. Some states use SSBG funds to support Home-Delivered Meals and Congregate Meals programs for the elderly.

Soda water A flavorless water with induced carbonation consumed plain or used as a mixer for alcoholic drinks or soda fountain confections; also known as club soda and seltzer.

Sodium The major positive ion (cation) in fluid outside of cells. The chemical notation for sodium is Na^+. When combined with chloride, the resulting substance is table salt.

Sodium bisulfite Sodium bisulfite is used as an anti-darkening agent when drying fruit. You may substitute sodium sulfite, or sodium or potassium metabisulfite. These ingredients may be obtained from some pharmacies. To pre-treat fruits, prepare a solution of one tablespoon of sodium bisulfite, or two tablespoons of sodium sulfite, or 4 tablespoons of sodium metabisulfite in one gallon of water. Place sliced fruit into the solution as soon as it is sliced. Soak slices for at least 5 minutes and halves for at least 12 minutes. After soaking is complete, drain the fruit and rinse with cold water. The fruit is now ready for drying.

Sodium nitrite A salt used in smoked or cured fish and in meat curing preparation. It acts as a preservative and colour fixative. Can combine with chemicals in the stomach to form nitrosamine, a carcinogenic substance.

Soluble fiber A type of dietary fiber found in psyllium, cereals, oatmeal, apples, citrus fruits, beans and other foods which increases the viscosity in the gut and acts to reduce high blood cholesterol levels which decreases the risk of cardiovascular disease.

Somatization Physical symptoms and no recognizable physical abnormality.

Sorbet A semi-frozen water ice, usually made with fruit, sugar syrup or a liqueur, traditionally served as a palate cleanser between courses but now eaten more commonly as a refreshing dessert.

Granita is a slightly coarser, crunchier Italian style of sorbet that doesn't require an ice-cream maker.

Sorrel The name sorrel is used to describe several related plants, including wild sorrel and French sorrel. Its name derives from the French for sour, in reference to the plant's characteristic acidity.

It's incredibly sour and it shouldn't be eaten in large quantities because it contains a high amount of oxalic acid. The leaves of the sorrel plant are the part used in cookery. They're bright green arrow-shaped leaves with a crisp texture.

Because of its bitter flavour sorrel is often combined with other ingredients. It can be eaten raw in salads or cooked in soups, purées and stuffings and goes particularly well with fish and egg dishes.

Soup kitchen A community food service and resource where meals are prepared and distributed on site.

Sour cream This is cream that has been processed commercially so as to be soured under ideal conditions. It contains about 20% butterfat, 7% milk solids, and the remainder is water.

Sour salt Sour salt is an old name for citric acid. This ingredient may be mentioned in old canning publications as substance to prevent fruit from darkening. A good substitute to prevent fruit from darkening is lemon juice or a commercial antioxidant like Fruitfresh®.

Sous-Chef This position means "the under chief" in French. This is person is second in command and takes responsibility for the kitchen operations if the chef is absent.

Soy protein The protein found in soybeans and soy-based foods which when consumed at the level of 25 grams per day may reduce the risk of heart disease.

Soy sauce Made from defatted soya beans fermented with salt, water and crushed barley or wheat, soy sauce (or soya sauce) forms a basic ingredient in Japanese, Chinese and other Asian cooking. It's either added to dishes during cooking or used as a table condiment. There are many varieties of soy sauce that vary in consistency and in strength of flavour.

Light soy sauce is quite thin and has a saltier flavour than dark soy. It's used to give flavour to dishes without darkening them, such as when stir frying vegetables or chicken, for instance. Dark soy is thicker in consistency and richer. It gives good colour to noodle dishes and its sweetness makes it a good dipping sauce.

The darkest and richest is Indonesian ketjap (or kecap), which is made from black soya beans. Tamari is a dark soy sauce that's made without wheat, and is therefore suitable for coeliacs. Soy sauce is a versatile store cupboard ingredient. It makes a great marinade or it can be splashed into stews or used in sauces for meat and vegetables.

Special milk program A USDA program that provides milk to children in schools and childcare institutions who do not participate in other child nutrition programs. The program reimburses schools for the milk they serve.

Specific nutritional treatment Actions recommended by peculiar situations of nutritional risk, such as anemia, goiter, vitamin A deficiency and other conditions.

Spelt Spelt (Triticum spelta) is an ancient type of wheat that's native to southern Europe, where it's been used for thousands of years. It has a mellow nutty flavour and is easily digestible, and has a slightly higher protein content than ordinary wheat. Spelt can be tolerated by many people with wheat intolerances.

Spelt is most often milled into spelt flour, which is available in health-food stores. It can be substituted for ordinary wheat flour in baked goods. Wholemeal spelt noodles and pasta can often be found in health-food shops, too.

Spina bifida Spina bifida is a birth defect in which the infant is born with the spinal cord exposed. These children can grow to adulthood although they often suffer from paralysis and other disabilities. Also, see "neural tube defects (NTDs)."

Spinal cord A column of nerve tissue that runs from the base of the skull down the back. It is surrounded by three protective membranes, and is enclosed within the vertebrae (back bones). The spinal cord and the brain make up the central nervous system, and spinal cord nerves carry most messages between the brain and the rest of the body.

Spinal muscular atrophy An inherited neuromuscular disorder that affects motor neurons, which control movement of voluntary muscles; three groups, based on age of clinical onset, are recognized

Sponge A batter to which yeast is added. This batter is so stiff that it does not drop from a spoon, but can be handled.

Spring water Water obtained from an underground source that flows naturally to the earth's surface.

Squamous cell A flat cell that looks like a fish scale under a microscope. Squamous cells cover internal and external surfaces of the body.

Squid A sea mollusc related to the cuttlefish and also known as calamari. Squid can be grilled or fried. Larger squid can be added to stews or stuffed or cooked in their own ink. Their shape makes them very good for stuffing with vegetables or other kinds of seafood. They're also very good deep-fried or stir fried.

Stanol/sterol esters A functional component found in wood oils, corn, soy and wheat which may reduce the risk of coronary heart disease by lowering blood cholesterol levels.

Staple crops Those crops which are most common in people's diets are considered staple crops.

Staple crops of greatest importance include rice, wheat and maize (corn). These three crops provide 60 percent of the world's food energy intake. And rice feeds almost half of humanity. Typically, staple crops are well adapted to the conditions in their source areas. For example, they may be tolerant of drought, pests or soils low in nutrients.

Star anise The fruit of a shrub native to the Far East (Illicium verum), star anise is shaped like an eight-pointed star and contains shiny seeds with an aniseed flavour, which comes from the essential oil, anethole. It's used widely in Chinese cooking and is one of the five spices in Chinese five-spice powder.

Statistical power A mathematical quantity that indicates the probability a study has of obtaining a statistically significant effect. A high power of 80 percent, or 0.8, indicates that the study if conducted repeatedly—would produce a statistically significant effect 80 percent of the time. On the other hand, a power of only 0.1 means there would be a 90 percent chance that the research missed the effect—if one exists at all.

Statistical significance The probability of obtaining an effect or association in a study sample as or more extreme that the one observed if there was actually no effect in the population. Based on the hypothesis that if there truly is no effect, the results of a study are unlikely to have occurred. A P value of less than five percent ($P<0.05$) means the result would occur less than five percent of the time if there were no effect, and is generally considered evidence of a true treatment effect or a true relationship.

Stearate A saturated fatty acid containing eighteen carbon atoms in its molecular "backbone" that is essentially neutral in effect on coronary heart disease in humans (i.e., doesn't appreciably increase low density lipoproteins in the bloodstream). Because of the heart disease neutrality and resistance to oxidation/breakdown, stearate containing oils are an excellent cooking oil choice.

Stearic acid Saturated fatty acid with eighteen carbon atoms (chemically octadecenoic acid); is present in most animal and vegetable fats.

$H_3C(CH_2)_{16}C(=O)\text{-}O\text{-}CH_2$
$HCOH$
$HC\text{-}R$
H

$R: \text{-}OH,\ \text{-}O\text{-}C(=O)(CH_2)_{16}CH_3$

Fig. Stearic acid

Steatorrhoea Excretion of faeces containing a large amount of fat, and generally foul-smelling. May be due to lack of bile, lack of lipase in the digestive juices, or defective absorption of fat. Treatment is by feeding low-fat diet. See also coeliac disease; sprue.

Steep The process of leaving a food to stand in water, either to soften it or to extract its flavour and colour. Also the preparation of fruit liqueurs by steeping fruit in spirit.

Sterols Alcohols derived from the steroids; including cholesterol, ergosterol in yeast (the precursor for synthetic vitamin D 2), sitosterol and stigmasterol in plants, and coprosterol in faeces.

Stilboestrol Synthetic substance with potent activity as female sex hormone; the first non-steroid compound developed to have oestrogen activity. Formerly widely used both clinically and for chemical caponization of cockerels and to stimulate the growth of cattle.

Stress The neurophysiological and subjective response to stimuli. In contrast to the common interpretation of the term "stress" as a psychological phenomenon, it should be understood as any real or perceived perturbation of an organism's homeostasis, or state of harmony or balance. Stress may disrupt the function of nerve and even immune cells in the GI tract and in the brain. The central stress system involves the release of chemical stress mediators in the brain, which in turn orchestrate an integrated autonomic, behavioural, neuroendocrine, and pain modulatory response.

This biological response in turn will alter the way the brain and the viscera (internal organs such as the gut/intestines) interact, and this altered brain-gut interaction can result in worsening of symptoms in functional GI disorders. For example, stress can increase GI symptoms by changing how the brain controls unwanted and painful sensation.

Stroke The sudden death of some brain cells due to a lack of oxygen when the blood flow to the brain is impaired by blockage or rupture of an artery to the brain. A stroke is also called a cerebrovascular accident or, for short, a CVA.

Strudel An Austrian dessert made from very thin layers of strudel pastry - similar to filo pastry - wrapped around a filling of fresh fruit, most famously apple, dried fruit and spices. Strudels are usually sweet but savoury versions can be made too.

Stunting Reduction in the linear growth of children, leading to lower height for age than would be expected, and generally resulting in lifelong short stature. A common effect of protein-energy malnutrition, and associated especially with inadequate protein intake.

Subscapular skinfold measure Measurement of the skin and subcutaneous fat layer below the shoulder blade, often used in conjunction with triceps skinfold and arm muscle circumference measurements to estimate fat stores

Substance 1. Material with particular features, as a pressor substance.

2. The material that makes up an organ or structure. Also known in medicine as the substantia.

3. A psychoactive drug as, for example, in substance abuse.

Sucralose Sucralose is the only low calorie sweetener that is made from sugar. It is approximately 600 times sweeter and does not contain calories. Sucralose is highly stable under a wide variety of processing conditions. Thus, it can be used virtually anywhere sugar can, including cooking and baking, without losing any of its sugar like sweetness.Currently, sucralose is approved in over 25 countries around the world for use in food and beverages. In the US, the FDA has been petitioned to approve the use of sucralose in 15 different food and beverage categories. sucrose Sucrose, a type of sugar, is a diglyceride composed of glucose and fructose. Also, see "carbohydrates."

Sucrose Sucrose (common name: table sugar, also called saccharose) is a disaccharide (glucose + fructose) with the molecular formula $C_{12}H_{22}O_{11}$. Its systematic name is β-D-fructofuranosyl α-D-glucopyranoside. It is best known for its role in human nutrition.

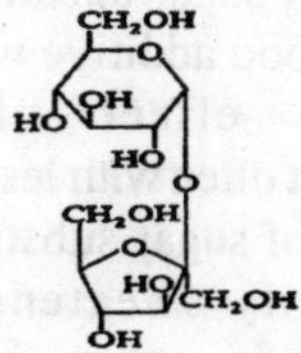

Fig. Sucrose

Sugar Although the consumer is confronted by a wide variety of sugars—sucrose, raw sugar, turbinado sugar, brown sugar, honey, corn syrup—there is no significant difference in the nutritional content or energy each provides, and therefore no advantage of one nutritionally over another. There also is no evidence that the body can distinguish between naturally occurring or added sugars in food products. sugar alcohols Ingredients used to add sweet flavors to food. Those often used instead of sugars include sorbitol, mamitol, and xylitol. Many fruits and vegetables contain sugar alcohols naturally. They're also found in some sugarless gum, hard candies, jams and jellies. Besides adding sweetness, sugar alcohols also add texture, help foods stay moist, prevent browning when food is heated and give a cooling effect to the taste of food. They supply four calories per gram, but are absorbed slowly and incompletely and thus require little or no insulin for metabolism. They are not cavity producing because they are not metabolized by bacteria that produce cavities.

Sugar alcohols Ingredients used to add sweet flavors to food. Those often used instead of sugars include sorbitol, mannitol, and xylitol. Many fruits and vegetables contain sugar alcohols naturally. They're also found in some sugarless gum, hard candies, jams and jellies. Besides adding sweetness, sugar alcohols also add texture, help foods stay moist, prevent browning when food is heated and give a cooling effect to the taste of food. They supply four calories per gram, but are absorbed slowly and incompletely and thus require little or no insulin for metabolism. They are not cavity-producing because they are not metabolized by bacteria that produce cavities.

Sugar substitute A sugar substitute, or artificial sweetener, is a food additive which attempts to duplicate the effect of sugar or corn syrup in taste, but often with less food energy.An important class of sugar substitutes are known as high intensity sweeteners. These are compounds whose sweetness is many times that of sucrose; accordingly, much less sweetener is required and energy contribution often negligible. The sensation of sweetness caused by these compounds (the "sweetness profile") is sometimes notably different from sucrose, so they are used in complex mixtures that achieve the most natural sweet sensation.

Sulfite Sulfites (also sulphite) are compounds that contain the sulfite ion SO_{32}". They are often used as preservatives in wines (to prevent spoilage and oxidation), dried fruits, and dried potato products.Sulfites occur naturally in almost all wines. In the US, those bottled after mid-1987 must have a label stating that they contain sulfites if they contain more than 10 parts per million. In the EU an equivalent regulation came into force in November 2005. Organic wines are not necessarily sulfite-free. Most beers no longer contain sulfites. Although shrimp is sometimes treated with sulfites on fishing vessels, the chemical may not appear on the label. In 1985, the United States federal government banned the addition of sulfites to most fresh fruits and vegetables, though fresh-cut potatoes and dried fruits are exceptions.

Sulphate The mineral sulphur occurs in foods and in the body in two main forms: as sulphates (salts and esters of sulphuric acid, H_2SO_4); and in the sulphur amino acids methionine and cysteine.

Sulphoraphane A functional component of cruciferous vegetables (e.g., broccoli, kale, horseradish) which provides the health benefits of neutralizing free radicals and possibly reducing the risk of cancer.

Sulphur An element that is part of the amino acids cystine and methionine and is therefore present in all proteins. It is also part of the molecules of vitamin B1 and biotin and occurs in foods and in the body as sulphates. Apart from these amino acids and vitamins, there appears to be no requirement for sulphur in any other form and no deficiency has ever been observed, although it is essential for plants. Not only was the old-fashioned remedy of sulphur and molasses (brimstone and treacle) quite unnecessary, but elemental sulphur is not used by the body.

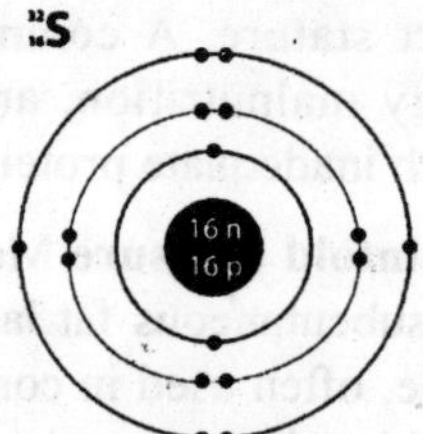

Fig. Sulphur

Sulphur dioxide (SO_2) Preservative used in gaseous form or as salts (sulphites) for fruit drinks, wine, comminuted meat, and as a processing aid to control physical properties of flour; also prevents enzymic and non-enzymic browning. Protects vitamin C but destroys vitamin B1. Prepared by ancient Egyptians and Romans by burning sulphur and used to disinfect wine.

Summer food service program (SFSP) This USDA program provides free meals primarily to children in low-income areas through sponsored programs when school is not in session.

Superglycerinated fats Neutral fats are triacylglycerols, i.e. with three molecules of fatty acid to each molecule of glycerol. Mono- and diacylglycerols (sometimes called mono- and diglycerides) are known as superglycerinated high-ratio fats or fat extenders.

Glyceryl monostearate (GMS) is solid at room temperature, flexible, and non-greasy; it is used as a protective coating for foods, as a plasticizer for softening the crumb of bread, to reduce spattering in frying fats, as an emulsifier and stabilizer. Glyceryl mono-oleate (GMO) is semi-liquid at room temperature.

Supervision of sibilings and contacts Careful supervision along with the ecessary treatment (food support or suplementation, growth evaluation, basic healthcare) for sibilings and mothers (considered "contacts") of children between the ages 6-23 months with malnutrition. Malnutrition in this age group can be indicative of malnourished mothers and sibilings, constituting nutritional risk groups.

Sur lattes With reference to wines, means storage 'on their side' so that the cork is kept moist and airtight.

Surfactants Surface active agents; compounds that have an affinity for fats (hydrophobic) and water (hydrophilic) and so act as emulsifiers, e.g. soaps and detergents. Used as wetting agents to assist the reconstitution of powders, including dried foods, to clean and peel fruits and vegetables, also in baked goods and comminuted meat products.

Surimi Water extract of minced flesh of low-oil fish (mostly myofibrillar protein) with gelling properties, used to prepare a range of foods. It is white, and relatively tasteless and odourless. Introduced from Japan into the United States in 1979, as the basis for seafood analogues but with broad potentialities.

Susceptor plates Special metallic films (usually powdered aluminium) deposited inside the packets of foods intended for microwave cooking; they concentrate the energy on the outside of the food and brown and crisp it.

Sussex bread Old English loaf made from wheat and rye flour mixed with grains, given to servants; now revived.

Sustagen Trade name for a food concentrate in powder form, also useable for tube feeding; mixture of whole and skim milk, casein, maltose, dextrins, and glucose.

Sweat A technique in which vegetables are cooked very slowly in a covered pan using just a small amount of butter or oil, so that they soften but don't brown. Sweating plays an important part in tenderising vegetables, especially finely diced onions, before other ingredients are added.

Sweet cicely A wild plant (Myrrhis odorata) with a smell of aniseed. The aniseed-flavoured leaves are used to flavour fruit cups, fruit salads, and cooked fruit; the main root can be boiled, sliced, and used in salads. Also known as sweet chervil.

Sweet potato A root vegetable that resembles a potato, although it's quite different in taste and texture (and isn't related to the potato). It has a pinkish-orange skin and deep orange flesh.

Sweet potatoes can be cooked in a variety of ways. They have a slightly sweet flavour and a lovely creamy flesh, much lighter and fluffier than the potato. They can be cooked in similar ways to the potato - baked, mashed, roasted or used in vegetable soups and bakes, or added to risottos, pasta dishes and curries.

Sweetness One of the five basic senses of taste.

Swells Infected cans of food swollen at the ends by gases produced by fermentation. A 'hard swell' has permanently extended ends. If the ends can be moved under pressure, but not forced back to the original position, they are 'soft swells'. 'Springers' can be forced back, but the opposite end bulges. A 'flipper' is a can of normal appearance in which the end flips out when the can is struck.

Hydrogen swells are harmless, and due to acid fruits attacking the can.

Swiss chard The spinach-like leaves and broad midrib of Beta vulgaris var. cicla, also known as leaf beet, leaf chard, sea kale beet, silver beet, white leaf beet, spinach beet. A 100-g portion (boiled) is a rich source of vitamin A (as carotene); a good source of vitamin C; a source of iron; supplies 18 kcal.

The term is also used for blanched summer shoots of globe artichoke and for inner leaves of cardoon, Cynara carduncula.

Syllabub A delicious old English dessert made with whipped cream, sherry or white wine and sugar, often infused with lemon. Syllabub dates back to the time of Elizabeth I. It should be served well chilled and can be decorated with finely chopped nuts and served with some small crisp tuile biscuits.

Syndrome A set of symptoms or conditions that occur together and suggest the presence of a certain disease or an increased chance of developing the disease.

Synergistic effect The effect achieved by the combination of two or more substances or organisms which neither alone could accomplish.

Systemic Affecting the entire body.

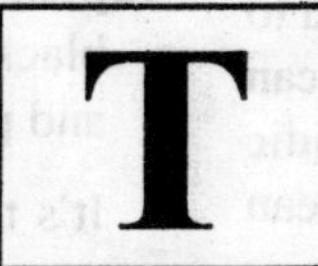

T cell T cells belong to group of white blood cells known as lymphocytes and play a central role in cell-mediated immunity. They can be distinguished from other lymphocyte types, such as B cells and NK cells by the presence of a special receptor on their cell surface that is called the T cell receptor (TCR). The abbreviation "T", in T cell, stands for thymus since it is the principal organ for their development.

T3 Tri-iodothyronine, one of the thyroid hormones.

T4 Thyroxine (tetra-iodothyronine), one of the thyroid hormones.

Tabasco Tabasco is the trade name of a range of hot, spicy chilli sauces made in the US state of Louisiana. The original Tabasco sauce is fiery red and made from a variety of chilli pepper called Tabasco, combined with vinegar and salt and matured in oak barrels. Other varieties include a milder green Tabasco sauce made from jalapepo peppers and green peppers. Just a few drops of Tabasco adds a spicy, chilli flavour to meats, sauces, burgers, salad dressings or cocktails.

Tachycardia Rapid heartbeat, as occurs after exercise; may also occur, without undue exertion, as a result of anxiety, and in anaemia and vitamin B1 deficiency.

Tagine The name 'tagine' pertains to both a dish and the implement it's cooked in. Tagines are meat and vegetable stews that are central to Moroccan cuisine. They're traditionally cooked in tagines, special earthenware dishes with conical-shaped lids.

Tagines are important in the cuisines of many other North African countries and throughout much of the Middle East. Lamb frequently features as the main ingredient and preserved lemons are often included.

Tagliatelle Long thin ribbons of pasta sold either in curled nests or straight, like spaghetti. Tagliatelle can be plain or green (flavoured with spinach) and is available fresh or dried. It goes well with thick creamy sauces that cling to the pasta well.

Talin Trade name for thaumatin, an extract of the berry Thaumatococcus danielli, about 3000 times as sweet as sucrose.

Tamari A type of soy sauce that's made without wheat and is therefore suitable for those with wheat allergies or coeliac disease. Tamari is dark in colour and has a rich flavour, making it useful in marinades and dressings. It's also good as a dip. If you can't find it, substitute dark soy sauce.

Tamarillo A red, egg-shaped tropical fruit about the size of a plum. It's sometimes called a tree tomato.

Tamarillo is usually eaten cooked and can be quite tart when raw, though a sprinkling of sugar can help. Avoid eating the skin, which is bitter, but use the flesh in ice creams or sorbets and serve cooked tamarillo with poultry or fish.

Tamarind A flavouring agent made from the fruit of the tamarind tree. The fruit is shaped like a long bean, inside which is a sour pulp. The pulp can be pressed to form a 'cake' or processed to make a paste. Small pieces of tamarind cake can be broken off and infused to create an acidic liquid flavouring used in Asian and Caribbean cooking.

Tamarind tastes a bit like a date but is less sweet (and more sour), and is sometimes known as the Indian date. It's an ingredient in Worcestershire sauce.

Tamarind juice is also available and some Asian supermarkets may sell tamarind pods, which can be eaten raw. Use tamarind to flavour meat and vegetable curries, chutneys and dhals.

Tandoori A tandoor is a tall, cylindrical clay oven found in countries stretching from the Arabian peninsula to India. Naan breads, as well as various meats and kebabs, are traditionally cooked in a tandoor. The term 'tandoori' pertains to dishes cooked in such a clay oven. In the UK, the word tandoori is frequently used to describe food that has been marinated in a spice paste made of ginger, cumin, coriander, paprika, turmeric and cayenne mixed with purıed garlic, purıed ginger, lemon juice, oil and, frequently, yoghurt. The paste coats the food, which turns a red-orange colour. It's then cooked in the tandoor (although for home cooks, a very hot oven will have to do). The tandoor imparts a wonderful smoky aroma to the food.

Tangerine A generic name given to numerous small orange citrus fruits, more commonly known as mandarins. Satsumas are simply a different variety and clementines are a hybrid between the tangerine and the sweet orange.

Tangerines begin to appear on shop shelves from autumn onwards and are often associated with Christmas. They're usually peeled and eaten raw but can also be used in fruit salads and for making jams and marmalades.

Tank culture It is another form of onshore farming. Tanks, usually made of steel and reinforced cement, or fiberglass in a variety of shapes, are used to contain populations of fish in water.

Tapenade Tapenade is a rich, soft paste made of black olives, capers, anchovies, mustard, basil and parsley.

It's traditionally spread on bread, but you can use tapenade in canapıs or starters such as crostini or bruschetta, or you can stir a little into pasta dishes or sauces, use it as a marinade for meat and also for adding to casseroles and stews. It can be bought ready-made in jars.

There are several varieties to choose from, based on different types of olives and with the addition of extra flavourings such as peppers, anchovies or sun-dried tomatoes.

Taramasalata A thick, creamy Greek dip made from olive oil, fish roe, breadcrumbs and seasonings. It's usually served as a mezze dish or as an hors d'oeuvre. It can be bought ready-made but avoid tubs of electric pink taramasalata with too much food colouring.

Tarragon An aromatic herb, often used in French cooking. Its long, soft green leaves have a distinctive aniseed flavour and can be used to flavour oils and vinegars. Dried tarragon retains much of the flavour of fresh, so it's fine to use if you can't find fresh. It's one of the herbs that makes up fines herbes and is also used in bıarnaise sauce. Tarragon is particularly good with chicken but also use it to flavour salads and egg dishes and as a flavouring for fish.

Tartare The term tartare can be used in two ways. Tartare sauce is made from mayonnaise, gherkins and capers and is the traditional accompaniment to fish. Steak tartare is made with minced beef served raw with egg yolk and seasoning.

Tarte tatin The name given to a classic French apple tart in which the fruit is cooked under a lid of pastry, but served upside down - with the pastry underneath and the fruit on top. It combines the taste of caramel with the flavour of apples cooked in butter and was made famous by the Tatin sisters who ran a hotel-restaurant in France in the early 1900s.

Many variations of the original apple 'upside-down' tart have since been developed, including savoury versions using shallots or onions.

Taste Taste belongs to our chemical sensing system, or the chemosenses. The complicated process of tasting begins when molecules released by the substances stimulate special cells in the mouth or throat. These special sensory cells transmit messages through nerves to the brain where specific tastes are identified.

Tea 1 A beverage prepared by infusion of the young leaves, leaf buds, and internodes of varieties of Camellia sinensis and C. assamica, originating from China. Green tea is dried without further treatment. Black tea is fermented (actually an oxidation) before drying; Oolong tea is lightly fermented. Among the black teas, Flowering Pekoe is made from the top leaf buds, Orange Pekoe from first opened leaf, Pekoe from third leaves, and Souchong from next leaves. See also caffeine; herb tea; xanthines.

2 An afternoon meal; may consist of a light meal (especially in southern Britain) or be a substantial meal (high tea) as in northern Britain.

Team nutrition A program of the Food and Nutrition Service at the USDA that provides schools with nutrition education materials for children and families; technical assistance materials for school food service directors, managers, and staff; and materials to build school and community support for healthy eating and physical activity. State agency partners provide training and technical assistance to support these programs in local schools.

Teaspoon An old-fashioned but convenient household measure. A teaspoon holds about 5 cc of liquid.

Teriyaki Usually, a Japanese dish consisting of beef, chicken or fish that has been marinated in a mixture of soy sauce, mirin, sugar, ginger and seasonings before being grilled or fried. However, the term can be used to describe the sauce itself or the cooked dish made with the sauce. The sugar in the marinade gives the cooked food a slight glaze.

Teriyaki sauce is made with the above ingredients and is sold in bottles, although it's easy to make your own. Teriyaki was traditionally used as a glaze for fish or meat after it had been cooked, but now is more commonly used for marinating the meat prior to cooking. The ingredients used in teriyaki sauce tend to be loosely interpreted by many chefs and can include a range of ingredients including sesame oil, honey and Tabasco.

Terrine This term usually describes a kind of pβtι and is also the term to describe the ovenproof dish that pβtι is cooked in - usually ceramic and similar to a loaf tin.

Tertiary care Medical care in a highly specialized centre.

Tetracyclines A group of closely related antibiotics including tetracycline, oxytetracycline (terramycin), and aureomycin. The last two are used in some countries for preserving food and as growth improvers, added to animal feed at the rate of a few mg per tonne.

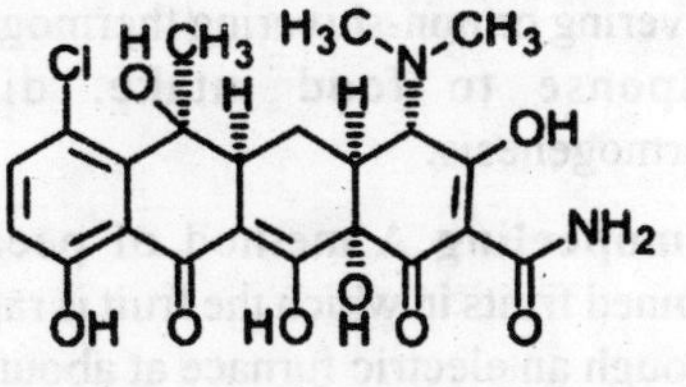

Fig. Tetracyclines

Texture Combination of physical properties perceived by senses of kinaesthesis (muscle-nerve endings), touch (including mouth feel), sight, and hearing. Physical properties may include shape, size, number, and conformation of constituent structural elements.

Texture profile Organoleptic analysis of the complex of food in terms of mechanical and geometrical characteristics, fat and moisture content, including the order in which they appear from the first bite to complete mastication.

The Butcher Commis The common cook under one of the Chef de Partie. This level of cook comprises the bulk of the kitchen staff

Therapeutic property Property of a specific food or drug see pharmaceutical products to perform curatively in correcting deviations or fully characterizes illnesses, as in the case of nutrition-related illnesses.

Therapeutic treatment Treatments adopted to correct clinical pathological situations. Actions destined toward curing diseases.

Thermal effect of food The increase in energy expenditure associated with the processes of digestion, absorption and metabolism of food; represents approximately 10% of a person's total energy expenditure and includes facultative thermogenesis and obligatory thermogenesis; often called diet induced thermogenesis (DIT).

Thermoduric Bacteria that are heat resistant but not thermophilic, i.e. they survive, but do not develop at, pasteurization temperatures. Usually not pathogens but indicative of insanitary conditions.

Thermogenesis Increased heat production by the body, either to maintain body temperature (by shivering or non-shivering thermogenesis) or in response to food intake, diet-induced thermogenesis.

Thermopeeling A method of peeling tough-skinned fruits in which the fruit is rapidly passed through an electric furnace at about 900°C then sprayed with water.

Thiaminase An enzyme present in many species of micro-organisms, plants, and fish which splits thiamin (vitamin B1), forming products that have anti-vitamin activity. Non-enzymic cleavage of thiamin, for example by polyphenols, is also sometimes called thiaminase action. Chastek paralysis in foxes and mink fed diets rich in raw fish, and blind staggers in horses and other animals eating bracken fern, are due to acute vitamin B1 deficiency caused by dietary thiaminase.

H
NH₂
S
CH₂—N⊕
CH₂—CH₃
CH₃
H₃C
N

Fig. Thiamin

Thrifty food plan A food plan based upon market baskets of food that people of a specific age and gender could consume at home to maintain a healthful diet that meets current dietary standards. The Thrifty Food Plan is the most economical of four food plans calculated by the USDA and is one factor used to determine the amount of a household's food stamp benefit allotments.

Thrombosis Thrombosis is the formation of a clot or thrombus inside a blood vessel, obstructing the flow of blood through the circulatory system. Thromboembolism is a general term describing both thrombosis and its main complication which is embolisation.

Thumb The short thick finger situated at an angle to the other fingers so it can be opposed to the them, making it possible to pick up and hold things. The thumb is analogous in position to the big toe (the great toe) and similarly has only two phalanges (all the other digits have three).

Thyme No kitchen should be without the heady, aromatic character of thyme. There are many different varieties, both cultivated and wild, but the most widely used is the common garden thyme (Thymus vulgaris). The intensely pungent flavour complements most meats, including chicken and game. Its robust nature means that it can withstand long cooking times and it's a good complement to slow-cooked dishes such as stews and daubes.

It's one of the herbs used in bouquet garni, along with parsley and bay. Its flavour also marries well with other robust and heady herbs such as rosemary and sage. Chop it up in stuffings for poultry or lamb or use it chopped in a marinade for olives. Add sprigs to marinades for meat, fish or vegetables or tuck a few sprigs with half a lemon and an onion inside a chicken before roasting.

Tibia length Measurement of the tibia; sometimes used as an estimator of stature

Timbale A layered dish cooked in a tall mould (which is also called a timbale) and then turned out onto a serving plate. Often made of rice layered with vegetables or perhaps slices of aubergine layered with other vegetables and tomato sauce.

Tiramisu An Italian dessert, similar to a trifle, made with Italian sponge biscuits or macaroons soaked in coffee, brandy or liqueur, with mascarpone cheese and chocolate. Tiramisu translates as 'pick me up'.

Tisane An infusion of fresh or dried herbs that's drunk hot. Most tisanes are made from medicinal plants. A wide range of herbal teas or tisanes are available to buy from health-food shops and supermarkets.

Tofu A delicate, versatile, semi-soft food made by adding mineral salt to soymilk, which solidifies it into a white "cake." Tofu has become increasingly more popular in the United States and is used in everything from soup to main course to dessert. Tofu has good calcium content, if processed with calcium. If processed with calcium, 1 cake of soft tofu (2-1/2 inches x 2-3/4 inches x 1 inch), has approximately 90 calories and 154 milligrams of calcium. A glass of milk has approximately 313 milligrams of calcium and 1/2 cup of cooked spinach has 100 milligrams.

Tongue From various animals, e.g. lamb, ox, sheep. A 150-g portion is an exceptionally rich source of iron, a rich source of protein, niacin, and vitamin B2; contains about 35 g of fat and supplies 450 kcal.

Tooth The structures within the mouth that allow for biting and chewing. Teeth have different shapes, depending on their purpose. The sharp canine and frontal teeth allow for biting, while the flattened, thick molars in the back of the mouth provide grinding surfaces for masticating food. All teeth have essentially the same structure a hard crown above the gum line, which is attached to two or four roots by a portion called the neck. The roots are covered with a very thin layer of bone, and keep the tooth embedded in the bones of the jaw. The exposed exterior of the tooth is covered with tough enamel. Under the enamel is a thick layer of dentin, and in the centre is the pulp. Blood vessels and nerves are found within the pulp.

Topside This is a prime lean cut of beef from the rear of the animal, usually sold rolled and tied with a layer of fat for roasting. It can also be pot-roasted, braised or boiled.

Tortilla A Spanish omelette made with eggs, potatoes, olive oil and salt. Sometimes other ingredients, such as peppers, chorizo, onion, tuna, asparagus and mushrooms, are added. It's cut into wedges and eaten hot or cold, similar to an Italian frittata. In Mexico, tortilla refers to a soft floury flatbread made from corn or wheat flour, or tortilla chips - the spicy triangular corn crisps served with salsa and guacamole.

Total Quality Management Total Quality Management (TQM) is a management strategy aimed at embedding awareness of quality in all organizational processes. TQM has been widely used in manufacturing, education, government, and service industries, as well as NASA space and science programs.Total Quality provides an umbrella under which everyone in the organization can strive and create customer satisfaction. TQ is a people focused management system that aims at continual increase in customer satisfaction at continually lower real costs.

Tournant The Relief cook. This term describes the cook in the kitchen who provides help to all the different cooks rather than having a specific job.

Toxicologist A scientist who studies the nature, effects and detection of poisons and the treatment of poisoning.

Toxicology The scientific study of the chemistry effects and treatment of poisonous substances.

Toxin A toxin (Gk. toxikon "(poison) for use on arrows,") is a poisonous substance produced by living cells or organisms. Toxins are nearly always proteins that are capable of causing disease on contact or absorption with body tissues by interacting with biological macromolecules such as enzymes or cellular receptors. Toxins vary greatly in their severity, ranging from usually minor and acute (as in a bee sting) to almost immediately deadly (as in botulinum toxin).

Traditional crop breeding For traditional crop breeding, breeders mix thousands of genes in order to transfer the protein products to enhance one or a few genetic traits. Therefore, the odds of something undesirable being transferred unintentionally are far greater in traditional breeding than in biotechnology.

Trans fat An unhealthy substance, also known as trans fatty acid, made through the chemical process of hydrogenation of oils. Hydrogenation solidifies liquid oils and increases the shelf life and the flavor stability of oils and foods that contain them. Trans fat is found in vegetable shortenings and in some margarines, crackers, cookies, snack foods and other foods.

Trans fatty acid A form of unsaturated fatty acid that is straight (rather than bent, i.e cis) at the double bond; not abundant in natural edible oils but occurring in ruminant fats and formed during some manufacturing processes.

Translational science Conversion of basic science discoveries into the practical applications that benefit people.

Tray culture A tray culture involves the use of a permanent structure for mollusks to attach themselves to. Trays are set underwater in calm bays or estuaries to stimulate the growth of clams, oyster, and other shellfish. Sometimes ropes or strings are hung into the water for mussels and scallops to grow on.

Triacylglycerols Compounds of glycerol and three fatty acids also called triglycerides; the main constituents of dietary and body fat.

Triglyceride Glyceride occurring naturally in animal and vegetable tissues; it consists of three individual fatty acids bound together in a single large molecule; an important energy source forming much of the fat stored by the body (hypernym) lipid, lipide, lipoid (substance-holonym) fat.

Triceps skinfold measure Measurement of the skin and subcutaneous fat layer around the triceps muscle, used with arm circumference measurement to estimate fat and muscle stores

Triglyceride The storage form of fat consisting of three fatty acids and glycerol.

Trigonelline A metabolite of niacin, chemically N-methylnicotinic acid, excreted in the urine in small amounts after consumption of relatively large amounts of nicotinic acid. It also occurs in some foods; it has no vitamin activity, but a considerable amount is converted to active niacin during the roasting of coffee.

Tripe The stomach of a cow, pig, sheep or ox - ox having arguably the best flavour. Tripe is usually sold specially prepared or cleaned for cooking and is very much an acquired taste. Depending on which animal it comes from, it will have a different appearance ('honeycomb' tripe is reckoned by some to be the best for cooking). A popular way of cooking it in the UK is with onions.

Trisomy 13 A genetic disorder in which an individual has an extra 13th chromosome, characterized by mental retardation and malformed ears in all patients, and in most patients cleft lip or palate, small mandible, polydactyly, cardiac defects, convulsions, renal anomalies, intestinal malrotation, and dermatoglyphic anomalies; the condition is usually fatal within several weeks or months of birth

Trisomy 18 A genetic disorder in which an individual has an extra 18th chromosome, characterized by mental retardation, abnormal skull shape, malformed ears, and cardiac defects; the condition is usually fatal within several weeks or months of birth

Trisomy 21 A genetic disorder in which an individual has an extra 21st chromosome, typically characterized by short stature, low muscle tone, cardiac problems, GI malformations and a distinct facial appearance; also called Down syndrome

Truffle By weight, this knobbly fungus is one of the most expensive foods in the world. Although attempts have been made to cultivate truffles, the majority are still found wild, growing around the roots of oak, chestnut, hazel and beech trees.

There are two main types black (Tuber melanosporum) and white (Tuber magnatum Pico). The finest black truffles are found in the Pιrigord region of France; the best white truffles (in fact they're more beige) in the Piedmont region of Italy. Truffles are sniffed out by pigs or dogs trained to recognise the smell.

Black truffles are peeled and can be used raw or lightly cooked, while white are just carefully wiped clean and should never be cooked. They have a distinct peppery taste and are usually sliced raw directly onto the dish. You can buy a special slicer that cuts razor-thin slices, or use a mandolin.

The truffle's unique aroma and taste does something magical to foods - shave it over pasta or add it to scrambled eggs, omelettes or risotto.

Truffle oil is the next best thing - a combination of olive oil and truffle extract that can be drizzled over pasta, risotto and salads or used in salad dressings and sauces. There's no substitute for the unique taste of a fresh truffle though.

The word truffle also refers to a chocolate confection, usually filled with cream flavoured with a liqueur, the shape of which resembles a freshly dug black truffle.

TSP Trade name for textured soya protein, prepared by extrusion through fine pores to give a fibrous, meat-like texture to the final product.

Tun Obsolete measure; a large cask holding 216 imperial gallons (972 litres) of ale; 252 gallons (1134 litres) of wine.

Turbot A fairly expensive flat sea fish with good-flavoured firm flesh, on a par with Dover sole. It's available as fillets, steaks or whole. Buy it whole when you can because the bones help to add flavour to the flesh, but the fillets are good for poaching or grilling and can be served with sauces such as parsley sauce or hollandaise

Turmeric A bright yellow spice that comes from the rhizome of a plant in the ginger family. It's sometimes available fresh, but is usually sold dried and ground, in powder form. Turmeric is often a component of curry powder and it's used on its own in many Asian dishes, including fish curries, dhals, pilafs as well as in many North African meat and vegetable dishes.

Turmeric also gives chutneys and pickles (such as piccalilli) their distinctive yellow tinge. It has a slight peppery aroma and a musky taste and is sometimes substituted for the more expensive saffron because it produces the same bright yellow colour, but it has a very different flavour.

Turner syndrome A disorder in females marked by the absence of one X chromosome, typically characterized by ovarian failure, genital tissue defects, cardiac problems, and short stature

Type 1 diabetes A disorder primarily caused by failure of the pancreas to release enough insulin, characterized by hypo- and hyperglycemia, glucosuria, water and electrolyte loss, ketoacidosis and coma; long-term complications can affect the nervous, renal and cardiovascular systems

Type 2 diabetes Previously known as "noninsulin-dependent diabetes mellitus" (NIDDM) or "adult-onset diabetes." Type 2 diabetes is the most common form of diabetes mellitus. About 90 to 95 percent of people who have diabetes have type 2 diabetes. People with type 2 diabetes produce insulin, but either do not make enough insulin or their bodies do not use the insulin they make. Most of the people who have this type of diabetes are overweight. Therefore, people with type 2 diabetes may be able to control their condition by losing weight through diet and exercise. They may also need to inject insulin or take medicine along with continuing to follow a healthy program of diet and exercise. Although type 2 diabetes commonly occurs in adults, an increasing number of children and adolescents who are overweight are also developing type 2 diabetes.

Tyramine The amine formed by decarboxylation of the amino acid tyrosine; chemically p-hydroxyphenylethylamine.

Tyrosinase Enzyme that oxidizes the amino acid tyrosine and other phenolic compounds to form brown and black pigments (melanin). Absent from albinos and the white areas of piebald animals. It is present in some fruits and vegetables, e.g. potato and apple, and is responsible for the dark colour produced when cut raw food or the juice is exposed to air.

Tyrosine A non-essential amino acid that can be formed in the body from the essential amino acid phenylalanine, hence it has some sparing action on phenylalanine. In addition to its role in proteins, tyrosine is the precursor for the synthesis of melanin (the black and brown pigment of skin and hair), and for adrenaline and noradrenaline.

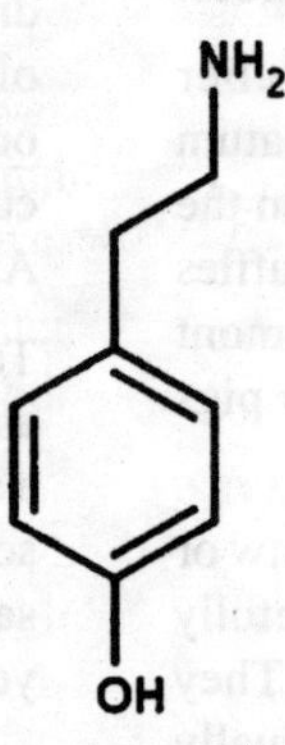

Fig. Tyramine

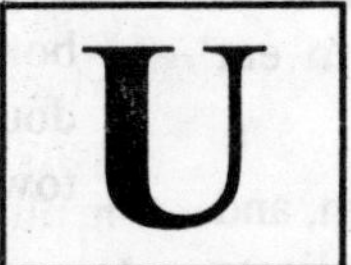

Ubiquinol An antioxidant produced by normal metabolism. Ubiquinol is the only known fat-soluble antioxidant synthesised by animal cells. It is believed to play an important role in cellular defence against oxidative damage. Ubiquinol can also contribute to the antioxidant defence system by regenerating the active form of vitamin E after that vitamin has reacted with a free radical. (The water-soluble vitamin C can also perform this function.).

Ugli fruit A hybrid of a grapefruit and a mandarin or tangerine. It has a distinctive, thick, mottled green and yellow skin that peels easily like tangerines. It tastes most like grapefruit but is slightly sweeter. Eat it as it is or use it in fruit salads, fruit fools and other fruit-based desserts.

Ulcer A crater-like lesion of the skin or a mucous membrane resulting from tissue death associated with inflammatory disease, infection, or cancer. Peptic ulcers affect regions of the gastro-intestinal tract exposed to gastric juices containing acid and pepsin: gastric in the stomach and duodenal in the duodenum. Treatment was formerly conservative, with a bland diet, followed if necessary by surgery; specific antagonists of histamine receptors have improved treatment enormously. May be caused or exacerbated by infection with Helicobacter pyloris.

Ultrasound An imaging method in which high-frequency sound waves are used to outline a part of the body.

Umami In addition to the four main taste components (sweet, sour, salty and bitter), there is the additional taste characteristic called "umami" or savory. One of the food components responsible for the umami flavor in foods is glutamate, an amino acid.

Uncooked roux It is a roux that is added at the end of cooking for a quick thickening.

Underwater weighing A research method for estimating body fat. A person is placed in a tank, underwater, and weighed. By comparing weight underwater with weight on land, one can get a very good measure of body fat.

Univariate analysis Techniques for studying the effects of a single factor on an outcome variable.

Unsaturated fat An unsaturated fat is a fat or fatty acid in which there is one or more double bond in the fatty acid chain. A fat molecule is monounsaturated if it contains one double bond, and polyunsaturated if it contains more than one double bond. Where double bonds are formed, hydrogen atoms are eliminated. Thus, a saturated fat is "saturated" with hydrogen atoms. The greater the degree of unsaturation in a fatty acid (ie, the more double bonds in the fatty acid), the more vulnerable it is to lipid peroxidation (rancidity). Antioxidants can protect unsaturated fat from lipid peroxidation.

Unleavened bread Bread that has been made without 'leavening' - that is, no raising agent such as yeast or baking powder.

Unleavened breads include chapattis and tortillas and they play an important role in Jewish ritual during Passover when it's forbidden to eat leavened bread.

Unmould To turn out a cake, jelly, ice cream, and so on, from a tin or mould. This can be a delicate operation needing a little gentle help. To unmould aspics and jellies, plunge the base of the mould in hot water for a few seconds. For sponge cakes the tin should initially be lined with greaseproof paper or greased and dusted with flour; turn out immediately after removing from the oven.

If the cake seems stuck in the tin, turn it over onto a plate and cover the base with a damp cloth, or place it immediately on a cold surface.

For ices, dip the mould briefly into cold water and then into lukewarm water. Loosen ice with knife blade, place plate on top of mould and turn over quickly.

Unsaturated fat A fat that is liquid at room temperature. Vegetable oils are unsaturated fats. Unsaturated fats include polyunsaturated fats, and monounsaturated fats. They include most nuts, olives, avocados, and fatty fish, like salmon.

Unsaturated fatty acid Fatty acid whose hydrocarbon chain contains at least one double bond. Monounsaturated fatty acids contain one double bond; polyunsaturated fatty acids contain tow or more.

Upper endoscopy Examination of the inside of the esophagus, stomach, and duodenum using an endoscope.

Urticaria Urticaria or hives is a relatively common form of allergic reaction that causes raised red skin welts. Urticaria is also known as nettle rash or uredo. These welts can be to 5 mm (0.2 inches) in diameter or more, itch severely, and often have a pale border. Urticaria is generally caused by direct contact with an allergenic substance, or an immune response to food or some other allergen. Hives can also be caused by stress.

USDA US Department of Agriculture.

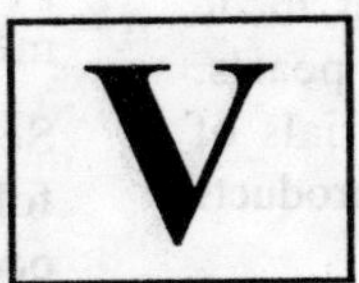

Vacherin A seasonal cows' milk cheese that's made during the winter months in France and Switzerland.

When it's fully ripe, after two to three months, the crust of this cheese encases a runny-textured cheese that has a mild, sweet and creamy taste. It's so soft that, traditionally, it's eaten with a spoon.

A vacherin is also a cold dessert made of a ring of meringue or almond paste filled with ice cream, so-called because its shape and colour are similar to the cheese.

Validity The extent to which a measure accurately reflects the concept that it is intended to measure.

Vanadium A mineral known to be essential to experimental animals, although sufficiently widespread for human dietary deficiency to be unknown. Its precise function is unknown, although it acts as an activator of a number of enzymes.

Vanilla pod The sweetly fragrant dried, cured pods of the vanilla orchid (Vanilla planifolia), which is native to Central America and Mexico. (There are other varieties from Tahiti and Hawaii.).

The pods can be used either whole or split to reveal the aromatic seeds, which can be scraped out and added to custards, sauces, and so on. The pods can then be stored in a sugar jar to impart their flavour, or they can be infused directly in custards, creams and milk puddings.

Vanilla extract is an alcoholic solution with the true flavour and aroma of vanilla pods. Those marked 'pure vanilla extract' are the best quality, if more expensive. Vanilla extract can be used as flavouring in place of the real thing, but avoid using products marked 'vanilla flavouring', which lacks the true flavour and aroma of vanilla.

Variable Any characteristic that may vary in study subjects, such as gender, age, body weight, diet, behaviour, attitude or other attribute. In an experiment, the treatment is called the independent variable; it is the factor being investigated. The variable that is influenced by the treatment is the dependent variable; it may change as a result of the effect of the independent variable.

Vector In medicine, a vector is a carrier. The best way to understand a vector is to recall its origin as a word. Vector is the Latin word for a "bearer." It is often an intermediary vehicle. For example, in malaria where the mosquito serves as a vector that carries and transfers the infectious agent (Plasmodium) injecting it with a bite. In molecular biology, a vector may be a virus (or a plasmid); a piece of foreign DNA is inserted in the vector genome to be carried and introduced into a recipient (host) cell. In physics, there are vectors but they go beyond the biomedical realm.

Veganism Veganism (also known as strict vegetarianism or pure vegetarianism) is a philosophy and lifestyle that avoids using animals and animal products for food, clothing and other purposes. In practice, a vegan (an adherent to veganism) commits to the abstention from consumption or use of all animal products, including meat, fish, poultry, honey, eggs and dairy products, as well as articles made of fur, wool, bone, leather, feathers, pearls, nacre, coral, sponges and other materials of animal origin. Many vegans also avoid products that have been tested on animals.

Vegetable butters Naturally occurring fats that melt rather sharply because they contain a preponderance of a single triacylglycerol. Cocoa butter from the cocoa bean, used in chocolate; Borneo tallow or green butter from the Malaysian and Indonesian plant, Shorea stenopiera, resembles cocoa butter; shea butter from the African plant, Butyrospermum parkii, softer than cocoa butter. Mowrah fat or illipt butter from the Indian plant, Bassia longifolia, used for soap and candles.

Vegetable cook or entremetier Prepares vegetables, soups, starches, and eggs. Large kitchens may divide these duties among the vegetable cook, the fry cook, and the soup cook.

Vegetable oils Oils obtained from vegetable sources, including soybeans, peanuts, cottonseeds and palms. Vegetable oils are generally high in unsaturated fats, with the exception of tropical oils, which are considered saturated. Vegetable oils are used in cooking, and in salad oils and dressings.

Vegetable shortening A vegetarian alternative to lard, this is a solid fat made from hydrogenated vegetable oils. It can be substituted for other fats in cooking and is often used in baking.

Vegetarian A person who does not include meat in her or his diet. Approaches to vegetarianism differ and are described by the following terms:

Lacto-ovo-vegetarian Person whose diet includes eggs and milk products, but no animal flesh (e.g., beef, pork, poultry, fish).

Lacto-vegetarian Person who chooses diet with dairy products, but not meat, poultry, fish or eggs.

Vegan or strict vegetarian Person whose diet includes only plant foods, excluding any animal meats or animal products (e.g., dairy). Vegans also avoid any foods that include animal products as ingredients such as baked goods made with eggs or butter.

Semi-vegetarian Person who most always follows vegetarian eating patterns, but may occasionally consume animal foods.

Verjus or verjuice Literally 'green juice', this is a sour juice made from sour grapes, crab apples or other unripe fruit. It was used a great deal in medieval European cookery and is undergoing a revival. It's used as a flavouring in certain condiments, and in cooking can be used in place of lemon juice. It's easier to find now and can be found in the speciality food section of most major supermarkets, or in specialist food shops.

Vermicelli Vermicelli is very fine, long strands of pasta - like a skinny spaghetti - often used in soups. The name means 'little worms' in Italian. It's available fresh or dried.

Dried vermicelli is usually sold boxed in coiled nests to prevent the delicate strands from breaking. Serve it with delicate oil-based or thin creamy sauces, because thick sauces will soak into the pasta and make it go soggy.

The term is also used to describe Asian noodles, which are also sold dried, and which come in varying widths, from very thin to wide.

Rice vermicelli can be used in soups or stir-fries, served cold in spicy Asian salads, or used as the basis for some sweets.

Very-low calorie diet A person following a VLCD eats or drinks a commercially prepared formula that has 800 calories or less, instead of eating food. A VLCD can allow a person to lose weight more quickly than is usually possible with low-calorie diets, but should only be used under the supervision of a health care provider.

Vichyssoise A velvety soup made from potatoes, leeks and cream, blended until smooth and served cold, garnished with chopped chives. The name is sometimes used to refer to any cold soup based on potatoes and another vegetable.

Videofluoroscopic swallowing study (VFSS) A radiologic procedure used to evaluate the swallowing mechanism; foods are mixed with barium and feeding is recorded and observed

Villi Tiny finger-like projections on the surface of the small intestine that help absorb nutrients.

Vinaigrette Also known as French dressing, vinaigrette is French for 'little vinegar'. It's a fairly thick salad dressing made from a mixture of olive oil, wine vinegar (red, white or balsamic) and salt and pepper to which various flavourings can be added, such as herbs, mustard, honey or chilli. The standard ratio is three parts oil to one part vinegar but it's best to experiment until you find a combination you like.

Drizzle it over raw or warm salads, or over salad starters such as avocado halves, or pan-fried asparagus.

There are plenty of ready-made bottled versions to try, but it's very quick and easy to make - just put all the ingredients in a jar and shake well. The word can also be used to describe dishes dressed with a vinaigrette sauce.

Vinegar Mother "Mother" of vinegar (cloudy vinegar) will naturally occur in vinegar products as the result of the vinegar bacteria itself. "Mother" is actually cellulose (a natural carbohydrate which is the fiber in foods such as celery and lettuce) produced by the harmless vinegar bacteria. Today, most manufacturers pasteurize their product before bottling to prevent these bacteria from forming "mother" while sitting on the grocery store shelf. After opening, you may notice "mother" beginning to form. Vinegar containing "mother" is not harmful or spoiled. Just remove the substance by filtering and continue to use the product. Shelf life is almost indefinite. Because of its acidic nature, vinegar is self-preserving and does not need refrigeration. White vinegar will remain virtually unchanged over an extended period of time and while some changes can be observed in other types of vinegars, such as colour changes or the development of a haze or sediment, this is only an aesthetic change, unless the vinegar has become contaminated. The product should be safe to use unless contaminated.

Vinegar–Cloudy Vinegar, especially cider or wine vinegar, may become cloudy and dark on storage. Cloudiness occurs when iron and tannins in the vinegar combine. Tannins are responsible for the stringent flavor in the vinegar. The reaction is more likely if vinegar is stored in a clear bottle and is exposed to light. Acidity of the vinegar is not affected by this colour reaction. Darkening of vinegar may also just be an effect of age. This low darkening is the same thing as the darkening of fruits with aging. Use as you would normally use vinegar.

Vinegar–Distilled Distilled or white vinegar is made form diluted distilled ethyl alcohol. It adds no colour to a food but may have a harsh acid taste. Vinegars usually have 4%-6% acetic acid, an organic acid responsible for the acidity of vinegar. It is formed when a microorganism called aceto-bacter aceti acts on ethyl alcohol in the presence of oxygen. While the acid is the same in vinegar from any source, the flavor, odor, and colour of the vinegar depend upon the materials from which it is made.

Vinegar–Malt Malt vinegar is made from barley malt or other cereals where starch has been converted to maltose. It is a two-fold fermentation process. Vinegar is made by 2 distinct biochemical processes, both the result of the action of microorganisms. The first process is brought about by the action of yeasts, which change natural sugars to alcohol under controlled conditions. This is called alcoholic fermentation. The second process results from the action of a group of bacteria upon the alcohol portion, converting it to acid. This is the acetic, or acid fermentation that forms vinegar. Malt vinegar has a heavy lemon-like flavor. It can be used instead of lemon in many dishes including sauces for fish.

Vintage The year of production of a wine, from the French vendage, for grape harvest. Used mainly for superior quality wines, when each year's production is matured separately. Ordinary and table wines (see wine classification) are not generally dated, and indeed the production from more than one year may be blended.

Violet The sweetly scented flowers of the wild violet (Viola odorata) are candied or crystallized and used as decorations in confectionery, or to make a sweet soufflι. The flowers can be used to flavour syrups, and both flowers and leaves can be used in salads.

Virus A simple, noncellular particle (entity) that can reproduce only inside living cells (of other organisms). The simple structure of viruses is their most important characteristic. Most viruses consist only of a genetic material—either DNA or RNA—and a protein coating. Viruses are "alive" in that they can reproduce themselves, but they have none of the other characteristics of living organisms. Viruses cause a large variety of significant diseases in plants and animals, including humans.

Visceral hypersensitivity (intestinal) Enhanced perception, or enhanced responsiveness within the gut — even to normal events.

Visceral Relating to the internal organs, such as the gut/intestines or bladder.

Vision The process of vision is mediated by a pigment derived from vitamin A bound to a protein (opsin). The pigments are variously known as visual purple (because of the colour), rhodopsin (in the rod cells of the retina) and iodopsin (in the cone cells). The action of light on rhodopsin causes a chemical change, with loss of the purple colour (known as bleaching), which results in the initiation of a nerve impulse from the retina to the brain.

Vitamers Chemical compounds structurally related to a vitamin, and converted to the same overall active metabolites in the body. They thus possess the same kind of biological activity, although sometimes with lower potency.

When there are several vitamers, the group of compounds exhibiting the biological activity of the vitamin is given a generic descriptor (e.g. vitamin A is the generic descriptor for retinol and its derivatives as well as several carotenoids).

Vitamin The word "vitamin" was coined in 1911 by the Warsaw-born biochemist Casimir Funk (1884-1967). At the Lister Institute in London, Funk isolated a substance that prevented nerve inflammation (neuritis) in chickens raised on a diet deficient in that substance. He named the substance "vitamine" because he believed it was necessary to life and it was a chemical amine. The "e" at the end was later removed when it was recognized that vitamins need not be amines.

Vitamin A deficiency Low vitamin A availability in hepatic deposits and diminished levels in the blood; may or may not presents signs and symptoms of the deficiency.

Vitamin A precursors Substances contained in plant foods carotenes that convert to vitamin A after being ingested.

Vitamin B1 Thiamin; essential for the liberation of energy from foods, especially carbohydrates, and for nerve conduction. Deficiency, especially when associated with a carbohydrate-rich diet, results in the disease beriberi—degeneration of the sensory nerves in the hands and feet fast spreading through the limbs, with fluid retention and heart failure. Relatively acute deficiency, especially associated with alcohol abuse, results in central nervous system damage, the Wernicke-Korsakoff syndrome.

Good sources are whole grain and enriched bread and cereals, meat (especially liver, kidney, and heart, and pork), yeast, potatoes, and peas; cooking losses can be as much as 50%.

Vitamin B12 A term that covers several chemically related compounds (cobalamins) essential for cell division in tissues where this process is rapid, e.g. in the formation of red blood cells. Deficiency leads to pernicious anaemia when immature red blood cells are released into the bloodstream, and there is degeneration of the spinal cord. This type of anaemia is the same as seen in folate deficiency. The absorption of vitamin B 12 requires a particular protein (called the intrinsic factor) which is secreted in the gastric juice and it is a shortage of this protein rather than a dietary deficiency of B 12 that is the more usual cause of the problem. However, B12 is found only in animal foods so vegans have to rely on special bacterial preparations. The deficiency can be treated with injections of B12.

Meat, eggs, and dairy produce are rich sources and dietary deficiency is improbable except among vegans.

Vitamin B13 Orotic acid, an intermediate in pyrimidine synthesis; there is no evidence that it is a dietary essential, and hence not a vitamin.

Vitamin B14 Not an established vitamin; name originally given to a substance found in human urine that increases the rate of cellproliferation in bone-marrow culture.

Vitamin B15 Pangamic acid; no evidence that it has any physiological function in the body, so not a vitamin.

Vitamin B16 This term has never been used.

Vitamin B17 Laetrile; there is no evidence that it has any physiological function in the body, so it is not a vitamin.

Vitamin B complex An old-fashioned term for the various B vitamins: vitamin B1, (thiamin), vitamin B2 (riboflavin), niacin, vitamin B6, vitamin B12, folate, biotin, and pantothenic acid. These vitamins occur together in cereal germ, liver, and yeast; function as coenzymes; and historically were discovered by separation from what was known originally as vitamin B; hence, they are grouped together as the B complex.

Vitamin C An antioxidant vitamin that protects cells from oxidative damage. Vitamin C is necessary for the production of collagen, hormones and neurotransmitters, it may have a role in fighting infection.

Vitamin content of foods According to the UK Code of Practice, no claims for the presence of a vitamin (or mineral) in. a food should be made unless the amount ordinarily consumed in a day contains onesixth of the daily requirements. No claim should be made that the food is a rich or excellent source unless half of the daily requirement is present; no reference to the prevention of disease unless the full day's requirement is present.

EU labelling regulations only permit claims to be made if a food provides more than 15%o of the labelling reference value per 100 g or 100 mL.

Vitamin D Calcium and phosphorus metabolism, aids bone growth and integrity, promotes strong teeth.

Vitamin E Antioxidant powers protect cell membranes, essential for red blood cells, aids cellular respiration and protects lung tisse from pollution. Vegetable oils, wheat germ, green leafy vegetables, seeds, nuts, seafood, apples, carrots and celery.

Vitamin F Sometimes used for the essential fatty acids.

Vitamin G Obsolete name for vitamin B 2.

Vitamin K Fat-soluble vitamin essential for the production of prothrombin and several other proteins involved in the blood clotting system, and the bone protein osteocalcin. Deficiency causes impaired blood coagulation and haemorrhage; sometimes called the antihaemorrhagic vitamin. Two groups of compounds have vitamin K activity: phylloquinones, found in all green plants, and a variety of menaquinones synthesized by intestinal bacteria. Dietary deficiency is unknown, except when associated with general malabsorption diseases. However, some newborn infants are at risk of developing haemorrhagic disease as a result of low vitamin K status, and it is general practice to give a single, relatively large dose of the vitamin by injection.

Vitamin L Factors extracted from yeast and thought at the time to be essential for lactation; they have not become established vitamins.

Vitamin M Obsolete name for folic acid.

Vitamin P Name given to a group of plant flavonoid substances (sometimes called bioflavonoids) which affect the strength of the walls of the blood capillaries: rutin (in buckwheat), hesperidin, eriodictin, and citrin (a mixture of hesperidin and eriodictin in the pith of citrus fruits). Now considered that the effect is pharmacological and that they are not dietary essentials; indeed, there is little evidence that they can be absorbed through the gut.

It was called vitamin P from the German permeabilitδts vitamin, because of the effect on capillary permeability and fragility.

Vitaminoids Name given to compounds with 'vitamin-like' activity; considered by some to be vitamins or partially to replace vitamins. Includes bioflavonoids (vitamin P), inositol, carnitine, choline, lipoic acid, and the essential fatty acids. With the exception of the essential fatty acids, there is no evidence that any of them is a dietary essential.

VO2 Max (Maximal oxygen consumption) The highest volume of oxygen a person can consume during exercise. Often used as a predictor of potential in endurance sports.

Vodka Made from neutral spirit, i.e. alcohol distillate mainly from potatoes, with little or no acid, so that there is no ester formation and hence no flavour. Polish vodka is flavoured with a variety of herbs and fruits.

Vol-au-vent A light, round bite-sized shell of puff pastry, sometimes with a pastry lid, with a delicate filling, served as a hot or cold starter or hors d'oeuvre. The filling is made of meat, seafood or vegetables, usually bound with a sauce. You can buy ready-made vol-au-vents from delis and larger supermarkets.

Votator Machine used for the continuous manufacture of margarine; the fat and water are emulsified, and the subsequent conditioning process carried out in the same machine.

Vulnerability Deals with the biological, occupational or social factors that increase the risks of nutritional damages.

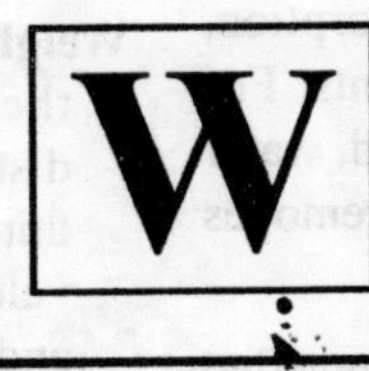

Wafer Very thin, crisp, sweet biscuit, served with ice cream etc. Wafer sandwich biscuits consist of several layers of wafer with a sweet or savoury cream filling.

Waffle Crisp, golden-brown pancake with deep indentations made by baking batter in a waffle iron which cooks both sides simultaneously.

Waist circumference A measurement of the waist. Fat around the waist increases the risk of obesity-related health problems. Women with a waist measurement of more than 35 inches or men with a waist measurement of more than 40 inches have a higher risk of developing obesity-related health problems, such as diabetes, high blood pressure, and heart disease.

Walnut A creamy-coloured nut with an edible light-brown skin enclosed in a knobbly beige shell. Walnuts are very versatile and good to cook with. Ground and chopped walnuts make a delicious addition to cakes, biscuits, buns and breads. The flavour is also exquisite in ice cream, toffee, fudge and other confectionery, such as walnut brittle or praline. New-season walnuts are delicious eaten with cheese, especially soft goats' cheese or cream cheese. Very young walnuts that are still green and in their shells can be salted and pickled to serve with a cheeseboard or with cold meats.

Walnuts have a short shelf life once shelled, so they're best kept in the fridge in an airtight container. For longer-term storage, it's best to buy walnuts in shells and shell them as you need them. If the shell is firmly sealed you can store them for a few months. Never keep nuts from one year to the next because the flavour and quality quickly deteriorate, and they may become rancid. Walnut halves or roughly chopped nuts can add crunch to salads laced with walnut oil dressing.

Add them to noodles, use with chicken in Chinese dishes, or chop them into stuffings. Push walnut pieces into dates as an after-dinner sweetmeat, or just enjoy a bowl of walnuts with a glass of tawny port.

Wasabi Although this bright green condiment is often referred to as 'Japanese horseradish', it isn't actually related to horseradish at all. It comes from the root of a perennial herb that grows in Japan and eastern Siberia.

Wasabi is a traditional accompaniment to sushi and sashimi, but it can also be used to make dressings and sauces. Fresh wasabi is rarely available outside Japan, but in the UK it's available in paste or powdered form. The latter is a better choice, because you can use it as you need it by mixing to a paste with water.

Water Although deficiencies of energy or nutrients can be sustained for months or even years, a person can survive only a few days without water. Experts rank water second only to oxygen as essential for life. In addition to offering true refreshment for the thirsty, water plays a vital role in all bodily processes. It supplies the medium in which various chemical changes of the body occur, aiding in digestion, absorption, circulation and lubrication of body joints. For example, as a major component of blood, water helps deliver nutrients to body cells and removes waste to the kidneys for excretion.

Water, demineralized Water that has been purified by passage through a bed of ion-exchange resin which removes mineral salts. Demineralized or de-ionized water is at least as pure as distilled water, and may be purer.

Waxing Coating fruits and vegetables with a thin layer of edible wax. In the case of apples and oranges this replaces the natural wax that is removed when the crop is washed; in the case of vegetables it is an addition; in both instances the waxing prevents loss of moisture, prolongs storage life, and improves the appearance.

Weaning The process of progressively developing a diet for infants and young children from one based on breast-milk or infant formula to one covering a wide range of textures and tastes. This weaning period usually starts sometime between four and six months of age.

Weaning foods Weaning foods are foods that are consumed during the weaning period. Commercial weaning foods are formulated to meet the dietary requirements of infants and children during the weaning process and are marketed for that age group. Products include follow-on formulas, ready-to-eat baby food, dried baby food, cereal-based weaning food including pastas, biscuits and rusks, milk-based desserts, and drinks.

Weight loss Weight loss is a decrease in body weight resulting from either voluntary (diet, exercise) or involuntary (illness) circumstances. Most instances of weight loss arise due to the loss of body fat, but in cases of extreme or severe weight loss, protein and other substances in the body can also be depleted. Examples of involuntary weight loss include the weight loss associated with cancer, malabsorption (such as from chronic diarrheal illnesses), and chronic inflammation (such as with rheumatoid arthritis).

Weight/age ratio percentiles Perccentile refers to the position of an individual in a given distribution of reference. Thus, the tenth and third percentiles, as used in the text, refer to those values of weight presented by, respectively, 10% and 3% of the children in the distribution of the anthropometric parameters of reference. In this way, a child whose weight is equal or inferior to these two limits has a greater possibility of presenting a nutritional disorder. In other words, it can be affirmed that the tenth or third percentile of weight/age ratio is the diving line represented graphically on the official growth. Visualization of the chart clarifies well the principle and application of tenth percentile and third percentile.

Weight-cycle Losing and gaining weight over and over again. Commonly called "yo-yo" dieting.

Welschriesling A grape variety widely used for wine making, although not one of the classic varieties. Also known as Italian riesling; the wines cannot legally be labelled simply riesling.

Welsh rarebit A traditional British speciality consisting of a slice of toasted bread covered with a mixture of Cheshire or cheddar cheese that has been melted in pale ale with English mustard, pepper and sometimes a dash of Worcestershire sauce. It's then grilled and served very hot so the cheese is bubbling and tinged with brown. The dish is also punningly called 'Welsh rabbit', and food historians continue to argue about which is the proper term.

WHA World Health Assembly. The governing body of WHO, the WHA determines WHO policies and programs and approves its budget. Delegates of member states hold their annual meeting in May.

Wheat The most important of the cereals and one of the most widely grown crops. Many thousand varieties are known but there are three main types: Triticum vulgare, used mainly for bread; Triticum durum (durum wheat), largely used for pasta; and Triticum compactum (club wheat), too soft for ordinary bread. The berry is composed of the outer, branny husk, 13% of the grain; the germ or embryo (rich in nutrients), 2%; and the central endosperm (mainly starch), 85%. See also flour, extraction rate.

Whelk Whelks are saltwater molluscs with grey or brownish shells. They resemble pointy snails. They're usually sold already cooked and shelled and can be eaten with a sprinkling of vinegar or with slices of bread and butter. The chewy flesh is quite juicy and salty. They're available year-round but are at their best from September to February.

If you do cook them from fresh, ensure you wash them thoroughly in several changes of water then leave them to soak for a couple of hours. They only need minimal cooking of about ten to 15 minutes in boiling salted water, otherwise the flesh will be rubbery.

Whey Protein Whey protein is a very high quality protein that is derived from sweet dairy whey. It has a very high biological value and many other attributes. We strongly recommend viewing of our FAQs section or a quick visit to www.whey-protein.com

Whipped butter Has air or nitrogen gas whipped into it to increase the volume, lighten the texture and make it easier to spread.

Whipping cream A lighter version of double cream with a fat content of over 35 per cent - the minimum amount necessary to allow it to stay firm once beaten. It's the fat globules that trap whisked air, creating the characteristic foam and texture of whipped cream. Whipping cream whips well without being quite as rich as double cream and also makes a slightly lighter pouring cream. It makes a good topping for desserts, meringues and puddings that need a slightly lighter touch.

White pudding Sausage made from white meat (chicken, rabbit, pork) cereal, and spices. The French version, boudin blanc, includes eggs and onions. Irish white pudding is made from flake or leaf lard and oatmeal, spiced; served sliced and fried.

Whiting A white round sea fish, whiting is a member of the cod family. It's more economical to buy than cod, although it has a relatively bland taste.

It's best bought fresh and eaten immediately otherwise it loses its flavour. It's light and easy to digest and it goes well with a variety of flavours. Whiting is also a good fish to use in fishcakes and fish mousses.

Who code The International Code of Marketing of Breast-milk Substitutes. Its aim is to contribute to safe and adequate nutrition for infants through the protection and promotion of breastfeeding and by ensuring the proper use of breast-milk substitutes, when needed, through adequate information and approriate marketing and distribution.

Who director-general The Director-General is the Secretariat's chief technical and administrative officer.

Who executive board The Executive Board is composed of 32 individuals technically qualified in the field of health. Its main functions are to give effect to the decisions and policies of the Health Assembly, to advise it and generally to facilitate its work.

Who secretariat The Secretariat is staffed by some 4,000 health and other experts in both professional and general service categories working at headquarters and in the six regional offices.

WHO The World Health Organization.

Whole grains The whole kernel of grain which includes the bran (outer shell), germ (nutrient rich core) and endosperm (starchy portion). The health benefit provided by whole grains is the reduced risk of cardiovascular disease which results from the combination of fiber, vitamins, minerals and phytochemicals found in whole grains.

Wholefoods Foods that have been minimally refined or processed, and are eaten in their natural state. In general nothing is removed from, or added to, the foodstuffs in preparation. Wholegrain cereal products are made by milling the complete grain.

WIC Food Package A group of foods specifically tailored to the nutritional needs of pregnant women, new mothers, and infants and young children that program participants are able to purchase with WIC benefits. WIC Food Package items include milk, cheese, juice, eggs, beans, peanut butter, iron-fortified cereal and infant formula. The nutritional content of the WIC Food Package is currently under review by the Institutes of Medicine and the USDA.

WIC Special Supplemental Nutrition Program for Women, Infants, and Children. Established in 1972, the WIC program provides food and nutrition education to improve the nutritional status of medically high-risk pregnant and lactating women and children up to 5 years of age from low-income families. The program is administered by the U.S. Department of Agriculture.

Williams syndrome A genetic disorder of chromosome 7 characterized by distinctive facial features, growth and developmental delays, varying degrees of learning disabilities, cardiac defects and sometimes hypercalcemia in infancy

Wilson's disease An inherited (autosomal recessive) disorder of copper storage, which leads to renal, cardiac, pancreatic and liver disease and central nervous system manifestation.

Wine Fermented juice from grapes (varieties of Vitis vinifera), also made with other fruits and even vegetables with the addition of sugar. Red wines are made by fermenting the juice together with the skins at 21-29 °C; white wines normally from white grapes by fermenting the juice alone at 15-17°C; rosı by removing the skins after 12-36 hours, or by mixing red and white wines.

Beverages made by fermenting other fruit ju:ces and sugar in the presence of vegetables, leaves, or roots are also called wines (elderberry, elder flower, parsnip, peapod, rhubarb, etc.), although the legal definition may be restricted to the fermented grape. See also alcoholic beverages.

White wines are graded as dry (0.6% sugars), to sweet (6% sugars), on a scale of 1 to 9. Red wines are graded from A (light and dry) to E (fullbodied and heavy). Wines generally contain 9-14% alcohol, dry wines 70 kcal (290 kJ), sweet wines 120 kcal (500 kJ), and about 1 mg of iron per 100 mL; there are only traces of vitamins.

Wine classification Many of the major wine-producing countries have legally enforced systems of classification of wines based on grape varieties used and regions of production. Other countries have a system of denomination of origin for wines grown in defined regions which may or may not reflect quality. The national classifications are as follows (in increasing order of quality for each country):

Wineberry Orange-coloured fruit of the Japanese and Chinese wild raspberry, Rubus phoenicolasius, and now also hybrids with European cultivated raspberries.

Wok Chinese vessel for stir frying; a shallow, bowl-shaped pan in which food can be fried rapidly in a small amount of oil over a high heat.

Worcestershire sauce A classic English bottled sauce that is said to have originated from an Indian recipe. It's a thin, spicy, dark-brown fermented sauce made from a variety of ingredients including anchovies, shallots, garlic, soy sauce, tamarind, salt and vinegar, which is then left to age in barrels.

The final sauce has a spicy, concentrated flavour, so you only need a dash. It can be used to give a little boost to meat stews and casseroles, pies, soups, sauces and marinades. Sprinkle it over sausages, steaks, chops and kebabs or use it as a table condiment or in drinks such as a classic Bloody Mary.

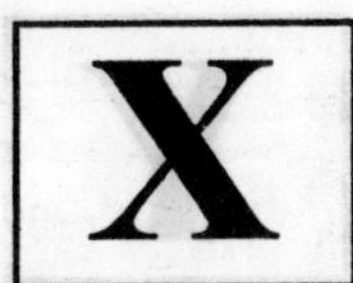

Xavier A cream soup or consommι thickened with arrowroot or rice flour and garnished with diced chicken.

Xenobiotics Synthetic chemicals believed to be resistant to environmental degradation. A branch of biotechnology called bioremediation is seeking to develop biological methods to degrade such compounds.

Xerophthalmia Ocular alterations resulting from vitamin A deficiency.

XO XO stands for 'extra old' and is used to show that a cognac has been aged for an extended period of time. The legal minimum for this designation is seven years old but most XO cognacs are much older than that, many ranging from 20 to 50 years old. The minimum age of the youngest cognac in the blend must be at least seven years old. The minimum age of VS (very special) cognac is two years old and that of VSOP (very superior old pale) is four years old.

XO sauce is also a sauce and condiment used in Chinese cooking. Ingredients include dried shrimp, dried scallops and garlic, along with other flavourings, often chillies. XO sauce can be used as a dip or in stir-fries.

Xylitol A five-carbon sugar alcohol found in raspberries, endive, lettuce, and formed in the body as an intermediate in glucose metabolism; 80-100% of the sweetness of sucrose; used in sugar-free hard sweets and gelatine gums. Apart from being of low cariogenicity, xylitol is said to have an effect in suppressing the growth of some of the bacteria associated with dental caries. See sugar alcohols; toothfriendly sweets.

Xylose Pentose (five-carbon) sugar found in plant tissues as complex polysaccharide; 40% as sweet as sucrose. Also known as wood sugar.

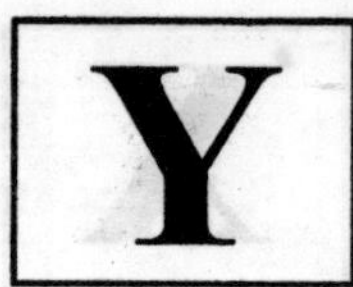

Yam The yam is a staple food in many tropical countries, particularly the Caribbean. Yams have brown tough skins and the flesh can vary in colour - anything from white to yellow to purple - depending on the variety.

Small yams can be cooked in their skins, but larger ones should be peeled and blanched for ten to 20 minutes in boiling salted water before being used. Yams can be used in the same way as potatoes or sweet potatoes.

Serve mashed yams with plenty of butter and seasoning as an accompaniment to meat or other vegetable dishes. Make yam chips or bake yams in their skins.

Yeast A microscopic living fungus that multiplies rapidly in suitable conditions. It's an essential ingredient for bread-making and brewing. When mixed with warm water, sugar and flour, yeast produces carbon dioxide, which causes dough to rise.

Yiu tiao Chinese; fried dough sticks, generally eaten for breakfast.

Yoghurt Yogurt is made from fermented milk and has a great many uses. It can be consumed as a drink (such as the Indian lassi) or eaten as a kind of relish (such as the Indian raita, a cooling mixture of yoghurt and cucumber), or made into a kind of cheese (such as labneh). It can also be used as a dressing or as a marinade to tenderise meats, as in tandoori chicken.

In western Europe yoghurt is perhaps most popular as a sweetened, fruity dessert or breakfast food. Yoghurt can be made from the milk of cows, sheep, goats, even mares, camels and female yaks; each has its own flavours and cooking properties. It's often used in northern Indian curries to give flavour and texture and to temper the heat of chillies.

Yoghurt is very digestible, even to people with lactose intolerance. It's also seen as a 'healthy' food in many parts of the world. Yoghurt can be used as a replacement for cream or crθme fraζche in most recipes. It's available with a wide range of fat contents, from full-fat with added cream to very low fat.

Yoghurt with a very low-fat content has a tendency to curdle when used in hot dishes, though, so allow the dish to cool first and don't let it boil once the yoghurt is added.

Yogurt A common dish made of milk curdled and fermented with a culture of Lactobacillus (the milk bacillus). The word was acquired in the 1620s from Turkey. It can be spelled myriad ways including yogurt, yoghurt, yaghourt, yooghurt, yughard, and yaourt. The most popular spellings in the Anglo-Saxon world are yogurt and yoghurt while in France one eats yaourt.

Z

Zabaglione A rich, foamy Italian dessert made by whisking egg yolks, Marsala wine and sugar together over a gentle heat. It's usually served barely warm. Some versions might have the addition of fresh fruit or fruit coulis. Zabaglione is quite similar to the French sabayon.

Zander A large freshwater game fish found in the rivers and lakes of continental Europe. If you happen to find some fresh zander (it isn't readily available in the UK) then you can cook it whole, stuffed and either poached or baked. It has firm flesh that has a tendency to dry out.

Zeaxanthin A type of carotenoid found in eggs, citrus fruits and corn which positively contributes to the maintenance of eye vision.

Z-enzyme Enzyme found associated with amylases, that attacks the few ί-1,3-links present in amylose. Pure, crystalline ί-amylase will convert only 70% of amylose to maltose; it requires the presence of the Z-enzyme for complete conversion.

Zest The outer rind of citrus fruit containing aromatic essential oils. Remove the zest carefully using a grater, potato peeler or zester, depending on the intended use. Take care not to remove any of the white pith with the zest, because it can be very bitter. The zest of citrus fruits can be used to add flavour to sweet or savoury dishes, or as a decoration or garnish. Lemon zest is a key ingredient in gremolata.

Zinc Essential for normal growth, development and immunity. Helps maintain skin, hair and bones. Keeps reproductive organs functioning and helps in the perception of taste and the ability to see at night.

Zollinger-Ellison syndrome (ZES) A rare disorder that causes tumors in the pancreas and duodenum. The tumors secrete a hormone called gastrin that causes the stomach to produce too much acid, which in turn causes stomach and duodenal ulcers (peptic ulcers).

Zucchini The Italian and American word for courgette. Zucchini are very versatile to cook with, but buy the younger, smaller ones, because older vegetables tend to have large, tough seeds and can be very watery.

Zymogens The inactive form in which some enzymes, especially the protein digestive enzymes, are secreted, being activated after secretion. Also called pro-enzymes, or enzyme precursors.

Zymotachygraph An instrument that measures the gas produced in a fermenting dough and the amount escaping from the dough, as an index of bread-making properties.